DATE DUE

BRODART   Cat. No. 23-221

Physical Consequences of Depression

Physical Consequences of Depression

Edited by

Jogin H. Thakore

Senior Lecturer in Psychiatry and Consultant Psychiatrist, Dublin, Ireland

WRIGHTSON BIOMEDICAL PUBLISHING LTD
Petersfield, UK and Philadelphia, USA

Editorial Office:

Wrightson Biomedical Publishing Ltd
Ash Barn House, Winchester Road, Stroud,
Petersfield, Hampshire GU32 3PN, UK
Telephone: 44 (0)1730 265647
Fax: 44 (0)1730 260368
E-mail: wrightson.biomed@virgin.net

British Library Cataloguing in Publication Data
Physical consequences of depression
    1. Depression, Mental – Physiological aspects
    I. Thakore, Jogin H.
    616.8'527

Library of Congress Cataloging in Publication Data
A catalog record for this book is available from the Library of Congress

ISBN 1 871816 44 0

Composition by Scribe Design, Gillingham, Kent
Printed in Great Britain by Biddles Ltd, Guildford

For
Shenaz, Adam and Nadia

Contents

Contributors

Alejandro Ayala, *Clinical Neuroendocrinology Branch, NIMH, 10 Center Drive, Bethesda, MD 20892, USA*

Per Björntorp, *Department of Heart and Lung Diseases, Sahlgren's University Hospital, University of Göteborg, SE 41345, Sweden*

George P. Chrousos, *Pediatric and Reproductive Endocrinology Branch, NICHD, Bethesda, MD, USA*

Giovanni Cizza, *Clinical Neuroendocrinology Branch, NIMH, 10 Center Drive, Bethesda, MD 20892, USA*

Marianne Daley, *Merck Research Laboratories, Rahway, NJ, USA*

E. Ronald de Kloet, *Division of Medical Pharmacology, LACDR/LUMC, PO Box 9503, Leiden, The Netherlands*

Roel H. DeRijk, *Laboratorium Rijngeest Groep, Endegeesterstraatweg 5, 2342 AJ Oegstgeest, The Netherlands*

Michael Deuschle, *Central Institute of Mental Health, 68159 Mannheim, Germany*

Timothy G. Dinan, *Department of Clinical Pharmacology and Therapeutics, University College, Cork, Ireland*

Elissa S. Epel, *Department of Psychiatry, School of Medicine, University of California, San Francisco, CA 94143, USA*

Philip W. Gold, *Clinical Neuroendocrinology Branch, NIMH, 10 Center Drive, Bethesda, MD 20892, USA*

Jane F. Gumnick, *Department of Psychiatry and Behavioral Sciences, Emory University School of Medicine, 1639 Pierce Drive, Suite 4000, Atlanta, GA 30322, USA*

Brian E. Leonard, *Pharmacology Department, National University of Ireland, Galway, Ireland*

Jonathan Mann, *Department of Psychiatry, Royal South Hants Hospital, Southampton, UK*

Onno C. Meijer, *Division of Medical Pharmacology, LACDR/LUMC, PO Box 9503, Leiden, The Netherlands*

Andrew H. Miller, *Department of Psychiatry and Behavioral Sciences, Emory University School of Medicine, 1639 Pierce Drive, Suite 4000, Atlanta, GA 30322, USA*

Charles B. Nemeroff, *Department of Psychiatry and Behavioral Sciences, Emory University School of Medicine, 1639 Pierce Drive, Atlanta, GA 30322, USA*

D. Jeffrey Newport, *Department of Psychiatry and Behavioral Sciences, Emory University School of Medicine, 1639 Pierce Drive, Atlanta, GA 30322, USA*

Bradley D. Pearce, *Department of Psychiatry and Behavioral Sciences, Emory University School of Medicine, 1639 Pierce Drive, Suite 4000, Atlanta, GA 30322, USA*

Victor I. Reus, *Department of Psychiatry, School of Medicine, University of California, 401 Parnassus Avenue, San Francisco, CA 94143-0984, USA*

Jogin H. Thakore, *Neuroscience Centre, St Vincent's Hospital, Richmond Road, Dublin 3, Ireland*

Marie-Therese Walsh, *Department of Psychiatry, Royal College of Surgeons in Ireland, St Stephen's Green, Dublin 2, Ireland*

Owen M. Wolkowitz, *Department of Psychiatry, School of Medicine, University of California, 401 Parnassus Avenue, San Francisco, CA 94143-0984, USA*

Preface

A question I struggled with for quite some time before I became committed to editing this volume was whether anyone would believe that depression had physical consequences. To publish a book that deals with topics in depression below the level of the neck seemed like a radical idea. To put it into perspective, depression has been regarded by some as a disease of the mind whose origins lie in their psychosocial environment, distant or present, others have contended that this illness has a firm biological basis, while a few brave souls have dared mention that both of these apparently opposing theories may play a role in the pathogenesis of this condition.

For the moment let us assume that depression is an 'organic disorder', to use a quaint but rather appropriate expression, which is linked to changes in a stress axis termed the hypothalamic–pituitary–adrenal (HPA) axis and that one consequence of such an abnormality is the development of somatic disorders. So far so good except for the fact that even within the biological camp there exists much controversy about whether certain forms of depression are linked to abnormalities of this stress axis.

However, the observations put forward in this book speak for themselves. Melancholic depression is categorically associated with certain physical illnesses which not only cause great suffering but can also significantly shorten life expectancy. Therefore, the various chapters will be of interest not only to my colleagues in psychiatry but also to general practitioners, epidemiologists and physicians. Leaving these specialists aside, much of what is written has a direct relevance to those in basic science as, in this instance, chance clinical observations may lead to the discovery of the mechanism by which they arose.

In order for those whose 'first language' is not the HPA axis I felt it necessary to have a section introducing this fascinating area from a systems perspective to a molecular level, which is written by two experts in their field, Charlie Nemeroff and Ron de Kloet. Brian Leonard finishes this section with an overview of the complex inter-relationship between the immune system and the HPA axis. The next part of the book deals with the physical problems that can occur in depression and, in essence, topics in this part range from the epidemiological relationship between depression and the metabolic syndrome (Per Björntorp), cardiovascular disorders (Michael

Deuschle), cancer (Andrew Miller and colleagues), bone mineral density (George Chrousos and colleagues) to metabolic abnormalities (Jonathan Mann and Jogin Thakore). The last section concerns itself with alternative mechanisms by which currently available antidepressants may work (Ted Dinan and Marie-Therese Walsh) and with novel antidepressant therapies which may soon be realised and which have as their primary mode of action an effect on the HPA axis (Owen Wolkowitz and colleagues).

Our book is not intended to be, nor can it be, the definitive text in this field as the area is still growing with new findings being reported at an astonishing rate. However, it is unique as it is the first time that such a collection of subjects has been gathered together under the rubric of depression.

Jogin H. Thakore

1

Hypothalamic–Pituitary–Adrenal Axis: Normal Physiology and Disturbances in Depression

D. JEFFREY NEWPORT and CHARLES B. NEMEROFF

Department of Psychiatry and Behavioral Sciences, Emory University School of Medicine, Atlanta, GA, USA

NORMAL HPA AXIS PHYSIOLOGY

It would be a misconception to construe this chapter as an introduction to the endocrinology of depression. In considering the hypothalamic–pituitary–adrenal (HPA) axis, our attention is naturally drawn to the end-product hormones of this system, i.e. the glucocorticoids, and their neurobiological effects. Teleologically, the purpose of this axis is to produce bioactive hormones which act upon target tissues throughout the body in an effort to preserve homeostasis during periods of stress. However, the HPA axis is not simply an endocrine system, but rather a neuroendocrine system. The hypothalamus, long considered the apex of the HPA axis, is in actuality a relay point for information exchange between several higher components of the central nervous system (CNS), and any of several peripheral endocrine axes including the HPA axis. In fact, the hypothalamus has numerous bidirectional communication pathways with the complex of CNS regions known as the limbic system. Consequently, the HPA axis in its broader sense might be better named the limbic–hypothalamic–pituitary–adrenal (LHPA) axis. Although we will adhere to the conventional nomenclature by referring to this system as the HPA axis, it is important to recognize that this axis interfaces in an intricate manner with extra-hypothalamic CNS structures.

The term limbic literally means 'border' and was first applied anatomically to the structures bordering the interface of the cerebrum with the lower and phylogenetically more primitive CNS regions, i.e. the midbrain and brain stem. We have since learned that the primary function of the structures in this region is the modulation of motivational drives and behaviour. Thus, the limbic system now refers more generally to all CNS regions intimately involved with the control of emotions and behaviour, the so-called extended amygdala. The most important components of the limbic system include the amygdala, the hippocampus, certain regions of the thalamus, and a ring of basilar areas of cerebral cortex including the cingulate gyrus, the orbitofrontal cortex, the parahippocampal gyrus, the nucleus accumbens/striatum, and the uncus.

Each of the limbic structures plays a relatively distinct role in the regulation of emotion and behaviour. In lower animals dependent upon a well-developed sense of smell to capture prey (or avoid predation), the amygdala primarily serves to facilitate the association of olfactory stimuli. In humans, the chief role of the amygdala is instead to modulate behavioural responses to emotionally-charged stimuli. Operating preconsciously to coordinate the interaction between thoughts and the environmental circumstance, the amygdala patterns the intensity and direction of human behavioural responses so that they are contextually appropriate to the situation.

Like the amygdala, the hippocampus also processes sensory input. However, the chief function of the hippocampus appears to be the consolidation of experiences into long-term memory. The ring of limbic cortex that encircles the subcortical limbic structures is perhaps the least understood component of the system. In general, it can be said to serve as an association area for behavioural control that serves to coordinate communication between the neocortex and the subcortical limbic structures. Although anatomically distinct from the remainder of the limbic system, the hypothalamus is physiologically the central component of the system. Neurons of the hypothalamus transmit signals in three directions: (1) downstream within the CNS to brain stem autonomic control regions such as the locus coeruleus, (2) upstream within the CNS to the limbic structures within the midbrain and cerebral cortex, and (3) outside the CNS via the infundibulum to the pituitary gland.

If we define stress as any environmental (either internal or external) perturbation that challenges an organism's maintenance of homeostasis, then the HPA axis is arguably the primary biological stress response system in mammalian species. Indeed, a wide array of environmental stressors induce the cascade of HPA axis activation. The catalogue of stressors that have demonstrated HPA axis activation in either human or animal studies include psychosocial stress, exposure to thermal extremes, infection and other disease states, surgery or anaesthesia, physical or emotional trauma, forced restraint, and the administration of certain pharmacological agents, e.g. adrenergic receptor agonists. Although other biological systems may participate in the stress response (e.g. infection invariably induces immune system activation), the HPA axis is unique in its reliable induction by such disparate stressors. Consequently, we can safely assume that HPA axis activation is crucial to the generic mammalian response to stress.

A cascade of biological events probably beginning in the hypothalamus and proceeding through the anterior pituitary gland and subsequently the adrenal cortex comprises what we collectively refer to as HPA axis activation. Within the context of the HPA axis (as opposed to the gonadal, thyroid or growth hormone axes), the pre-eminent hormone hierarchically, secreted by hypothalamic neurons, is corticotrophin-releasing hormone (CRH). CRH is a 41 amino acid neuropeptide that was first chemically characterized in the early 1980s (Spiess *et al.*, 1981; Vale *et al.*, 1981). It is well established as the primary secretagogue stimulating HPA axis activity. CRH functions as both a neurotransmitter and hormone. By definition, neurotransmitters are substances secreted by neurons for communication with *immediately adjacent cells*. The neighbouring cells, typically other neurons, possess receptors for the neurotransmitter and transduce the biological response. In its communication *within the CNS*, neuronally-secreted CRH functions as a classic neurotransmitter substance. CRH serves as a neurotransmitter in both hypothalamic and extra-hypothalamic regions.

Hormones, in contrast to neurotransmitters, are secreted by cells to facilitate communication with *distant cells*. Hormones are released directly into the circulatory system where they are transported to distant parts of the body to exert their effects. In its interaction *outside the CNS* (i.e. with the pituitary gland), CRH secreted by hypothalamic neurons acts as a neurohormone, i.e. it is manufactured and released from neurons directly into a circulatory system. The axonal processes of parvocellular CRH hypothalamic neurons project mainly to the median eminence, an enlarged area of the infundibulum below the hypothalamus. The median eminence is adjacent to an extensive capillary bed that flows into a venous network known as the hypothalamic–hypophysial portal system. This portal system connects the hypothalamus and the anterior pituitary gland where another capillary bed enables hormones to cross readily between the circulatory system and the secretory cells of the anterior pituitary. CRH secreted from terminals of hypothalamic neurons in the median eminence travels via this portal system to the pituitary gland. The anterior pituitary, or adenohypophysis, is comprised of several secretory cell types. At the anterior pituitary, CRH acts upon the corticotrophs, one group of pituitary secretory cells that comprise approximately 20% of the gland's overall volume. When the pituitary corticotrophs are activated by CRH, these cells increase the production and release of adrenocorticotrophic hormone (ACTH). Although other peptides including vasopressin, oxytocin and somatostatin may alter ACTH release, CRH is by far the greatest physiological regulator of ACTH secretion.

ACTH is a 39 amino acid-containing peptide that is actually derived from a larger precursor molecule, pro-opiomelanocortin (POMC). Cleavage of POMC produces three bioactive peptides: ACTH, β-endorphin, and melanocortin. Consequently, stress exposure typically induces parallel increases in serum concentration of ACTH and β-endorphin. Once secreted from the anterior pituitary gland, ACTH released into the systemic circulation acts at the adrenal cortex to stimulate the production and release of glucocorticoids.

The glucocorticoids are a family of adrenal steroid hormones that are all derived from cholesterol. Cortisol comprises 95% of the circulating glucocorticoids in humans while corticosterone and a handful of other related substances comprise the remaining 5%. Over 90% of the circulating glucocorticoids are bound to cortisol binding globulin (CBG) and other plasma proteins leaving less than 10% in the unbound bioavailable state. However, stress not only increases glucocorticoid release but also decreases circulating CBG levels, thereby increasing glucocorticoid bioavailability through at least two distinct mechanisms.

Glucocorticoids were named due to the fact that their best documented metabolic effect is to increase glucose production. Glucose is a ready cellular energy source that can quickly be used. Teleologically, it makes sense to increase this fuel supply in the context of environmental stress that may require swift adaptive responses. However, increasing the availability of an immediate energy source comes at a price. Cortisol induces the production of glucose in several ways: (1) by triggering the catabolic mobilization of protein stores from muscle and activating hepatic enzymes that convert these proteins into glucose; (2) by converting glycogen into glucose; (3) by increasing the availability of a secondary energy source via the mobilization of fatty acids from adipose tissues. Thus, HPA axis activation sacrifices muscle mass, glycogen stores and adipose tissue in order to provide ready energy sources during stress.

The catabolic effects of HPA axis activation may be critical and therefore biologically adaptive in enabling the organism to meet the challenges of a stressor. However, unbridled HPA axis hyperactivity can lead to a depletion of protein, glycogen and fat that may have adverse consequences and thus be maladaptive. Therefore, negative feedback mechanisms that serve to decrease HPA axis activity once sufficient glucocorticoid release has been attained are crucial to the normal physiology of this system. Glucocorticoid receptors at all levels of the HPA axis including the hippocampus, hypothalamus, pituitary and adrenal glands mediate the negative feedback effect. When the cascade of HPA axis activation elevates the circulating concentration of cortisol, it acts upon target tissues throughout the body to produce the biological effects described above. Some of the cortisol, however, acts at these feedback sites. Cortisol feedback at the hypothalamus reduces CRH release, at the pituitary inhibits ACTH release, and at the adrenal gland inhibits further cortisol release. Cortisol feedback at the hippocampus inhibits CRH secretion from the hypothalamus by an activation of hippocampal neurons that send efferents to the hypothalamus. In addition, there are other feedback (short and ultrashort) and feedforward mechanisms that render the HPA axis an exquisitely tuned and balanced stress response system.

HPA AXIS PATHOPHYSIOLOGY IN DEPRESSION

An enormous research database has accumulated regarding the pathophysiology of depression. The bulk of this literature addresses the putative role of alteration in monoamine systems, including norepinephrine (NE), serotonin (5HT), and to a lesser extent, dopamine (DA), in depression. Moreover, synaptic modulation of one or more of these neurotransmitters remains the prevailing pharmacodynamic mechanism of all currently marketed antidepressant medications. In recent years, however, attention has increasingly shifted to alterations in endocrine and immune system function in patients with depression, and the underlying CNS substrates mediating these effects. Giving rise to the burgeoning new fields of psychoneuroendocrinology and psychoneuroimmunology, this research also promises to provide novel insights into the pathophysiology of depression and other major stress-related psychiatric disorders.

Although several neuroendocrine axes have been studied in depressed patients, the most intensely scrutinized has undoubtedly been the HPA axis. Investigation of the HPA axis' role in the pathophysiology of depression commenced over 40 years ago when it was first reported that depressed patients have higher circulating concentrations of cortisol (Board et al., 1957; Sachar et al., 1970; Carpenter and Bunney, 1971). At about the same time, the dexamethasone suppression test (DST), the first test to provide a functional assessment of HPA axis activity, was developed by Liddle and other endocrinologists to aid in the diagnostic assessment of Cushing's syndrome. Dexamethasone, a synthetic analogue of cortisol, is used in the DST to evaluate suppressibility of HPA axis activity via the negative feedback mechanism. In healthy volunteers, dexamethasone activates the negative feedback loop and thus suppresses the release of ACTH and therefore cortisol, causing the circulating concentrations of these two hormones to fall. However, dexamethasone does not suppress cortisol release in many depressed patients, indicating that the HPA feedback mechanism is dysfunctional.

There was early excitement that cortisol nonsuppression in the DST might be a clinically useful diagnostic test representing a laboratory evaluation of depression (Carroll, 1968). However, its purported lack of specificity and sensitivity led in the 1980s to the DST becoming a major point of controversy (Arana and Mossman, 1988). Cortisol nonsuppression in the DST has not proven to be the definitive biological state marker for depression. Consequently, the test has little routine clinical utility. In our view, this conclusion probably misses the more significant point in that the DST, in addition to other measures of HPA activity, reliably demonstrates an association between HPA axis hyperactivity and the clinical severity of depression (Evans and Nemeroff, 1983; Krishnan et al., 1983; Schatzberg et al., 1984; Arana et al., 1985). Moreover, in difficult diagnostic conundra such as depression in comorbid states, adolescence, and in so-called 'masked' depression, the DST is often a helpful diagnostic adjunct.

Literally hundreds of studies have confirmed these early reports of HPA axis hyperactivity in depressed patients, but what is the ultimate cause of the observed hypercortisolaemia? One plausible theory is that the ACTH receptors at the adrenal glands of depressed patients may be up-regulated and thus hypersensitive to ACTH stimulation. Indeed, exogenous administration of pharmacological doses of ACTH in the ACTH stimulation test (another functional assay of HPA axis activity) demonstrates an exaggerated cortisol response in some depressed patients. However, the adrenal secretion of cortisol elicited by lower physiological doses of ACTH after pre-treatment with dexamethasone to suppress the pituitary release of endogenous ACTH is not altered in depressed patients (Krishnan *et al.*, 1990). It does not appear, therefore, that adrenocortical responsivity *per se* is appreciably altered in depressed patients.

Another theory is that adrenal gland enlargement during depression may increase the capacity for cortisol release. In fact, anatomical studies of depressed patients utilizing either post-mortem dissection from suicide victims or *in vivo* structural imaging demonstrate not only adrenal gland enlargement (Amsterdam *et al.*, 1987; Zis and Zis, 1987; Nemeroff *et al.*, 1992; Szigethy *et al.*, 1994; Rubin *et al.*, 1995), but pituitary enlargement as well (Krishnan *et al.*, 1991). Adrenal enlargement may indeed be at least partly responsible for the hypercortisolaemia commonly witnessed in depressed patients, but further investigation is needed. Future studies combining volumetric pituitary and/or adrenal imaging with low dose (i.e. physiological dose) CRH and/or ACTH stimulation may help clarify the relative contribution of glandular hypertrophy to HPA axis hyperactivity.

Although the impact of pituitary and adrenal enlargement upon other measures of HPA axis hyperactivity has not been resolved, recent data suggest that hypersecretion of CRH is likely to be the predominant cause of HPA axis hyperactivity in depression. Several lines of evidence in both animal and human studies indicate that many depressed patients hypersecrete CRH. First, intracerebral administration of CRH to laboratory animals produces behavioural changes, such as decreased appetite, disrupted sleep, and diminished libido, that are homologous to depression in humans (Sutton *et al.*, 1982; Dunn and Berridge, 1990). Second, behavioural changes similar to depression are witnessed in transgenic mice that either over-express CRH (Heinrichs *et al.*, 1997) or under-express a certain class of CRH receptor (Contarino *et al.*, 1999). Third, basal concentrations of CRH have repeatedly been shown to be elevated in the CSF of depressed patients (Nemeroff *et al.*, 1984; Arato *et al.*, 1987; Banki *et al.*, 1987; France *et al.*, 1988; Risch *et al.*, 1992). Fourth, depressed patients typically exhibit a blunted ACTH response after exogenous administration of CRH. This blunting of the ACTH response in the CRH stimulation test is thought to be a consequence of CRH receptor down-regulation at the pituitary which is, in turn, secondary to chronic CRH hypersecretion (Gold *et al.*, 1984; Holsboer *et al.*, 1984; Amsterdam *et al.*, 1988; Kathol *et al.*, 1989; Young *et al.*, 1990). It should be noted, however, that pretreatment with metyrapone (a potent inhibitor of cortisol production that presumably abolishes HPA axis negative feedback) before CRH administration increases the ACTH response in depressed patients (von Bardeleben *et al.*, 1988; Lisansky *et al.*, 1989; Young *et al.*, 1995). This may indicate that mechanisms other than CRH receptor down-regulation may, at least in part, underlie the blunted ACTH response to CRH stimulation, but metyrapone's acute effects on glucocorticoid receptor density (Rupprecht *et al.*, 1991) make these data difficult to interpret. Fifth, depressed suicide victims demonstrate a reduction in the density of CRH receptors in the frontal cortex (Nemeroff *et al.*, 1988), presumably due to chronic CRH hypersecretion, a finding recently replicated in a completely novel set of samples (Hucks *et al.*, 1997). Finally, perhaps the most definitive evidence comes from two studies by Raadsheer and colleagues of changes in the hypothalamus of depressed patients (Raadsheer *et al.*, 1994; Raadsheer *et al.*, 1995). These studies demonstrated a greater than 200% increase in the number of hypothalamic CRH-secreting neurons in patients who had died with untreated depression, suggesting that neurons which do not typically secrete CRH do so in depressed patients. Their second study documented marked increases in hypothalamic CRH mRNA expression in depressed patients compared with controls.

A critical question is whether CRH hypersecretion occurs only during a depressive episode or exists prior to the clinical manifestation of the illness. This question is important for at least two reasons. First, this is important to our understanding of the pathophysiology of depression. If CRH hypersecretion is a trait dependent variable in depressed patients, i.e. they hypersecrete CRH both prior to depression and when they are not depressed, then alterations in CRH secretion may be a permissive factor in the risk for becoming depressed. In this case, other factors may be involved in triggering an episode of illness. If, however, CRH hypersecretion is state dependent and occurs only during episodes of illness, then it is critical and perhaps even necessary for the development of the disorder. This is no small matter, and other combinations and permutations are possible. However, if CRH hypersecretion is state dependent, then a next major step in studying the neurobiology of depression is to investigate the mechanisms that induce persistent CRH hypersecretion. If CRH hypersecretion is largely trait dependent, then our next step is to determine why someone who chronically hypersecretes CRH suddenly becomes depressed. This question is also important from a clinical standpoint. If CRH hypersecretion is trait dependent, then it may afford an opportunity to devise a screening test that reliably identifies those at risk for becoming depressed. If it is state dependent, then we may ultimately be able to devise tests to guide medication selection or to monitor treatment response.

A definitive answer to the state v. trait question could be obtained by measuring CRH neuronal activity in healthy volunteers who had never been depressed but are at risk, and then repeating the measure if and when any of those subjects ever become depressed. Unfortunately, such research would be costly, unwieldy, and is unlikely ever to be undertaken. Moreover, patients at risk may hypersecrete CRH at baseline. Short of this, assessing CRH activity during an episode of depression and repeating that measure once the depression has resolved can provide some insight. These studies do exist. In fact, both the elevation of CRH concentration in CSF (Nemeroff *et al.*, 1991; Veith *et al.*, 1992; DeBellis *et al.*, 1993) and the blunting of the ACTH response to the CRH stimulation test (Amsterdam *et al.*, 1988) have been shown to normalize when depression resolves in response to antidepressant medication or electroconvulsive therapy. This suggests that CRH hypersecretion is likely to be a state dependent variable in patients with depression. It can be argued however that indirect effects of these somatic therapies upon HPA axis activity in depressed patients may confound these results. In other words, did the CRH hypersecretion resolve because the depression remitted or because the patient was treated with an antidepressant (a fine distinction but a fair and important one nonetheless)? Although HPA axis activity has been demonstrated to remain normal in successfully treated patients even after the course of antidepressant medication has been discontinued(Thakore *et al.*, 1997), a more satisfying answer to this question will no doubt be provided when future studies investigate HPA axis activity before and after a successful non-pharmacological treatment (e.g. psychotherapy, rapid transcranial magnetic stimulation).

BEYOND HPA AXIS CHANGES IN DEPRESSION

As the pivotal biological system responsible for integrating the mammalian stress response, it is unlikely that the activity of the HPA axis is insulated from interaction with other biological systems. Indeed, there is increasing evidence that complex, interdependent interactions exist between the HPA axis and other neural and endocrine systems. Furthermore, it is unlikely that this key stress response system functions aberrantly in depression but is not impacted in other stress-related disorders. Again, there is growing evidence of HPA axis dysfunction in other psychiatric and medical illnesses. A comprehensive review of other neurobiological changes in depression or HPA axis changes in other disorders is beyond the scope of this discussion. However, it is clearly of interest to go beyond a limited discourse of the HPA axis in depression. In so doing, we gain a better glimpse of the broader context in which the neuroendocrinology of depression will emerge, and will perhaps be better equipped to anticipate future directions in multi-system research.

Looking beyond depression, patterns of HPA axis activity have been investigated in a host of other psychiatric and medical disorders. Of particular interest are the HPA axis changes commonly reported in post traumatic stress disorder (PTSD). PTSD, like depression, is a stress-related psychiatric disorder that is associated with well-documented changes in HPA axis activity. Like patients with depression, those with PTSD appear to hypersecrete CRH as evidenced by elevated levels of CRH in CSF (Bremner et al., 1997; Baker et al., 1999) and a blunted ACTH response after exogenous CRH administration (Smith et al., 1989; Heim et al., 1997). However, the similarities may end here. Numerous studies, although not all, (Pitman and Orr, 1990; Lemieux and Coe, 1995; Liberzon et al., 1999) indicate that baseline urinary and plasma cortisol concentrations in patients with PTSD are decreased (Mason et al., 1986; Yehuda et al., 1990; Yehuda et al., 1995b; Boscarino, 1996; Goenjian et al., 1996; Heim et al., 1997; Jensen et al., 1997; Kellner et al., 1997; Kellner and Yehuda, 1999) despite the apparent hypersecretion of CRH. This is initially counter-intuitive. However, evidence that glucocorticoid receptors are up-regulated (Yehuda et al., 1991; Yehuda et al., 1996) and that cortisol concentrations are 'super-suppressed' in the DST (Stein et al., 1997) suggest a plausible mechanism. The low cortisol concentrations in patients with PTSD may be a consequence of exaggerated HPA axis negative feedback (Yehuda, 1998; Bremner et al., 1999).

There is an important point to be made in comparing the HPA axis changes associated with depression with those that occur in PTSD. Two psychiatric disorders that share certain phenomenological features and that are both related to stress apparently result in very distinct patterns of dysfunction within the HPA axis. Further complexity is provided by the common comorbidity of depression and PTSD. This concatenation of findings illustrates that we too readily rely on simplistic models of HPA axis function that are clearly lacking. If depression and PTSD demonstrate similar aberrations at the apical levels of the HPA axis but distinctly different activity at its lower levels, then there must be a complex system of homeostatic mechanisms regulating HPA axis activity that has not yet been elucidated.

In studying depression, it is also important to avoid the mistaken assumption that changes in HPA axis function are independent of, and unrelated to, alterations in other biological systems. Furthermore, one should not be fooled into thinking that cross-system interactions are unidirectional and straightforward. For example, it was long assumed that hyperactivity of the HPA axis suppresses immune function. After all, synthetic glucocorticoids are routinely used to suppress immune responses in patients with allergic reactions and autoimmune disorders. However depressed patients exhibit signs of both immunosuppression and immunoactivation which defy simple explanation (Miller, 1998). Cellular immunity studies in depressed patients incorporating cellular enumeration and immune cell proliferative responses have on the whole indicated a pattern of cellular immunosuppression.

Decreased natural killer cell activity arguably has been the most consistent finding. However, certain components of the humoral immune system often appear to be activated as part of an acute phase response in depressed patients. Indeed, depressed patients have exhibited increases in concentrations of a variety of acute phase proteins (e.g. α_1-acid glycoprotein) and proinflammatory cytokines (e.g. IL-1, IL-2, and IL-6).

How can evidence of immunosuppression be reconciled with the apparently contradictory evidence of immunoactivation? It may be that the stress associated with depression elicits bidirectional, homeostatic interactions between the endocrine and immune systems. For example, increased CRH secretion has been associated with humoral immunoactivation as evidenced by increased proinflammatory cytokine release. Cytokines may in turn augment HPA axis function by promoting additional CRH release and by inducing glucocorticoid resistance that impairs HPA axis negative feedback. Conversely, HPA hyperactivity also elicits immunosuppression as evidenced by decreased natural killer cell activity. Clearly the interaction between the immune system and the HPA axis is complex and interdependent. It is this intricate cross-system coordination that will undoubtedly drive future multi-system neurobiological research.

THE HPA AXIS AND THE DIATHESIS/STRESS MODEL OF DEPRESSION

Stress plays a seminal role in the pathogenesis of depression and, in fact, many other psychiatric disorders. Stressful life events clearly trigger episodes of psychiatric illness (Kendler *et al.*, 1999) and for that matter a variety of medical illnesses (Hurst *et al.*, 1976; Elliot, 1989; Levenson and Bemis, 1991; Adler and Hillhouse, 1996). Nevertheless, some individuals can tolerate greater magnitudes or more prolonged stress without becoming ill. Others unfortunately have a constitutional predisposition rendering them highly vulnerable to stress-induced illness. This predisposition to illness, known as a diathesis, serves as the foundation for the widely accepted diathesis/stress model of depression (Alloy *et al.*, 1988; Robins and Block, 1989; Monroe and Simons, 1991; Metalsky and Joiner, 1992; Spangler *et al.*, 1993; Coyne and Whiffen, 1995; Flett *et al.*, 1995; Hilsman and Garber, 1995; Brent *et al.*, 1996; Nemeroff, 1998a; Burke and Elliott, 1999).

What is the source of this diathesis? Proponents of the diathesis/stress model typically posit that both genetic (i.e. inherited) and epigenetic (i.e. acquired) factors contribute to the vulnerability to stress-induced illness. This of course extends the discussion to the often contentious nature v. nurture debate in which the relative contribution of inheritance and environment is deliberated. The diathesis/stress model affords opportunity for a balance between these two disparate views and can be used as a comprehensive schema with which to organize the primary concepts regarding the inherited and non-inherited mechanisms by which a person becomes vulnerable to illness.

There is certainly a genetic component to the diathesis for depression. Concordance rates for major depression among monozygotic twins are twice that of dizygotic twins (Nurnberger *et al.*, 1986; Torgersen, 1986; McGuffin and Katz, 1989). Nevertheless, it has been difficult to identify the gene or genes, much less their products, that underlie the biological substrates that mediate the genetic contributions to the diathesis for depression. Most psychiatric geneticists are by now reconciled to the fact that the genetic contribution to depression and other psychiatric illnesses is not a single gene inherited by Mendelian transmission. To be certain, this would probably have been readily detectable long ago by linkage analysis. It is more likely that the genetic component of the constitutional predisposition to depression in certain individuals arises either from complex polygenic patterns of inheritance or even more complicated epigenetic modification of genotypic risk (Plotsky and Nemeroff, 1998).

There is also clear epidemiological evidence of a considerable environmental contribution to the risk for depression. The epigenetic contribution to the diathesis can in fact emanate from biological, psychological, familial, or social stressors. Thus, stress plays a bifurcated role in the pathogenetic mechanism (Richters and Weintraub, 1990). A life stressor coincident with an episode of depression serves as a precipitant to its onset. However, when stress antedates an episode of depression (particularly during childhood development), the stress is likely to serve a more formative role in shaping the predisposition to future illness. Although there is evidence that the predominant epigenetic contributions to the diathesis occur during the maturational processes of childhood (thereby interfering with normal development), the diathesis is never fixed. Ongoing stress during adulthood may in fact be 'bad for the brain' and continue to modify the predisposition to illness (Bremner, 1999). Theoretically, this vulnerability to illness should be quantifiable both by psychological and biological measures. It is this conviction that the diathesis for illness may be measurable that drives an expanding line of research into the persistent sequelae of adverse early life experiences. Building upon the existing literature regarding normal HPA axis physiology and HPA axis dysfunction in depression and other illnesses, these studies have understandably initially investigated the impact of early life stress upon HPA axis function with intriguing results.

The bulk of the extant data regarding the developmental effects of early life stress is derived from the animal literature. Numerous stress paradigms have been implemented in young animals, but the two that produce the most robust findings are the maternal/social deprivation studies and the variable foraging studies. In rodent maternal deprivation studies, rat pups are separated from their mother for a prescribed interval (or repeated intervals) prior to weaning. The separated pups are not only deprived of maternal care during the period of the separation, but maternal behaviour typically remains deranged even after the pups are returned (Huot et al., 1997). Maternal deprivation produces abrupt increases in HPA axis activity as indicated by elevations in the serum concentrations of corticosterone (the rodent equivalent to cortisol) (Schanberg and Kuhn, 1985; Pauk et al., 1986; Pihoker et al., 1993) and ACTH, (Walker et al., 1991) in conjunction with findings suggestive of CRH hypersecretion (Pihoker et al., 1993).

Of paramount relevance to the diathesis/stress model is the finding that the HPA axis changes induced by maternal deprivation persist into adulthood. When exposed to a stressor during adulthood, rats that were maternally deprived as pups exhibit a variable pattern of changes in ACTH and corticosterone responses (Ladd et al., 1996; Workel et al., 1997; van Oers et al., 1998). Furthermore, maternally deprived adult rats demonstrate increases in hypothalamic expression of CRH mRNA in the hypothalamus and increased CRH concentrations in the median eminence, indicating that CRH hypersecretion probably underlies the persistent alterations in HPA axis activity (Plotsky et al., 1993).

Maternal deprivation studies have also been conducted in non-human primates, though these are perhaps better termed social deprivation studies because they separate the young animal not only from mother but also from the social group as a whole. The earliest reports from this model emphasized the homology of the behavioural response of the separated animal to depression in humans (Harlow and Harlow, 1962). Subsequent experimental refinements in which the infant's mother was replaced with a series of incrementally more realistic maternal surrogates (Harlow et al., 1971) provided an opportunity for a scalar assessment of varying degrees of early life social deprivation.

Unfortunately, HPA axis function has had relatively limited investigation in socially deprived primates. Monkeys raised in total isolation do exhibit higher basal cortisol concentrations than those raised apart from their mothers with a group of age-matched peers; however, no differences in the cortisol response to a novel situation have been found (Sackett, 1973). A surprising study reported that basal concentrations of ACTH and ACTH/cortisol responses to stress were higher in mother-reared monkeys than peer-reared monkeys (Clarke, 1993). The implications of these findings are unclear.

Recognizing that the total and prolonged social isolation implemented in these studies has few if any parallels in humans, other studies have utilized a briefer (typically 24 hour) maternal separation. One such study placed the young non-human primates into one of four experimental conditions: total isolation, remaining with mother, placed with a peer of the same group, or placed with a peer from another group (Gunnar et al., 1980). Thirty minutes after separation, the isolated infant and the infant placed with a strange peer exhibited hypercortisolaemia, but one day later only the isolated infant had a demonstrable elevation in cortisol concentration. Thus, the presence of peer-aged conspecifics modulated the HPA axis response to separation. It is also possible to vary the mode of maternal separation. For example, another study placed the infants into one of three conditions: total isolation, remaining with mother, separated from mother but able to see her (Levine et al., 1985). In this study, the totally isolated infants had the highest plasma cortisol concentrations while there were no detectable differences in the cortisol concentrations of the other two groups. A similar study in which infants were totally isolated, left with mother, or placed in an adjacent cage with mother in full view produced elevations in plasma cortisol that were greatest in the total isolates and at an intermediate level in those separated but able to see their mother (Wiener et al., 1990).

Primate variable foraging studies represent an incremental advance in early life stress research. These paradigms avoid direct human contact with the young animal by instead modulating an environmental stressor that does not directly stress the infant but instead renders more difficult the mother's ability to provide adequate maternal care. The purpose is not to starve the animals but to increase the work of parenting while permitting adequate nutrition of both mother and infant. This model utilizes three foraging conditions: low foraging demand (LFD), high foraging demand (HFD), and variable foraging demand (VFD). In the LFD condition, food can always be readily obtained with minimal maternal effort. HFD mothers, however must always perform a task such as digging through wood chip bedding to procure food. Finally, in the VFD condition, the amount of maternal effort necessary to obtain food is unpredictable.

Adult primates that were raised under VFD conditions exhibit higher CSF CRH concentrations than either the HFD and LFD groups (Coplan et al., 1996). However, the VFD offspring exhibit lower CSF cortisol concentrations than the comparator groups (Coplan et al., 1996), a finding that is strikingly similar to HPA axis changes reported in PTSD (Yehuda et al., 1995a; Yehuda, 1998; Bremner et al., 1999). A subsequent study demonstrated that somatostatin, a peptide whose release is potentiated by CRH but that itself suppresses HPA axis activity, is also elevated in adult primates raised under VFD conditions (Coplan et al., 1998). Consequently, somatostatin hypersecretion could potentially explain the conundrum in some disorders of hypocortisolaemia in the context of CRH hypersecretion.

Human research into the impact of early life stress upon HPA axis function is in its infancy. Two recent studies do warrant mention. Both studies compared measures of HPA axis activity in four groups of adult women: healthy volunteers, women exposed to significant early life stress, women exposed to significant early life stress who fulfilled criteria for major depression at the time of the study, and women had major depression at the time of the study but were not exposed to early life stress. Early life stress

PHYSICAL CONSEQUENCES OF DEPRESSION

in these studies was defined as repeated moderate to severe sexual or physical abuse. In the first study, the subjects underwent CRH and ACTH
hormonal challenge tests (Heim *et al.*, 2001). The patients who had been
abused, but were not depressed, exhibited an exaggerated ACTH response
but a blunted cortisol response to CRH stimulation. By contrast, both
depression groups (abused and non-abused) demonstrated both a blunted
ACTH and a blunted cortisol response to exogenous CRH administration.
In the ACTH stimulation test, survivors of child abuse exhibited a diminished cortisol response. These findings suggest that traumatic early life
experiences may precipitate a persistent sensitization of the anterior pituitary
with a counter-regulatory adrenocortical adaptation.

Table 1. Summary of persistent HPA axis changes related to early life stress.

	CRF Stimulation Test		Psychosocial Stress Test	
	ACTH	Cortisol	ACTH	Cortisol
Early life stress only	↑	↑	↑	0
Early life stress and depression	↓	↓	↑↑	↑
Depression only	↓	↓	0	0

↑: greater response than controls.
↓: smaller response than controls.
0: response does not differ from controls.

In the accompanying study, the same subjects participated in a standardized laboratory psychosocial stressor protocol in which they were asked to
perform a series of mental tasks in front of a small audience (Heim *et al.*,
2000). In this study, the abused/depressed group exhibited the most robust
increases in ACTH and cortisol responses. Meanwhile, the abused/non-
depressed group also demonstrated an increased ACTH, but a normal cortisol, response to the stressor. Interestingly, HPA axis responses in the
depression only group were indistinguishable from those of the healthy
volunteers. Consistent with the first study, the psychosocial stress appears to
demonstrate in the abused/non-depressed group a pattern of sensitization at
the level of the anterior pituitary associated with an adrenal adaptation. The
findings from the abused/depressed group raise two interesting points. First,
the adrenal adaptation appears to be lost when survivors of child abuse
become depressed. Second, a more intriguing point arises when we compare
the pituitary responses of this group in the two companion studies.
Exogenous administration of CRH exhibited a blunted ACTH response in
this group; however, the most marked ACTH response to the psychosocial
stressor was seen in this same group. How are we to understand this apparent contradiction? If CRH is not driving the ACTH response to the
psychosocial stressor (as the results of the CRH stimulation test would

suggest), then what biological process is inducing the release of ACTH in the depressed/abused group? There is presently no clear answer to this question, though potentiation of CRH release by vasopressin is one possibility.

These represent the first human studies to move beyond the neuroendocrinology of depression to address instead the neurobiology of its diathesis. The importance of this line of research should not be underestimated. First, this research has the potential to answer questions not only about the pathophysiology of depression and other psychiatric disorders but also about the pathogenesis of those illnesses. Second, as further studies more clearly characterize the neurobiology of diathesis, the possibility of finding biological markers not only for current illness but for the risk of illness becomes plausible. Such markers would be useful in screening at-risk populations. Finally, improved understanding of the neurobiology of diathesis may ultimately inform treatment selection for children exposed to early life stress before the neurobiological changes that convey the risk for adulthood psychopathology are in place.

THE HPA AXIS AND THE PSYCHOPHARMACOLOGY OF DEPRESSION

HPA axis research in depressed patients has uncovered a wealth of information regarding the neurobiology of the disorder; however, it has to date produced little of direct clinical relevance. None of the HPA axis hormonal assays including the DST, the ACTH and CRH stimulation tests, or the dexamethasone–CRH stimulation test has demonstrated the degree of specificity or sensitivity necessary to be of clinical value in the diagnosis of depressed patients. Furthermore, all of the current antidepressant treatment modalities continue to act primarily upon biogenic amine systems.

Our failure thus far to identify a definitive biological marker for depression coupled with our inability to utilize biological measures to guide rational antidepressant selection speaks of the complexity of the pathophysiology of depression. Indeed, biologically, depression is surely a heterogeneous syndrome. Consequently, a better understanding of how a particular stressor precipitates a depressive syndrome may lead to more diagnostic clarity and more specifically targeted therapies.

These shortcomings may, at least in part, be ripe for change. Future advances in the treatment of stress-related illnesses including depression and PTSD are likely to focus on agents that directly modulate CRH activity (Nemeroff, 1998b, Holsboer, 1999). Indeed, the efficacy of serotonergic antidepressants in treating stress-dependent illness may depend upon serotonin/CRH interactions at the locus coeruleus and other CNS sites (Curtis and Valentino, 1994; Price et al., 1998). A number of CRH receptor antagonists currently in testing loom on the horizon (Owens and Nemeroff, 1999a; Owens and Nemeroff, 1999b); they appear to possess both antidepressant and anxiolytic properties.

The spectrum of application for CRH antagonists may indeed be quite broad. In addition to treating psychiatric illness, CRH antagonists may provide a means to circumvent the development of a diathesis for stress-induced illness in children exposed to the stress of child abuse or other childhood traumatic experiences. If adverse early life experiences induce a diathesis to subsequent psychopathology and persistent changes in CRH neuronal circuits and the HPA axis activity are the biological substrate for that diathesis, then CRH receptor antagonists may avert the psychiatric liability of early life stress before the ultimate development of stress-related illness.

ACKNOWLEDGEMENTS

The authors are supported by NIMH MH-42088 and MH-39415, an Established Investigator Award from NARSAD (C.B. Nemeroff), and the American Psychiatric Association/Lilly Psychiatric Research Fellowship (D.J. Newport).

REFERENCES

Adler, C.M. and Hillhouse J.J. (1996). Stress, health, and immunity: A review of the literature. In: Miller, T.W. (Ed.), *Theory and Assessment of Stressful Life Events*. International Universities Press, Madison, CT, pp. 109–138.

Alloy, L., Hartlage, S. and Abramson, L. (1988). Testing the cognitive diathesis-stress theories of depression: Issues of research design, conceptualization, and assessment. In: Alloy, L. (Ed.), *Cognitive Processes in Depression*. Guildford Pess, New York: pp. 31–73.

Amsterdam, J., Maislin, G., Winokur, A. *et al.* (1988). The oCRH test before and after clinical recovery from depression. *J Affect Disord* **14**, 213–222.

Amsterdam, J., Marinelli, D., Arger, P. and Winokur, A. (1987). Assessment of adrenal gland volume by computed tomography in depressed patients and healthy volunteers. *Psychiatry Res* **21**, 189–197.

Arana, G., Baldesarrini, R. and Ornsteen, M. (1985). The dexamethasone suppression test for diagnosis and prognosis in psychiatry. *Arch Gen Psychiatry* **42**, 1192–1204.

Arana, G. and Mossman, D. (1988). The DST and depression: Approaches to the use of a laboratory test in psychiatry. *Neurol Clin* **6**, 21–39.

Arato, M., Banki, C., Nemeroff, C. and Bissette, B. (1987). Hypothalamic-pituitary-adrenal axis and suicide. *Ann N Y Acad Sci* **487**, 263–270.

Baker, D.G., West, S.A., Nicholson, W.E. *et al.* (1999). Serial CSF corticotropin-releasing hormone levels and adrenocortical activity in combat veterans with posttraumatic stress disorder. *Am J Psychiatry* **156**, 585–588.

Banki, C., Bissette, G., Arato, M., O'Connor, L. and Nemeroff, C. (1987). Cerebrospinal fluid corticotropin-releasing factor-like immunoreactivity in depression and schizophrenia. *Am J Psychiatry* **144**, 873–877.

Board, F., Wadeson, R. and Persky, H. (1957). Depressive affect and endocrine function: Blood levels of adrenal cortex and thyroid hormones in patients suffering from depressive reactions. *Arch Neurol Psychiatry* **78**, 612–620.

Boscarino, J. (1996). Posttraumatic stress disorder, exposure to combat, and lower plasma cortisol among Vietnam veterans: Findings and clinical implications. *J Consult Clin Psychol* **64**, 191–201.

Bremner, J.D. (1999). Does stress damage the brain? *Biol Psychiatry* **45**, 797–805.

Bremner, J., Licinio, J., Darnell, A. *et al.* (1997). Elevated CSF corticotropin-releasing factor concentrations in posttraumatic stress disorder. *Am J Psychiatry* **154**, 624–629.

Bremner, J., Southwick, S. and Charney, D. (1999). The neurobiology of posttraumatic stress disorder: An integration of animal and human research. In: Saigh, P. and Bremner, J. (Eds), *Posttraumatic Stress Disorder: A Comprehensive Text*. Allyn & Bacon, Needham Heights, MA, pp. 103–143.

Brent, D., Mortiz, G. and Liotus, L. (1996). A test of the diathesis-stress model of adolescent depression in friends and acquaintances of adolescent suicide victims. In: Pfeffer, C. (Ed.), *Severe Stress and Mental Disturbance in Children*. American Psychiatric Press, Washington, pp. 347–360.

Burke, P. and Elliott, M. (1999). Depression in pediatric chronic illness: A diathesis-stress model. *Psychosomatics* **40**, 5–17.

Carpenter, W. and Bunney, W. (1971). Adrenal cortical activity in depressive illness. *Am J Psychiatry* **128**, 31–40.

Carroll, B. (1968). Pituitary-adrenal function in depression. *Lancet* **556**, 1373–1374.

Clarke, A. (1993). Social rearing effects on HPA axis activity over early development and in response to stress in rhesus monkeys. *Dev Psychobiol* **26**, 433–446.

Contarino, A., Dellu, F., Koob, G.F. *et al.* (1999). Reduced anxiety-like and cognitive performance in mice lacking the corticotropin-releasing factor receptor 1. *Brain Res* **835**, 1–9.

Coplan, J., Andrews, M., Rosenblum, L. *et al.* (1996). Persistent elevations of cerebrospinal fluid concentrations of corticotropin-releasing factor in adult non-human primates exposed to early-life stressors: Implications for the pathophysiology of mood and anxiety disorders. *Proc Nat Acad Sci USA* **93**, 1619–1623.

Coplan, J., Trost, R., Owens, M. *et al.* (1998). Cerebrospinal fluid concentrations of somatostatin and biogenic amines in grown primates reared by mothers exposed to manipulated foraging conditions. *Arch Gen Psychiatry* **55**, 473–477.

Coyne, J. and Whiffen, V. (1995). Issues in personality as diathesis for depression: The case of sociotropy:dependency and autonomy:self-criticism. *Psychol Bull* **118**, 358–378.

Curtis, A. and Valentino, R. (1994). Corticotropin-releasing factor neurotransmission in locus coeruleus: A possible site of antidepressant action. *Brain Res Bull* **35**, 581–587.

DeBellis, M., Gold, P., Geracioti, T., Listwak, S. and Kling, M. (1993). Fluoxetine significantly reduces CSF CRH and AVP concentrations in patients with major depression. *Am J Psychiatry* **150**, 656–657.

Dunn, A. and Berridge, C. (1990). Physiological and behavioral responses to corticotropin-releasing factor administration. Is CRF a mediator of anxiety or stress responses? *Brain Res Rev* **15**, 71–100.

Elliott, G. (1989). Stress and illness. In: Cheren, S. (Ed.), *Psychosomatic Medicine: Theory, Physiology, and Practice*. International Universities Press, Madison, CT, pp. 45–90.

Evans, D. and Nemeroff C. (1983). Use of the dexamethasone suppression test using DSM-III criteria on an inpatient psychiatric unit. *Biol Psychiatry* **18**, 505–511.

Flett, G., Hewitt, P., Blankstein, K. and Mosher, S. (1995). Perfectionism, life events, and depressive symptoms: A test of a diathesis-stress model. *Curr Psychol Dev Learn Personal Soc* **14**, 112–137.

France, R., Urban, B., Krishnan, K. *et al.* (1988). CSF corticotropin-releasing factor-like immunoreactivity in chronic pain patients with and without major depression. *Biol Psychiatry* **23**, 86–88.

Goenjian, A., Yehuda, R. and Pynoos, R. (1996). Basal cortisol and dexamethasone suppression of cortisol among adolescents after the 1988 earthquake in Armenia. *Am J Psychiatry* **153**, 929–934.

Gold, P., Chrousos, G., Kellner, C. *et al.* (1984). Psychiatric implications of basic and clinical studies with corticotropin-releasing factor. *Am J Psychiatry* **141**, 619–627.

Gunnar, M.R., Gonzalez, C.A. and Levine, S. (1980). The role of peers in modifying behavioral distress and pituitary-adrenal response to a novel environment in year-old rhesus monkeys. *Physiol Behav* **25**, 795–798.

Harlow, H. and Harlow, M. (1962). The effect of rearing conditions on behavior. *Bull Menninger Clin* **26**, 213–224.

Harlow, H., Harlow, M. and Suomi, S. (1971). From thought to therapy: Lessons from a primate laboratory. *Am Scientist* **59**, 538–549.

Heim, C., Ehlert, U. and Rexhausen, J. (1997). Psychoendocrinological observations in women with chronic pelvic pain. In: Yehuda, R. and McFarlane, A. (Eds), *Psychobiology of Posttraumatic Stress Disorder*. New York Academy of Sciences, New York, pp. 456–458.

Heim, C., Newport, D., Heit, S. *et al.* (2000). Increased pituitary-adrenal and autonomic responses to stress in adult women after sexual and physical abuse in childhood. *JAMA* **284**, 592–597.

Heim, C., Newport, D., Bonsall, R., Miller, A. and Nemeroff, C. (2001). Altered pituitary-adrenal axis responses to provocative challenge tests in adult survivors of childhood abuse: The role of comorbid depression. *Am J Psychiatry* **158**, 575–581.

Heinrichs, S.C., Min, H., Tamraz, S. and Carmouche, M. (1997). Anti-sexual and anxiogenic behavioral consequences of corticotropin-releasing factor overexpression are centrally mediated. *Psychoneuroendocrinology* **22**, 215–224.

Hilsman, R. and Garber, J. (1995). A test of the cognitive diathesis:stress model of depression in children: Academic stressors, attributional style, perceived competence, and control. *J Personal Soc Psychol* **69**, 370–380.

Holsboer, F. (1999). The rationale for corticotropin-releasing hormone receptor (CRH-R) antagonists to treat depression and anxiety. *J Psychiatric Res* **33**, 181–214.

Holsboer, F., Von Bardeleben, U., Gerken, A. and Muler, D. (1984). Blunted corticotropin and normal cortisol response to human corticotropin-releasing factor in depression. *New Engl J Med* **311**, 1127.

Hucks, D., Lowther, S., Crompton, M., Katona, C. and Horton, R. (1997). Corticotropin-releasing factor binding sites in cortex of depressed suicides. *Psychopharmacology* **134**, 174–178.

Huot, R., Smith, M. and Plotsky, P. (1997). *Alterations of Maternal-infant Interaction as a Result of Maternal Separation in Long Evans Rats and its Behavioral and Neuroendocrine Consequences*. International Society of Psychoneuroendocrinology, XXVIIIth Congress, San Francisco, CA.

Hurst, M.W., Jenkins, C.D. and Rose, R.M. (1976). The relation of psychological stress to onset of medical illness. *Ann Rev Med* **27**, 1–31.

Jensen, C., Keller, T. and Peskind, E. (1997). Behavioral and plasma cortisol responses to sodium lactate infusion in post-traumatic stress disorder. In: Yehuda, R. and McFarlane, A. (Eds), *Psychobiology of Posttraumatic Stress Disorder*. New York Academy of Sciences, New York, pp. 444–447.

Kathol, R., Jaeckle, R., Lopez, J. and Mullter, W. (1989). Consistent reduction of ACTH responses to stimulation with CRF, vasopressin and hypoglycemia in patients with depression. *Br J Psychiatry* **155**, 468–478.

Kellner, M., Baker, D and Yehuda, R. (1997). Salivary cortisol in Operation Desert Storm returnees. *Biol Psychiatry* **42**, 849–850.

Kellner, M. and Yehuda, R. (1999). Do panic disorder and posttraumatic stress disorder share a common psychoneuroendocrinology? *Psychoneuroendocrinology* **24**, 485–504.

Kendler, K., Karkowski, L. and Prescott, C. (1999). Causal relationship between stressful life events and the onset of major depression. *Am J Psychiatry* **156**, 837–841.

Krishnan, K., France, P., Pelton, S. *et al.* (1983). What does the dexamethasone suppression test identify? *Biol Psychiatry* **20**, 957–964.

Krishnan, K., Ritchie, J., Saunders, W., Nemeroff, C. and Carroll B. (1990). Adrenocortical sensitivity to low -dose ACTH administration in depressed patients. *Biol Psychiatry* **27**, 930–933.

Krishnan, K., Doraiswamy, P., Lurie, S. *et al.* (1991). 'Pituitary size in depression.' *J Clin Endocrinol* **72**, 256–259.

Ladd, C., Owens, M. and Nemeroff, C. (1996). Persistent changes in corticotropin-releasing factor neuronal systems induced by maternal deprivation. *Endocrinology* **137**, 1212–1218.

Lemieux, A. and Coe, C. (1995). Abuse-related post-traumatic stress disorder: Evidence for chronic neuroendocrine activation in women. *Psychosom Med* **57**, 105–115.

Levenson, J.L. and Bemis, C. (1991). The role of psychological factors in cancer onset and progression. *Psychosomatics* **32**, 124–132.

Levine, S., Johnson, D.F. and Gonzalez, C.A. (1985). Behavioral and hormonal responses to separation in infant rhesus monkeys and mothers. *Behav Neurosci* **99**, 399–410.

Liberzon, I., Abelson, J.L., Flagel, S.B., Raz, J. and Young, E.A. (1999). Neuroendocrine and psychophysiologic responses in PTSD: A symptom provocation study. *Neuropsychopharmacology* **21**, 40–50.

Lisansky, J., Peake, G.T., Strassman, R.J. and Qualls, C. (1989). Augmented pituitary corticotropin response to a threshold dosage of human corticotropin-releasing hormone in depressives pretreated with metyrapone. *Arch Gen Psychiatry* **46**, 641–649.

Mason, J., Giller, E., Kosten, T., Ostroff, T. and Podd, L. (1986). Urinary free cortisol levels in post-traumatic stress disorder patients. *J Nerv Ment Dis* **174**, 145–149.

McGuffin, P. and Katz, R. (1989). The genetics of depression and manic-depressive disorder. *Br J Psychiatry* **155**, 294–304.

Metalsky, G. and Joiner, T. (1992). Vulnerability to depressive symptomatology: A prospective test of the diathesis-stress and causal mediation components of the hopelessness theory of depression. *J Personal Soc Psychol* **63**, 667–675.

Miller, A. (1998). Neuroendocrine and immune system interactions in stress and depression. *Psychiatr Clin North Am* **21**, 443–463.

Monroe, S. and Simons, A. (1991). Diathesis/stress theories in the context of life stress research: Implications for the depressive disorders. *Psycholog Bull* **110**, 406–425.

Nemeroff, C. (1998a). The neurobiology of depression. *Sci Am* **278**, 28–35.

Nemeroff, C. (1998b). Psychopharmacology of affective disorders in the 21st century. *Biol Psychiatry* **44**, 517–525.

Nemeroff, C., Widerlov, E., Bissette, G. *et al.* (1984). Elevated concentrations of CSF corticotropin-releasing factor-like immunoreactivity in depressed patients. *Science* **226**, 1342–1344.

Nemeroff, C., Owens, M., Bissette, G. and Andorn, A. (1988). Reduced corticotropin releasing factor binding sites in the frontal cortex of suicide victims. *Arch Gen Psychiatry* **45**, 577–579.

Nemeroff, C., Bissette, G., Akil, H. and Fin, M. (1991). Neuropeptide concentrations in the cerebrospinal fluid of depressed patients treated with electroconvulsive therapy: Corticotropin-releasing factor, beta-endorphin and somatostatin. *Br J Psychiatry* **158**, 59–63.

Nemeroff, C., Krishnan, K., Reed, D. *et al.* (1992). Adrenal gland enlargement in major depression: A computed tomographic study. *Arch Gen Psychiatry* **49**, 384–387.

Nurnberger, J., Goldin, L. and Gershon, E. (1986). Genetics of psychiatric disorders. In: Winokur, G. and Clayton, P. (Eds), *The Medical Basis of Psychiatry*. W.B. Saunders, Philadelphia, pp. 486–521.

Owens, M. and Nemeroff, C. (1999a). Corticotropin-releasing factor antagonists in affective disorders. *Exp Opin Investigat Drugs* **8**, 1849–1858.

Owens, M. and Nemeroff, C. (1999b). Corticotropin-releasing factor antagonists: Therapeutic potential in the treatment of affective disorders. *CNS Drugs* **12**, 85–92.

Pauk, J., Kuhn, C., Field, T. and Schanberg, S. (1986). Positive effects of tactile vs. kinesthetic or vestibular stimulation on neuroendocrine and ODC activity in maternally deprived rat pups. *Life Sci* **39**, 2081–2087.

Pihoker, C., Owens, M., Kuhn, C., Schanberg, S. and Nemeroff, C. (1993). Maternal separation in neonatal rats elicits activation of the hypothalamic-pituitary-adreno-cortical axis: A putative role for corticotropin-releasing factor. *Psychoneuroendocrinology* **7**, 485–493.

Pitman, R. and Orr, S. (1990). Twenty-four hour cortisol and catecholamine excretion in combat-related posttraumatic stress disorder. *Biol Psychiatry* **27**, 245–247.

Plotsky, P. and Nemeroff, C. (1998). Molecular mechanisms and regulating behavior. In: Jameson, J. (Ed.), *Principles of Molecular Medicine*. Humana Press, Totoaw, NJ, pp. 979–987.

Plotsky, P., Thrivikraman, K. and Meaney, M. (1993). Central and feedback regulation of hypothalamic corticotropin-releasing factor secretion. In: Chadwick, D., Marsh, J. and Ackrill, K. (eds), *Symposium on Corticotropin-Releasing Factor*. John Wiley, Chichester, pp. 59–84.

Price, M., Curtis, A., Kirby, L., Valentino, R. and Lucki, I. (1998). Effects of corticotropin-releasing factor on brain serotonergic activity. *Neuropsychopharmacology* **18**, 492–502.

Raadsheer, F., Hoogendijk, W., Stam, F., Tilders, F. and Swaab, D. (1994). Increased number of corticotropin-releasing hormone expressing neurons in the hypothalamic paraventricular nucleus of depressed patients. *Neuroendocrinology* **60**, 436–444.

Raadsheer, F., van Keerikhuize, J., Lucassen, P. and Hoogendijk W. (1995). Corticotropin-releasing hormone mRNA levels in the paraventricular nucleus of patients with Alzheimer's disease and depression. *Am J Psychiatry* **152**, 1372–1376.

Richters, J. and Weintraub, S. (1990). Beyond diathesis: Toward an understanding of high risk environments. In: Rolf, J., Masten, A. and Cicchetti, D. (Eds), *Risk and Protective Factors in the Development of Psychopathology*. Cambridge University Press, New York, pp. 67–96.

Risch, S., Lewine, R., Kalin, N. *et al.* (1992). Limbic-hypothalamic-pituitary-adrenal axis activity and ventricular-to-brain ratio studies in affective illness and schizophrenia. *Neuropsychopharmacology* **6**, 95–100.

Robins, C. and Block, P. (1989). Cognitive theories of depression viewed from a diathesis-stress perspective: Evaluations of the models of Beck and of Abramson, Seligman, and Teasdale. *Cogn Ther Res* **13**, 297–313.

Rubin, R., Phillips, J., Sadow, T. and McCracken, J. (1995). Adrenal gland volume in major depression: Increase during the depressive episode and decrease with successful treatment. *Arch Gen Psychiatry* **52**, 213–218.

Rupprecht, R., Kornhuber, J., Wodarz, N. and Lugauer, J. (1991). Disturbed glucocorticoid receptor autoregulation and corticotropin response to dexamethasone in depressives pretreated with metyrapone. *Biol Psychiatry* **29**, 1099–1109.

Sachar, E.,Hellman, L., Fukushima, D. and Gallagher, T. (1970). Cortisol production in depressive illness. *Arch Gen Psychiatry* **23**, 289–298.

Sackett, G. (1973). Adrenocortical and behavioral reactions by differentially raised rhesus monkeys. *Physiol Psychol* **1**, 209–212.

Schanberg, S. and Kuhn, C. (1985). The biochemical effects of tactile deprivation in neonatal rats. *Persp Behav Med* **2**, 133–148.

Schatzberg, A., Rothschild, A., Bond, T. and Cole, J. (1984). The DST in psychotic depression: Diagnostic and pathophysiologic implications. *Psychopharmacol Bull* **20**, 362–364.

Smith, M., Davidson, J. and Ritchie, J. (1989). The corticotropin releasing hormone test in patients with post-traumatic stress disorder. *Biol Psychiatry* **26**, 349–355.

Spangler, D., Simons, A., Monroe, S. and Thase, M. (1993). Evaluating the hopelessness model of depression: Diathesis-stress and symptom components. *J Abnorm Psychol* **102**, 592–600.

Spiess, J., Rivier, J., Rivier, C. and Vale, W. (1981). Primary structure of corticotropin-releasing factor from ovine hypothalami. *Proc Nat Acad Sci USA* **78**, 6517–6521.

Stein, M., Yehuda, R. and Koverola, C. (1997). Enhanced dexamethasone suppression of plasma cortisol in adult women traumatized by childhood sexual abuse. *Biol Psychiatry* **42**, 680–686.

Sutton, R., Koob, G. and LeMoal, M. (1982). Corticotropin releasing factor produces behavioral activation in rats. *Nature* **297**, 331–333.

Szigethy, E., Conwell, Y., Forbes, N., Cox, C. and Caine, E. (1994). Adrenal weight and morphology in victims of completed suicide. *Biol Psychiatry* **36**, 374–380.

Thakore, J., Barnes, C., Joyce, J., Medbak, S. and Dinan, T. (1997). Effects of antidepressant treatment on corticotropin-induced cortisol responses in patients with melancholic depression. *Psychiatry Res* **73**, 27–32.

Torgersen, S. (1986). Genetic factors in moderately severe and mild affective disorders. *Arch Gen Psychiatry* **43**, 222–226.

Vale, W., Spiess, J., Rivier, C. and Rivier, J. (1981). Characterization of a 41-residue ovine hypothalamic peptide that stimulates secretion of corticotropin and beta-endorphin. *Science* **213**, 1394–1397.

van Oers, H., DeKloet, E. and Levine, S. (1998). Early versus late maternal deprivation differentially alters the endocrine and hypothalamic responses to stress. *Brain Res* **111**, 245–252.

Veith, R., Lewis, N., Langohr, J. *et al.* (1992). Effect of desipramine on cerebrospinal fluid concentrations of corticotropin-releasing factor in human subjects. *Psychiatry Res* **46**, 1–8.

von Bardeleben, U., Stalla, G.K., Mueller, O.A. and Holsboer, F. (1988). Blunting of ACTH response to human CRH in depressed patients is avoided by metyrapone pretreatment. *Biol Psychiatry* **24**, 782–786.

Walker, C., Scribner, K., Cascio, C. and Dallman, M. (1991). The pituitary-adreno-cortical system of neonatal rats is responsive to stress throughout development in a time-dependent and stressor-specific fashion. *Endocrinology* **128**, 1385–1395.

Wiener, S.G., Bayart, F., Faull, K.F. and Levine, S. (1990). Behavioral and physio-logical responses to maternal separation in squirrel monkeys (*Saimiri sciureus*). *Behav Neurosci* **104**, 108–115.

Workel, J., Oitzl, M., Ledeboer, A. and DeKloet, E. (1997). The Brown Norway rat displays enhanced stress-induced ACTH reactivity at day 18 after 24 h maternal deprivation at day 3. *Brain Res* **103**, 199–203.

Yehuda, R. (1998). Psychoneuroendocrinology of post-traumatic stress disorder. *Psychiatr Clin North Am* **21**, 359–379.

Yehuda, R., Southwick, S., Nussbaum, G. *et al.* (1990). Low urinary cortisol excre-tion in patients with posttraumatic stress disorder. *J Nerv Ment Dis* **178**, 366–369.

Yehuda, R., Lowy, M. and Southwick, S. (1991). Increased lymphocyte glucocorticoid receptor number in post-traumatic stress disorder. *Am J Psychiatry* **149**, 499–504.

Yehuda, R., Giller, E., Levengood, R., Southwick, S. and Siever, L. (1995a). Hypothalamic-pituitary-adrenal functioning in post-traumatic stress disorder. In: Friedman, M., Charney, D. and Deutch, A. (Eds), *Neurobiological and Clinical Consequences of Stress: From Normal Adaptation to Post-Traumatic Stress Disorder*. Lippincott-Raven, Philadelphia, pp. 351–365.

Yehuda, R., Kahana, B., Binder-Byrnes, K. *et al.*(1995b). Low urinary cortisol excre-tion in Holocaust survivors with posttraumatic stress disorder. *Am J Psychiatry* **152**, 982–986.

Yehuda, R., Boisoneau, D. and Lowy, M. (1996). Dose-response changes in plasma cortisol and lymphocyte glucocorticoid receptors following dexamethasone admin-istration in combat veterans with and without post-traumatic stress disorder. *Arch Gen Psychiatry* **52**, 583–593.

Young, E., Watson, S. and Kotun, J. (1990). Beta-lipotropin-beta-endorphin response to low-dose ovine corticotropin releasing factor in endogenous depression. *Arch Gen Psychiatry* **47**, 449–457.

Young, E.A., Akil, Y., Haskett, R.F. and Watson, S.J. (1995). Evidence against changes in corticotroph CRF receptors in depressed patients. *Biol Psychiatry* **37**, 355–363.

Zis, K. and Zis, A. (1987). Increased adrenal weight in victims of violent suicide. *Am J Psychiatry* **144**, 1214–1215.

2

Brain Corticosteroid Receptors: Targets for Treatment of Depression

ROEL H. DeRIJK[a], ONNO C. MEIJER[b] and E. RONALD de KLOET[b]

aLaboratorium Rijngeest Groep, Oegstgeest, and bDivision of Medical Pharmacology, LACDR/LUMC, Leiden, The Netherlands

INTRODUCTION

Mammalian organisms show in response to real or imagined environmental challenges a spectrum of autonomic, endocrine and behavioural reactions which serve to promote adaptation. A common endocrine feature of this stress response is the activation of the hypothalamic–pituitary–adrenal (HPA) axis, which leads to an increase in circulating corticosteroid concentrations, i.e. corticosterone in rodents or cortisol in the case of primates and man. Corticosteroids modulate gene transcription in peripheral target tissues via binding to nuclear receptors, which are also present in the brain, where they exert genomic control over the activity of neurons and neuronal networks underlying behavioural adaptation and homeostatic control. The corticosteroids have two modes of operation which are mediated by two types of corticosteroid receptors in the brain: the mineralocorticoid receptors (MRs) and glucocorticoid receptors (GRs). They permit in the *proactive* mode the expression of a particular behaviour aimed to limit homeostatic disturbance. An example of this proactive mode of operation is the role of corticosteroids in the synchronization and coordination of circadian events such as food intake and sleep-related events. In the *reactive* mode, they facilitate the recovery of homeostasis after stress. For example, under these conditions the hormones promote information storage which can be retrieved in the appropriate context in order to cope with a next encounter (de Kloet *et al.*, 1998b, 1999).

Recent prospective studies indicate that stressful life events may precipitate depression in vulnerable individuals (Kendler *et al.*, 1999). Depression is characterized by specific changes in the functioning of neuropeptides and neurotransmitters, such as corticotrophin-releasing hormone (CRH), serotonin (5HT) and norepinephrine (NE). In the acute phase, at least 50% of depressed patients are impaired in the control of the HPA axis activity and display hypercorticism. Data are emerging which show that vulnerability to depression is related to dysregulation of the HPA axis following stress, i.e. the set-point of the HPA axis is changed following stress. Basal levels of cortisol are increased particularly in the evening, while HPA activity escapes suppression by dexamethasone. Increased CRH expression is observed in the brain. Together with elevated cortisol levels, such symptoms are indicative of resistance to glucocorticoid feedback. During antidepressant treatment normalization of enhanced HPA activity precedes full remission. In addition, preliminary data indicate that probands of depressive patients who are at risk of developing this mental disorder, have a premorbid changed set-point of the HPA axis (Holsboer et al., 1995; Holsboer and Barden, 1996).

Several factors may explain how dysregulation of the HPA axis in the depressed patients increases vulnerability to depression. On the one hand genetic factors are critical. These may be multiple genes encoding proteins involved in neuronal plasticity and adaptation which are essential for health but become a vulnerability factor upon dysregulation of the HPA axis. On the other hand, developmental and experience-related factors are involved as well as cognitive and non-cognitive inputs, which potentially can change the set-point of the HPA axis. It is thought that the set-point in certain individuals is (more) labile and sensitive to stress.

In this chapter we focus on the action of cortisol mediated by its nuclear receptors in the brain because this stress hormone is linked to the pathogenesis of depression. A fundamental issue for understanding the role of cortisol in the pathogenesis of depression is how cortisol action in the brain may shift from protection to damage and increase vulnerability to the disease; what is the cause and what are the consequences? We conclude by indicating the cortisol receptors in the brain as potential targets for therapeutic agents.

CORTISOL RECEPTORS IN THE BRAIN

Corticosteroid hormones are lipophilic molecules that diffuse readily through the plasma membrane of cells to bind to their receptors. Two receptor types are present in the brain that mediate the effects of corticosteroids: MRs and GRs (de Kloet et al., 1998). These receptors have been identified in the brain of rodents, monkeys and man. They differ in affinity for corticosteroids and in their regional distribution in the brain. MRs bind corticosteroids with a very high affinity (Kd = 0.5 nM), which implies that they are already occupied to a considerable extent under basal trough conditions. The expression of cortisol-binding MRs is limited and particularly high in limbic brain structures such as the hippocampus. GRs have a somewhat lower affinity for cortisol (Kd = 2.5–5 nM), and become highly occupied when hormone levels increase above basal levels, i.e. at the circadian peak of cortisol secretion and after stress-induced activation of the HPA axis. GRs are expressed much more widely than MRs, and are found in particularly high concentrations in the hippocampus, catecholaminergic neurons in the brain stem, and in nuclei that are part of the HPA axis, such as the hypothalamic paraventricular nucleus (PVN) and also, outside the brain, in the pituitary.

Activation of brain corticosteroid receptors is not only regulated by the secretion of hormone from the adrenal glands, but also at several other levels. First, synthetic glucocorticoids such as dexamethasone are substrates for the P-glycoprotein transporter, which is expressed in the blood–brain barrier, and thus access of these compounds to the brain is relatively poor. Corticosterone, the main glucocorticoid in rodents easily penetrates the brain. Second, the enzyme 11β-hydroxy steroid dehydrogenase (11β-HSD) type 2 converts cortisol and corticosterone to their inactive 11-dehydro metabolites in mineralocorticoid target tissues. Conversely, the 11β-HSD type 1 isoform that is often colocalized with GRs, can catalyse the reverse reaction and generate cortisol from cortisone within a target cell. This reaction takes place in the liver, and may also be relevant for certain areas in the brain.

GRs and MRs are members of the steroid hormone receptor superfamily, and accordingly act as transcription factors to change the expression levels of target genes. Binding of hormone leads to conformational changes in the receptor protein and subsequent translocation of the receptor from the cytosol to the nucleus of the cell, where genomic effects take place (Figure 1). These have a relatively slow onset (minutes to hours) and long duration. Examples of the transcriptional regulation by corticosteroids are the GR-mediated suppression of CRH synthesis in the PVN, and MR-mediated suppression of the $5HT_{1A}$ receptor in hippocampus, as well as stimulation of tyrosine amino transferase in the liver. The effects of cortisol are dependent on the receptor type that is present in the cell. DNA binding properties of MRs and GRs are similar but not identical: GR is often a more potent inducer of gene expression than MR. Repression of transcription via MR and GR often does not depend on binding of the (hormone-activated) receptor to the DNA, but rather on inhibitory interactions with other transcription factors, such as the immediate early gene product AP-1. As an interesting consequence, some of the genomic effects of corticosteroids can be expected to only take place depending on the presence of these other factors. In the case of repression of gene expression, MRs and GRs differ substantially, and it is likely that a number of genes are influenced in a differential manner via MRs or GRs.

Recently, it has been shown in cultured fibroblasts that the antidepressant drug desipramine can induce translocation of GRs to the nucleus, independent of the presence of hormone (Pariante et al., 1997). When the cells were

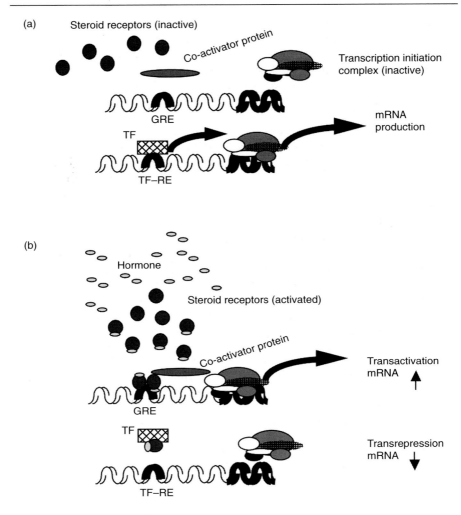

Figure 1. Mechanisms of corticosteroid receptor action on gene transcription. (a) In the absence of hormone. Glucocorticoid responsive element (GRE)-dependent target genes in the nucleus are not stimulated, while other transcription factors (TF) can bind to their response elements (TF–RE) to recruit the RNA polymerase containing pre-initiation complex to stimulate the synthesis of mRNA. (b) The hormone activated steroid receptors are present in the nucleus. They can (i) bind to their response elements in the DNA (GRE) to stimulate transcription. This mode of action involves interactions with so called co-activator proteins. (ii) The steroid receptors interfere with transcription activation by interactions with other transcription factors (transrepression). The latter mechanism may or may not involve interaction of the steroid receptor with the DNA. The interaction of the steroid receptors with other proteins in the cell constitutes a molecular basis for the conditional or context-dependent effects of corticosteroid hormones.

co-incubated with desipramine and dexamethasone, a potentiation of transcriptional activation was observed. Earlier observations also suggested that desipramine can influence the activity of (unidentified) transcription factors: desipramine treatment of cultured cells which contain a reporter gene driven by the promoter of the GR gene leads to higher transcription levels of the promoter, and to higher levels of the endogenous GR protein (Pepin *et al.*, 1992).

Expression levels of MRs and GRs are also regulated by antidepressants *in vivo*. In rats the expression levels of MRs and GRs can be elevated by treatment with antidepressant drugs, e.g. chronic (2–3 weeks) administration of tricyclic antidepressants or the monoamine oxidase (MAO) inhibitor moclobemide, and electroconvulsive treatment (ECT). The responsivity of MRs and GRs varies – moclobemide seems to increase brain MR expression specifically (Barden *et al.*, 1995), ECT induces both MR and GR protein in the hippocampus (Przegalinski *et al.*, 1993), while chronic treatments with amitriptyline or desipramine have been reported to either increase specifically GR binding (Przegalinski and Budziszewska, 1993), or mRNA of both MR and GR mRNA (Seckl and Fink, 1992). In addition, selective serotonin reuptake inhibitors (SSRIs) like citalopram and fluoxetine are also effective in changing MR or GR mRNA levels (Brady *et al.*, 1992; Seckl and Fink, 1992), but these effects seem to be less robust as compared with the other treatments. However, some specific noradrenaline reuptake inhibitors (oxaprotiline) have been reported to be without effect (Budziszewska and Lason, 1994; Eiring and Sulser, 1997). Interestingly, it has been shown that the regulation of GRs by desipramine is gender-dependent and does not occur in female rats, although the related compound imipramine was effective in both sexes (Peiffer *et al.*, 1991). Thus, although most antidepressant treatments enhance expression of brain corticosteroid receptors in the rat, not all of them do, and the mechanism by which this occurs may not primarily be dependent on changes in synaptic transmission.

CORTISOL ACTION IN THE BRAIN: MOLECULAR/CELLULAR EFFECTS

Effects on the hippocampus

Corticosteroids are potent modulators of cellular activity in the brain but in a permissive fashion: by themselves corticosteroids do not change firing frequency or membrane potential of neurons, but they do change the excitability of cells, e.g. the response to neurotransmitters. The steroids directly influence the synthesis of mRNA and protein of 'target genes', but to see the effects of these changes in protein status the neurons need to be activated. These effects have been best studied in the rodent hippocampus, a brain structure thought to be involved in learning, mood and affect. Its principal cell types express both MRs and GRs.

The effects of corticosteroids on neuronal excitability in the hippocampus depend on the relative occupation of the two receptor types. Under conditions of predominant MR activation, i.e. at the circadian trough at rest, neuronal excitability is relatively high, so that excitatory inputs to the hippocampal CA1 area result in considerable excitatory hippocampal output. In contrast, additional GR activation, e.g. following acute stress, generally depresses the transiently activated CA1 hippocampal output. A similar effect is seen after adrenalectomy (ADX), indicating a U-shaped dose response dependency of these cellular responses to corticosteroids (Joels and de Kloet, 1994).

The U-shaped dose–response effect of corticosteroids on neuronal excitability as determined by differential MR and GR activation is reflected in a number of parameters. For example, Ca currents and Ca-dependent effects are small under conditions of predominant MR occupation and elevated when GRs become activated in addition (Joels and de Kloet, 1994). Responses to both excitatory (glutamatergic) and inhibitory (GABA-ergic) inputs are maintained at a stable level when MRs are predominantly activated, i.e. with low corticosteroid levels. When GRs become occupied additionally as a consequence of rising corticosteroid levels, excitatory transmission (and thus CA1 hippocampal output) is reduced. At very high steroid levels inhibitory networks are also impaired. Hippocampal neurons also receive considerable input mediated by other neurotransmitters. High corticosteroid levels, occupying GRs, reduce the β-adrenergic receptor-mediated excitation of the CA1 hippocampal area, again leading to a reduction in responsiveness of the hippocampal neurons (Joels and de Kloet, 2000). Also the $5HT_{1A}$ receptor-mediated hyperpolarization of CA1 pyramidal cells is small under conditions of low corticosteroid levels (predominant MRs), and high when both MRs and GRs are occupied (Joels and de Kloet, 1992).

The relatively high excitability with predominant MR activation is reflected in long-term plastic changes involving this hippocampal network. In electrophysiological studies the role of corticosteroids has been extensively studied in long-term potentiation (LTP) and long-term depression (LTD), two phenomena that refer, respectively to the strengthening and weakening of synaptic contacts, upon repeated stimulation (Bliss and Collingridge, 1993). Synaptic strength is most pronounced with moderate corticosteroid levels, so that most of the MRs and only some of the GRs are activated, for example during the mildly stressful conditions in the context of a learning paradigm (Diamond et al., 1992; Shors and Dryver, 1994). When animals are subjected to a severe stressor, which results in extensive GR occupation, subsequent LTP induction is impaired, while LTD is enhanced (Xu et al., 1997). Likewise, if animals are subjected to novel information out of the context of the behavioural paradigm, the induction of LTP is prevented (Diamond *et al.*, 1994). The depotentiation could provide the means to erase synaptic strengthening installed by information that is no longer relevant to the situation. The point where LTP is impaired and LTD is facilitated does not merely depend on corticosteroid receptor dependency, but also on the recent history of synaptic plasticity and synaptic inputs related to previous events (de Kloet *et al.*, 1999).

Importantly, all these differential effects on excitability are brought on within hours. When corticosteroid levels are elevated for days or weeks (for example as a consequence of chronic stress) the neuronal physiology changes in a different, but less well-understood way. Under these conditions, many transmitter responses are small, in spite of the high occupation of GRs. Apparently some form of desensitization for GR-mediated effects occurs. Cellular responses under these conditions appear to be governed by MR-mediated effects – the balance between the two types of corticosteroid responses is disturbed. Also, under these conditions the apical dendrites of pyramidal neurons in the CA3 field show atrophy, i.e. they become shorter and have fewer branching points. This is correlated with impaired hippocampus-dependent learning, which may be caused by the morphological changes in CA3, but also by other physiological effects on these or other hippocampal neurons. Interestingly, treatment with the antidepressant tianeptine, a specific serotonin reuptake *enhancer*, prevents and even reverses dendritic atrophy, but SSRIs are not effective (Margarinos *et al.*, 1999).

Neurotransmitter systems

Many neurotransmitter systems are affected by corticosteroids. The activity of dopaminergic and serotonergic cells in lower brain areas, and the release of these transmitters in the brain are increased after stress. Blockade of GRs, which normally become activated as a consequence of the stress-induced activation of the HPA axis, prevents the increase in neurotransmitter release. For serotonergic neurons, corticosteroids are presumed to act on the activity of the rate-limiting enzyme for serotonin synthesis (tryptophan hydroxylase), and via attenuation of negative feedback inhibition by serotonin in the serotonergic neurons in the midbrain. Again, these are permissive effects, as corticosteroids do not change levels of dopamine or serotonin under basal conditions, but are necessary for stress-induced changes to occur (de Kloet *et al.*, 1998b).

Neuronal and behavioural responses to serotonin and dopamine receptor activation also depend on activation of corticosteroid receptors. Effects of dopamine agonists like apomorphine are stimulated by corticosteroids via GRs, and sensitization to repeated treatment with drugs that increase dopaminergic transmission, such as cocaine, depends on GR activation. In case of the serotonergic projections to the hippocampus, a coordinate regulation via MRs and GRs is present: as described above, the hyperpolarization response of hippocampal $5HT_{1A}$ receptors is low under basal conditions, when corticosteroid levels are low (Joels and de Kloet, 1992). In addition in rat, MRs in certain hippocampal areas (i.e. dentate gyrus) suppress expression of the $5HT_{1A}$ receptor, over a longer time range, but leave the expression of $5HT_{1A}$ mRNA in CA1 unaffected. Thus, a situation of predominant MR occupation is associated with low responses to serotonin in the hippocampus. In contrast, GR activation is necessary for increased release of serotonin upon stress, and

Figure 2. MR and GR regulation of the HPA axis, synaptic strength, 5HT neurotransmission and behaviour. This figure depicts a schematic representation of the HPA axis, together with several conditional effects of corticosteroids on processes involved in behaviour.

HPA axis: Schematic view of the HPA axis, showing the hippocampus, the PVN, the pituitary gland and the adrenals. A major inhibitory tone (GABA) to the PVN is enhanced by excitatory hippocampal output (Glu). In addition, elevated levels of corticosteroids exert negative feedback by means of GRs (black squares) in the anterior pituitary corticotrophs and the CRH neurons of the PVN. MRs (black stars) mediate potentiation of hippocampal output and thus enhance neural inhibition of the HPA axis, while GRs in the hippocampus dampen hippocampal output which thus leads to HPA axis disinhibition (van Haarst *et al.*, 1997). GRs also mediate the activation of ascending aminergic input (NE from the locus coeruleus, LC) and 5HT from the raphe nucleus (RN) to the PVN from brain stem.

Synaptic strength: LTP is induced optimally when corticosteroid levels are mildly elevated, that is, when MRs and some GRs are activated. In contrast, high levels of corticosteroids, occupying most GRs, not only inhibit LTP, but induce LTD. These data point to a bell-shape dose-dependency for LTP in the hippocampus (de Kloet *et al.*, 1999).

5HT neurotransmission: In the dorsal raphe nucleus (DRN), acute GR activation leads to a decrease in responsiveness to 5HT; this GR-mediated desensitization of somatic 5HT (inhibitory) autoreceptors will therefore enhance 5HT output (5HT neurotransmission, left panel: DRN feedback sensitivity). However, at the same moment when both MRs and GRs are activated in the hippocampus, hippocampal 5HT responsiveness (right panel: hippocampal 5HT responsiveness) actually enhances, leading to increased hyperpolarization. Since treatment of ADX rats with MR occupying doses of corticosterone leads to inhibition of hippocampal 5HT responsiveness, a U-shaped curve emerges (Joels and de Kloet, 1994; Meijer and de Kloet, 1998).

Behaviour: Inhibition of GRs (anti GR) immediately after acquisition on day 1 resulted in impaired performance in the Morris water maze as tested 24 hours later (right graph, GR block: consolidation). Following exposure to a learning task, the Morris water maze, application of a MR antagonist i.c.v. 15 minutes prior to the retrieval session on day 2 changed the swim pattern (left panel, MR block: swim pattern). Treated rats (anti MR) approach the former platform position directly. The rats spend less time searching in its vicinity, but instead search for an escape route from the whole pool. These MR- and GR-mediated effects on information processing facilitate behavioural adaptation (Oitzl and de Kloet, 1992; de Kloet *et al.*, 1999).

for increased postsynaptic responses to $5HT_{1A}$ receptor activation (Joels and de Kloet, 1992) (Figure 2). Interestingly, down-regulation of $5HT_{1A}$ mRNA expression is further enhanced under these conditions in the dentate gyrus, while some but not all reports also describe small reductions in $5HT_{1A}$ mRNA in CA1.

However, when corticosteroid levels are chronically elevated to levels in the GR-occupying range, *hypo*responses to serotonin are observed in hippocampal CA1 neurons (Karten *et al.*, 1999), to serotonin in hippocampal-associated behaviours (Meijer *et al.*, 1998) and in endocrine challenge tests

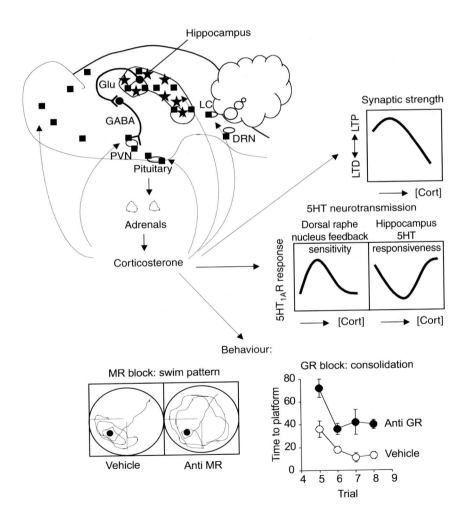

(Meijer and de Kloet, 1998). It is unclear which molecular changes underlie the transition from stimulatory to inhibitory effects of high levels of corticosteroids on serotonergic transmission. It is also unclear which mechanism underlies the striking regional difference in responsiveness of 5HT$_{1A}$ receptor expression in the hippocampus.

In contrast to the increased responsiveness of hippocampal neurons to 5HT, in the dorsal raphe nucleus, a decrease in responsiveness is observed after acute GR activation. This desensitization of the 5HT$_{1A}$ autoreceptors in the midbrain as a consequence of acute GR activation has an interesting parallel in the theory formation around the mechanisms of SSRIs. These compounds are thought to increase serotonergic tone in the brain by eventual down-regulation of the same population of presynapic 5HT$_{1A}$ autoreceptors upon chronic treatment (Blier and Montigny, 1994; Artigas et al., 1996). Thus, chronic treatment with SSRIs has an effect on serotonergic neurons comparable to acute GR activation, namely the desensitization of 5HT somatic autoreceptors.

GRs are abundantly present in the majority of the neurons in the midbrain norepinephrine cell groups. Although studies with adrenalectomized rats show a permissive function of corticosteroids for norepinephrine cells during ontogeny and stress (e.g. in relation to memory formation), the effects of GR activation in these cells and their postsynaptic targets are not as clear as for other transmitters. Postsynaptically, corticosteroids region-dependently regulate adrenergic receptor expression, e.g. induce the inhibitory α2 receptor in the hypothalamic paraventricular nucleus. In the hippocampus, the electrophysiological effects of norepinephrine are attenuated via a GR-dependent mechanism. Stress levels of corticosteroids reduce the cyclic AMP generation induced by norepinephrine acting via β-adrenergic receptors in the hippocampus (de Kloet et al., 1998b).

In addition to the classical neurotransmitter systems, many peptidergic systems are controlled via corticosteroid receptors, both at the level of peptide synthesis, and at the level of postsynaptic receptors. These peptides are involved in many aspects of brain function, including hypothalamic control of the HPA axis and regulation of metabolism and feeding. The best-studied examples are pro-opiomelanocortin (POMC)-derived peptides, CRH, and arginine vasopressin (AVP), because of their critical role in activation of the HPA axis. Both CRH and AVP mRNA levels are suppressed by corticosteroids in the parvocellular division of the PVN, presumably via GR activation. However, this type of regulation is cell-type dependent, as in the amygdala CRH mRNA is up-regulated by corticosteroids (Schulkin et al., 1998). Other peptide targets of corticosteroid receptors include neuropeptide Y and dynorphin in the hippocampus and preproenkephalin, neurokinin A and preprodynorphin in the caudate-putamen and nucleus accumbens (de Kloet et al., 1998b).

CORTICOSTEROID RECEPTORS IN NEUROENDOCRINE REGULATION AND BEHAVIOUR

Role of corticosteroid receptors in behaviour

Corticosteroids have been tightly linked to stress and it is therefore not surprising that these hormones have profound effects on behaviour. However, corticosteroids do not necessarily cause a behavioural change, but rather influence information processing and thereby affect the likelihood that a particular stimulus elicits an appropriate behavioural response. For example, the corticosteroid actions on hippocampal cell function show several features that are relevant to modulation of learning and memory processes. LTP for instance is considered a model for learning and memory processes and it is evident that predominant MR activation results in completely different actions than concomitant MR and GR activation. The relative activation of MR and GR therefore seems to be an important determinant of limbic activity. The MR- and GR-mediated action depends, however, on many factors, including the regulation of receptor expression, the affinity of the receptors, the interaction with proteins such as transcription factors, co-activators and co-repressors (Meijer et al., 2000) and of course the circulating levels of corticosteroids. The corticosteroid actions may also be influenced by the nature of prior or concomitant activation of specific afferent pathways. These phenomena could contribute to the contextual dependence observed in behavioural responses.

It is known that processing of information depends crucially on hippocampal functions associated with the recognition of goals and the evaluation of the outcome of actions (Gray and McNaughton, 1983). Behavioural studies have indeed shown that MR- and GR-mediated actions affect different aspects of information processing. Following exposure of animals to the so-called Morris water maze task, in which animals are trained to find a submerged platform, GR antagonists administered intracerebroventricularly (i.c.v.) during the acquisition phase interfere with consolidation of the newly acquired information. Accordingly, this GR antagonist treatment and consequent blockade of the central GRs has resulted the next day in impaired retention of the task (Oitzl and de Kloet, 1992). Since treatment before the retrieval test is ineffective, this finding demonstrates that hippocampal GRs rather promote the storage than the retrieval of information, provided the information is congruent with the context of the behavioural test. Likewise, glucocorticoids have appeared to be relevant in the consolidation of conditioned behaviours measured in passive and active avoidance assays (de Kloet et al., 1998b), and of acquired immobility as measured in the Porsolt test (Korte et al., 1996a; de Kloet et al., 1988a), which is a laboratory test to monitor potential antidepressant activity.

The MR antagonist does not affect the consolidation of new information, since blockade of hippocampal MRs during the acquisition phase does not affect retention of the learned behaviour when tested 24 hours later. Rather the MR antagonist changes the search and exploration pattern of animals once the previously used escape route has been removed (Figure 2). The rats still head directly to the place where they had learned to locate the underwater platform in the Morris water maze (hence consolidation is undisturbed). Subsequently, the rats explore other areas rather than remaining there as the controls do. This has led to the conclusion that MR-mediated effects are concerned with the interpretation of environmental information and the selection of the subsequent behavioural response to cope with the challenge (Oitzl and de Kloet, 1992; Oitzl et al., 1994). The activation of GRs on top of already activated MRs within the context of a behavioural task is a prerequisite for optimal memory. A similar conclusion was reached in studies with young chicks showing that a GR-mediated mechanism enhanced the long-term retention for an aversive stimulus in a passive avoidance learning paradigm, while the application of the MR antagonist changed the chicks' pecking pattern, indicating an effect of the MRs on their behavioural reactivity (Sandi and Rose, 1994; Loscertales et al., 1997).

Taken together these effects mediated by MRs and GRs eliminate behaviour that is no longer relevant and thus favour behaviour that is most relevant to adapt to the novel situation. When corticosterone is administered or rats are exposed to stress prior to the retrieval test, the time spent in the former platform quadrant is also reduced (de Quervain et al., 1998). At first sight this could be interpreted as a deficit entirely due to altered GR function. Yet, the unrelated stressor led to a change in exploratory behaviour and the behavioural response to the novel situation (no platform) that is very similar to the previously observed pattern after blockade of brain MR (Oitzl and de Kloet, 1992; Oitzl et al., 1994). In our view, the GR activation due to an unrelated stressor disrupts the function of MRs during the retrieval process. Chronically elevated corticosterone impairs learning and memory processes, while chronic blockade of the GRs facilitates the acquisition of a learning task (Oitzl et al., 1998). These effects of chronic and acute MR- and or GR-blockade relate not only to cognitive functions, but also to impulse control (Haller et al., 1998), fear and anxiety (Korte et al., 1995, 1996b). MR antagonists appear to have anxiolytic activities, but anxiolytic activity involving GRs was observed only when the assay system took cognitive functions into account. These experiments clearly demonstrate that MR- and GR-mediated effects are different, but interact and proceed in a co-ordinate manner, linked in time to the particular stage in information processing.

Neuroendocrine implications

Every disturbance, either real or imagined, evokes an autonomous, neuroendocrine and behavioural response, which serves to restore homeostasis and to facilitate adaptation. The neuroendocrine stress response is shaped by the

HPA axis, which secretes as endproduct the corticosteroids by the adrenal cortex. The central drive to the HPA axis occurs by the parvocellular CRH neurons of the hypothalamic PVN. Circuits innervating the PVN are activated in stressor-specific fashion (Herman and Cullinan, 1997). Furthermore, depending on the nature and the duration of the stimulus a cocktail of secretagogues is secreted at the median eminence into the portal system. The main PVN stress peptides are CRH and AVP, but their action is modulated by numerous peptidergic co-secretagogues, which in concert stimulate in response to stress the corticotrophic cells in the pituitary gland to release adrenocorticotrophic hormone (ACTH) from the POMC precursor into the circulation. ACTH in turn acts at the adrenal glands both to stimulate the synthesis and secretion of corticosteroids and the growth of adrenocortical cells. Corticosteroid secretion is therefore a rather stereotypical response to stress capable of co-ordinating and synchronizing numerous processes in the body and brain. However, at the target level the steroids have an enormous diversity, since their action is mediated by the co-ordinate action of MRs and GRs, and depends on the cellular context in which these receptors operate.

In concert with other components of the stress response cortisol displays two modes of operation. In the first 'proactive' mode cortisol maintains basal activity of the HPA axis and controls the sensitivity or threshold of the HPA response to stress. This action mediated by MRs involves processes in higher brain regions concerned with interpretation of novel information and selection of an appropriate response to cope with the challenge. The substrate of this MR-mediated action is the limbic circuitry, which exerts an overall inhibitory influence over the HPA axis. This is a trans-synaptic influence involving various inputs to a GABA-ergic hypothalamic network inhibiting the CRH neurons (Figure 2). Since the excitatory tone of the hippocampus is enhanced via MRs, this offers a satisfactory explanation of how the hippocampus maintains an inhibitory tone. A testable prediction is that the central application of MR antagonists would disinhibit the HPA axis both under basal conditions and in response to novelty. This is indeed observed. A synthetic MR antagonist or MR antisense applied i.c.v. elevates basal and stress-induced corticosterone secretion (Dallman et al., 1989; Ratka et al., 1989; Bradbury et al., 1994; Oitzl et al., 1995; Reul et al., 1997; Spencer et al., 1998). Likewise, the administration of spironolactone to human subjects also elevates circulating corticosterone (Dodt et al., 1993; Deuschle et al., 1998).

In the second 'reactive' mode the stress-induced elevated corticosteroid concentrations occupy increasingly the GRs in addition to the MRs. Corticosteroids feed back on brain and body in order to facilitate recovery, to restore homeostasis and to promote behavioural adaptation. Negative feedback control of the HPA axis response is exerted at the level of the PVN and the pituitary gland during stress levels of endogenous corticosteroids. These sites, and in particular the pituitary corticotrophs, are also the principal targets for synthetic glucocorticoids such as dexamethasone. Corticosteroids also feed back on the neuronal circuits that process information originally responsible for the activation of the HPA axis. These include among others the ascending aminergic pathways transmitting stressful visceral information, cognitive stress via the limbic inputs and circadian inputs generated by the nucleus suprachiasmaticus (SCN). The current evidence suggests an interesting twist in the story of corticosteroid feedback. While the steroids exert an unequivocal negative feedback directly via negative glucocorticoid responsive elements (nGREs) on the CRH and AVP genes in the PVN, the hormones actually sensitize and activate the aminergic inputs. They also suppress the excitatory output of the hippocampus which signals via an inhibitory GABA-ergic signal to the PVN, ultimately resulting in disinhibition. However, when the corticosteroids are effective in facilitating adaptive behaviour these influences cease to drive the CRH neurons and the HPA axis.

CRH is is not only central in the activation of the HPA axis, but also is involved in the organization of the autonomic and behavioural response to stress. CRH administration to laboratory animals induces arousal, a number of fear-related behavioural responses, inhibition of sleep, appetite and sexual activity. Moreover, blockade of CRH by means of central application of an antiserum or a CRH receptor antagonist has an anxiolytic effect. Corticosteroids, while decreasing CRH mRNA expression in the PVN, increase CRH mRNA expression in the central nucleus of the amygdala and in other extrahypothalamic regions such as the locus coeruleus (Schulkin *et al.*, 1998). This phenomenon adds to the apparent positive feedback effect of corticosteroids on the ascending aminergic projections originating from the locus coeruleus (Gold and Chrousos, 1998) as well as the raphe 5HT neurons and the adrenergic A2 neurons.

Depressed patients display feedback resistance to corticosteroids. The principal feature of this feedback resistance in CRH neurons is the disturbed balance between GR function, on the one hand, and the drive by excitatory inputs on the other. One way in which this can be disturbed is by a local GR deficit. This deficit can be congenital as is the case in transgenic mice, with decreased GR in the brain. Such mice show hypercorticism, cognitive impairment and metabolic disturbance resembling the symptomatology of Cushing's disease (Holsboer and Barden, 1996). Feedback resistance can also be acquired as is the case after local administration of glucocorticoid antagonists. If RU 486 (mifepristone, a GR antagonist) is infused chronically into the cerebral ventricles, within 4 days the animals show enhanced corticosterone levels at the circadian peak and in response to stress (van Haarst *et al.*, 1996). Basal trough corticosterone levels are not changed, but the amplitude of the corticosterone response is enhanced, apparently because the capacity of the adrenals to secrete corticosterone is also increased as well (van Haarst *et al.*, 1996). A third approach is through impairment of corticosteroid synthesis after administration of 11β-hydroxylase blocker metyrapone, which results in enhanced ACTH and CRH responses to stress (Dallman *et al.*, 1991).

Reset of feedback sensitivity occurs when the input from multiple sensory signalling pathways converging on CRH neurons becomes disproportionate. This occurs, for example, when chronic physical stressors activate brain stem aminergic neurons and thus stimulate CRH and AVP synthesis directly through α1-adrenergic receptors (Herman and Cullinan, 1997). Disproportionate input to CRH neurons can also be due to environmental changes, emotion, arousal or cognitive stimuli, which may become particularly potent chronic stressors under conditions of uncertainty, lack of control or poor predictability of upcoming events. Such conditions can be created in models of psychosocial stress in rats housed in mixed-sex groups in a complex environment resulting in a sustained HPA activation in subordinates. The elevated glucocorticoid levels caused by such chronic physical and psychological stressors produce tolerance to elevated glucocorticoids, through down-regulation of GRs in the CRH/AVP neurons (Makino *et al.*, 1995; Herman and Cullinan, 1997). The lower GR number then transduces the reduced magnitude of signal relative to the glucocorticoid elevation, leading to further dysregulation of the HPA axis.

Resistance to glucocorticoid feedback at the level of the CRH neurons would cause increased HPA activity and hypercorticism. As an unfortunate consequence, the rest of the body including the brain and the neural stress response circuitry suffers from glucocorticoid overexposure. Importantly, glucocorticoid elevation synergizes with stress-induced activation of serotonergic, dopaminergic and noradrenergic neurons in the brain stem, and thus increases the sensitivity of limbic-forebrain areas to aminergic inputs (de Kloet *et al.*, 1998b). These include direct aminergic input to the CRH/AVP neurons as well as indirect afferent inputs to these CRH neurons via the hippocampus. Moreover, the amygdaloid CRH system involved in stress-related behaviours is also activated by chronic stress and corticosterone (Schulkin *et al.*, 1998). By these mechanisms the feedback resistance at the level of the CRH neurons is increasingly reinforced.

The reverse occurs in situations where feedback inhibition of corticosteroids is enhanced, so that the organism suffers from hypocorticism which is centrally regulated. How such enhanced feedback inhibition at the level of the PVN is achieved is not known. It may be through synergy of GR with intracellular signalling mechanisms in the PVN, or via MR-enhanced, neurally mediated, tonic inhibitory input from the hippocampus on HPA activity. Alternatively, reduced adrenocortical output may also be caused by a deficit in the CRH drive, or by altered sympathetic outflow diminishing adrenal sensitivity to ACTH. Interestingly, in group-housed rats, a subgroup of chronically stressed subordinate animals displays a reduced corticosterone response to restraint stress (Albeck *et al.*, 1997). Using this type of psychosocial stressors, future studies may reveal how chronic stress results in pathology characteristic of stress-related disorders.

CORTICOSTEROIDS AND DEPRESSION

HPA axis and CRH in depression

In the acute state, about 50% of patients suffering from depression have a hyperactive HPA axis resulting in increased plasma concentrations of cortisol (Checkley, 1996) and hypertrophy of the adrenals as observed by magnetic resonance imaging (MRI). Furthermore, negative feedback is impaired. This can be tested by administration of the synthetic corticosteroid dexamethasone in the evening, which suppresses in the control persons the morning increase in ACTH and cortisol (de Kloet *et al.*, 1998b). Depressed patients typically escape the dexamethasone suppression, indicating GR-resistance at the level of the pituitary. Alternatively an increased drive of the HPA axis will interfere with dexamethasone-induced suppression. This increased drive to pituitary ACTH release could be due to CRH and/or vasopressin. For instance, administration of CRH induces signs reminiscent of depression, which include decreased libido, reduced slow wave sleep, reduced appetite, increased anxiety and impaired psychomotor activity. Together with findings of increased CRH concentrations in the CSF of depressed patients, this has led to the so-called CRH hypothesis of depression, in which an increased CRH drive is central in the pathogenesis of depression. CRH projections originating from the amygdala, the PVN and the bed nucleus of the stria terminalis (BNST) terminate in the locus coeruleus and may underlie the enhanced arousal in response to emotional stressors (Chrousos and Gold, 1992). The assumption has been made that the reciprocal activation of the CRH system and the norepinephrinergic locus coeruleus system as the core of the central stress system is not sufficiently restrained in depression (Chrousos and Gold, 1992; Gold and Chrousos, 1998).

Close examination of the ACTH and cortisol responses to synthetic ovine CRH administration to depressed patients gave biochemical support for the existence of two subgroups. First, melancholic patients showing a normal ACTH but high cortisol response as compared with healthy controls. These findings are consistent with an CRH *hyper*drive and the clinical features of (physiological) hyperarousal and fear. Secondly, a group of patients showing a relatively low ACTH together with low cortisol, designated as atypical depressed patients. Their clinical features are characterized by profound inertia and fatigue. These findings can be explained by a CRH *hypo*drive (Gold and Chrousos, 1998). In addition to the interaction with norepinephrine in the locus coeruleus, CRH also strongly interacts with other monoamine systems, such as the 5HT system at the level of the raphe nucleus, which also innervates the forebrain and the hippocampus. An increase in CRH drive by continuous infusion seems to interfere with the 5HT regulation in the hippocampus (Holsboer, 1999). Thus a dysregulation of centrally released CRH will also affect 5HT neurotransmission.

To further study the role of the PVN in the regulation of the HPA axis, a combination of dexamethasone suppression (administration in the evening) and CRH stimulation (administration next afternoon) is used (Heuser et al., 1994). In depressed patients this test reveals impaired glucocorticoid feedback both at the level of the pituitary and the PVN. Importantly, seemingly healthy probands of the depressed patients also showed enhanced escape and mild hypercorticism using the combined dexamethasone–CRH test. If indeed these relatives develop the disease at a later stage, this finding would support the involvement of genetic factors (Holsboer and Barden, 1996; Modell et al., 1998). The observed escape from dexamethasone suppression could result from AVP colocalized with CRH in the parvocellular neurons of the PVN, since CRH and AVP strongly synergize in inducing the release of ACTH. Indeed, post-mortem studies have shown an increased expression of CRH and AVP in the parvocellular neurones in the PVN of patients with depression (Purba et al., 1996). In addition, the plasma levels of AVP are elevated in patients with major depression during the acute phase (van Londen et al., 1997), although it is not yet clear to what extent AVP of a magnocellular PVN source contributes to the disease. Prolonged continuous stress, and also several single stressors even separated by long time intervals have been shown to increase AVP expression in PVN–CRH neurones (De Goeij et al., 1991), which indicates a further link between changes in HPA axis regulation and stress (Kendler et al., 1999). Irrespective of a role for AVP, the central question in the CRH hypothesis of depression is why the CRH response following stress is not properly restrained, but results in a CRH hyperdrive.

Cortisol and depression

As a consequence of increased activation of the HPA axis, hypercorticism will occur and this has been observed in the majority of depressed patients in the acute phase. Prolonged elevated levels of corticosteroids are associated with behavioural symptoms such as mood lability, depression, disturbed sleep, cognitive disturbances and even psychosis in patients, although the relation between elevated levels of cortisol and these symptoms is not completely clear yet. Administration of corticosteroids to healthy individuals results in identical but reversible defects. Cushing's disease patients provide an unfortunate natural model of prolonged cortisol exposure. However, depending on the cause of the hypercorticism, Cushing's disease patients can have low or high levels of CRH. It has been found that approximately 50% of the Cushing's disease patients with a positive psychiatric diagnosis fulfilled the criteria for atypical depression, which was thought to be associated with low levels of CRH (Dorn *et al.*, 1995). In any case, Cushing's disease patients share many psychiatric defects with depressed patients including decreases in affect, disturbed sleep, attentional deficits, fatigue and loss of energy, irritability, loss of memory and cognitive defects. Finally, usage of inhibitors of cortisol production, such as aminoglutethimide, ketoconazole and metyrapone, in depressed patients resulted in decreases in plasma cortisol levels and improvement in mood, insomnia, anxiety, diurnal variation, paranoia and obsessive compulsiveness (Ghadirian *et al.*, 1995), while a normalization in the dexamethasone suppression test occurred (Murphy *et al.*, 1998).

A dysregulation of the HPA axis, for example measured as a post-treatment escape from the dexamethasone suppression test, is an indicator of poor outcome of treatment (Ribeiro *et al.*, 1993). Moreover, patients with increased HPA axis functioning are less responsive to cognitive therapy (Thase *et al.*, 1996). These latter data emphasize the context-dependent action of steroids and suggest that cognitive therapy should be accompanied by drug-induced normalization of the HPA axis. Cognitive and memory effects have been described, which were induced by physiological stress levels of corticosteroids in seemingly healthy humans. This has been determined by reversible decreases in verbal declarative memory (Newcomer *et al.*, 1999). Stress-induced levels of cortisol also affect declarative memory, although the timing of the stress-induced increase in cortisol was found to be crucial in the induced memory defect (Lupien *et al.*, 1997). Again these data should be considered from the viewpoint that elevated corticosteroids and stress *out of context* may impair behaviour (de Kloet *et al.*, 1999). In conclusion, elevated levels of corticosteroids may contribute to the appearance of psychiatric symptoms observed in affective disorders, while normalization of the steroid levels is associated with amelioration of the symptoms. These steroid-dependent changes in mood and mental performance are thought to be governed by MRs and GRs in hippocampus because of their key role in aspects of declarative memory and neuroendocrine regulation of the HPA axis.

Antidepressants and HPA axis regulation

The previous section indicates a causative role of corticosteroids and corticosteroid receptors in the pathogenesis and pathology of depression. In the 1950s, however, it was thought that malfunctioning aminergic transmission was the cause of depression. This hypothesis was largely based on the direct effects of antidepressants on monaminergic transmission. Considerable evidence is now available to support a pivotal role of the 5HT system in depression and other affective disorders. More recently, Blier and Montigny have focused on somatic $5HT_{1A}$ receptors, e.g. in the dorsal raphe nucleus which is thought to be supersensitive to 5HT induced feedback, thereby decreasing 5HT turnover in target tissue such as the hippocampus and the forebrain (Blier and Montigny, 1994; Artigas et al., 1996). $5HT_{1A}$ agonists can increase the activity of these 5HT neurons, possibly by a desensitization of the somatic $5HT_{1A}$ receptors. In addition, corticosteroids regulate the activity of the raphe–hippocampal system in various ways. Under physiological fluctuations of corticosteroid concentrations, predominantly MR-mediated effects suppress the activity of the raphe–hippocampal system: postsynaptic hippocampal $5HT_{1A}$ receptors are down-regulated while the neuronal response to 5HT is attenuated (Meijer and de Kloet, 1998). Transiently increased concentrations of corticosteroids, as induced by stress, resulting in occupation of both MRs and GRs, allow increased activity of the raphe–hippocampal 5HT system. Stimulatory actions of elevated levels of corticosteroids involve increased responsiveness of neurons to 5HT, attenuated auto-inhibition of 5HT and a permissive effect on stress-induced 5HT release. These findings suggest regulation of the 5HT-system by a balance of MR-induced inhibition and GR-regulated activation, in line with the proposed *proactive* and *reactive* function of these receptors.

Under (pathological) conditions of chronically elevated corticosteroid concentrations, 5HT transmission is impaired. In rats injected daily for 3 weeks with a high dose of corticosterone the $5HT_{1A}$ receptor-mediated membrane hyperpolarization of hippocampal CA1 neurons gradually was attenuated. The expression of $5HT_{1A}$ receptors was not altered in these cells, but MRs were significantly reduced (Karten et al., 1999). In the case of depression, patients having elevated levels of cortisol showed a reduced prolactin response to D-fenfluramine, a specific 5HT releasing agent (Cleare et al., 1996). Application of the cortisol synthesis inhibitor ketoconazole normalized the blunted prolactin response to D-fenfluramine and alleviated the depression in the same patients (Thakore and Dinan, 1995). Thus, sustained stress or sustained increase in plasma cortisol concentrations inhibit the dynamics of the 5HT-system. Chronic stress may induce an imbalance between the MR- and GR-mediated actions, leading to a relative dominance of MR-mediated suppressive effect on the activity of the raphe–5HT system. This faulty cortisol–5HT system interplay, which is stressor driven, could underlie the pathogenesis of a subgroup of depression (van Praag, 1996).

Most antidepressants have been shown to increase the expression of the GRs and/or MRs (Barden et al., 1995; Holsboer and Barden, 1996). Importantly, SSRIs such as fluoxetine and citalopram have also been shown to increase GR and or MR expression in the hippocampus in rats treated for several weeks (Brady et al., 1992; Seckl and Fink, 1992). Therefore, the normalizing effects of antidepressants, both tricyclic antidepressants (TCAs) and SSRIs, on the activity of serotonergic neurons could at least in part be due to their effects on GRs and MRs. A further causative relationship between antidepressants and HPA axis functioning follows from longitudinal studies which showed that a return to dexamethasone suppressibility of morning plasma cortisol precedes resolution of depressive psychopathology (Holsboer and Barden, 1996). Also, antidepressants sometimes reduce CRH levels in the human spinal fluid suggesting that long-term administration of antidepressants may suppress the HPA axis, raising the possibility that lowering the HPA axis activity and the clinical response are causally related. Moreover, the effects of antidepressants on monaminergic systems are exerted within hours, while the clinical effects are not reached before several weeks. This time-path closely follows the effects of antidepressants on central MR and GR expression and normalization of the HPA axis activity. Finally, it is of note that the desipramine concentration needed for maximum effects on MR and GR-expression was in the range of 10^{-8} M, which corresponds to the plasma concentrations needed to achieve clinical efficacy. Thus antidepressants might elevate mood in depressive patients through their long-term effects on HPA axis regulation.

Anti-glucocorticoid treatment in depression

Since elevations of plasma cortisol are not epiphenomena but could be causative in the pathology and pathogenesis of depression, it seems obvious to aim treatment at reducing plasma cortisol levels or inhibit its actions. Lowering of plasma cortisol levels can be achieved through blockade of enzymes involved in the synthesis of cortisol at the level of the adrenal glands. Drugs used are ketoconazole, metyrapone and aminoglutethimide; all inhibitors of cortisol production. Across several studies using cortisol synthesis inhibitors, in approximately two-thirds of the patients a significant reduction of depressive symptoms was noted, ranging to relief of the symptoms (Wolkowitz and Reus, 1999). In different studies a decrease in insomnia, irritability, anxiety and neuroticism was observed, while libido, strength, concentration and cognitive performances were improved. Although these findings are impressive and are strong evidence for a central role of cortisol and corticosteroid receptors in the pathology of this mental disease, use of these drugs is hampered by severe side-effects, such as nausea, diarrhoea and headache.

An additional approach to block effects of endogenous cortisol is to use MR or GR antagonists (Table 1). The application of RU38486, a specific GR antagonist, has revealed improvement of three out of four patients (Murphy et al., 1993). This indicates deleterious effects of cortisol mediated through the GRs during the course of depression. However, long-term treatment with RU 38486 results in activation of the HPA axis as indicated by increases in urinary free and plasma cortisol and a decreased sensitivity to dexamethasone (Lamberts et al., 1991). In contrast, usage of spironolactone, an MR antagonist, in combination with amitriptyline, resulted in a less favourable

Table 1. Central MR and GR directed treatment of depression.

Treatment:	RU 28318 (MR antagonist/spironolactone)
Study:	Patients (2 × 15) were treated with amitriptyline with or without 100 mg spironolactone. Cotreatment with spironolactone was less effective compared with amitriptyline alone as measured after 4 weeks (Holsboer, 1999).
Treatment:	RU 38486 (GR antagonist/mifeprestone)
Study:	Four treatment-resistant patients were given RU 38486 (200 mg/day) for three weeks. The mean Hamilton Depression Rating Scale (HDRS) fell for 3 patients (Murphy *et al.*, 1993). Study was not completed because of shortage of RU 38486 (Murphy, 1997).
Treatment:	Dexamethasone
Studies:	(i) In a randomized double-blind study 4 mg/day of oral dexamethasone for 4 days was shown to induce a decrease in the HDRS in 37% of patients compared with 6% in the placebo-treated group, as determined 14 days later (Arana *et al.*, 1995). Effects of the dexamethasone treatment were modest: HDRS fell from 26.5 to 19.2 (n = 12). (ii) 10 treatment-resistant patients were treated with 3 mg/day of oral dexamethasone for 4 days while remaining on sertraline or fluoxetine (Dinan *et al.*, 1997); 6 patients showed a significant improvement (50% reduction in HDRS), which lasted for at least for 3 weeks.

Comment: One study has been performed using spironolactone in combination with amitryptiline, resulting in worsening of the symptoms, indicating a role for the MRs in depression. Blockade of central GRs was beneficial for patients, indicating a role for GRs in depression. Two studies using dexamethasone both showing improvement, suggest that lowering of central cortisol has a beneficial effect during depression. All studies are consistent with the suggestion that central MRs and GRs are involved in the pathogenesis of depression.

response compared with patients treated with amitriptyline alone (Holsboer, 1999). This could well be due to the activation of the HPA axis through spironolactone by decreasing the tonic inhibition exerted by the central MRs.

INDIVIDUAL DIFFERENCES IN VULNERABILITY TO DEPRESSION

A fundamental issue in the research of depression is why some individuals are susceptible to depression, while others under comparable conditions stay healthy. Of great importance for this question are the original observations of Henry and Stephens (1976) who demonstrated that individuals with extreme differences in stress reactivity co-exist in a normal population. In response to stressor, one population displays a *fight/flight* response. The individual will defend its territory vigorously, but will flee after psychosocial defeat. The sympathetic nervous response dominates, as exemplified by high blood pressure and marked adrenaline responses. The behaviour is viewed as expression of lack of control and directed by influences from the amygdala. On the other hand, in the same population the *conservation withdrawal response* is also observed which is predominantly governed from the hippocampus. The main characteristics are the parasympathetic response and elevated corticosteroid levels.

Research with genetically selected lines has shown that the genotype is an important determinant for these two different stress reaction patterns. One way to guide genetic selection is based on the response to apomorphine, which allows the discrimination of apomorphine susceptible and unsusceptible rat lines, which show pronounced behavioural and HPA differences (Rots *et al.*, 1996). Bohus *et al.* (1987) selected two different mouse lines on the basis of aggressive behaviour, i.e. the short attack latency mice (SAL) and the long attack latency mice (LAL). The SAL lines are fight/flight animals. These are animals that cope actively with stress and are at best in a stable environment, when their corticosterone level is low and testosterone is high. LAL mice are passive and most successful under changing conditions requiring a large adaptive capacity. Their corticosterone levels are high in response to stress. That their corticosteroid levels are high is not so much a sign of loss of control, but as noted by Bohus *et al.* (1987) a survival strategy of equal evolutionary success as the active copers.

Passive and active coping co-exist in all mammals, including man. In view of their diametrically opposed stress reaction patterns one might expect that under conditions of stress this also has consequences for stress-related disorders. The active animals are, because of their high sympathetic tone, susceptible to cardiovascular dysregulation. The passive animals display, because of their high corticosteroid levels, a predisposition to reduce immune responses, enhanced vulnerability to substance dependence and neuropsychiatric disorders such as depression.

The impact of a stressor thus depends on the nature of the stimulus, the genetic background of the individual and subjective issues such as the context of the event and previous experiences. In particular early life experiences appear to cause persistent changes in stress reaction patterns. These changes induced by early life events manifest themselves in the way the situation is experienced as stressful, and in the magnitude and the duration of the stress response.

In rats it has been known for more than 40 years that handling the animals during the first 2 weeks of life (during the stress hyporesponsive period) causes diminished emotional and adrenocortical reactivity in later life (Levine, 1967). Further research revealed that this persistent effect develops because the mother engages in increased care upon the return of the animal after the handling procedure (Meaney *et al.*, 1988; Frances *et al.*, 1999). In contrast, deprivation of animals from maternal care for a much longer period than the daily 15 minutes has completely different consequences for coping with stress (Rots *et al.*, 1996; Workel, 1999). For instance around mid-life deprived animals display hypercorticism and an altered MR/GR balance in the hippocampus, while their cognitive behaviour is slightly impaired. In subsequent studies it appeared that in the deprived animals features of the ageing process were enhanced. Thus, behaviourally, the deprived animals either aged successfully or became senile, at the expense of the average performance, which was the prevalent phenotype of the control mother-reared animals.

In collaboration with Levine's group we have identified several factors that are of relevance for the organization of the stress response system during development (van Oers *et al.*, 1998). The HPA axis response to stress is dramatically enhanced after 24 hours maternal deprivation of the infant rat.

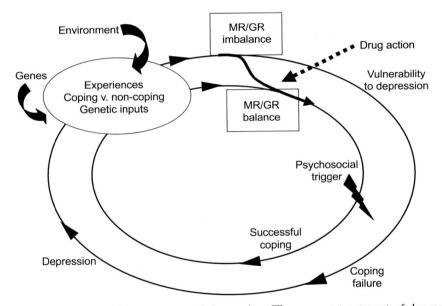

Figure 3. Corticosteroid receptors and depression. The current treatment of depression with tricyclic antidepressants and SSRIs is predominantly symptomatic. Future medication is expected to be aimed towards treatment of causality, eventually resulting in prevention. In this article we advocate the view that pharmacotherapy should be directed towards recovery from an imbalance in MR- and GR-mediated actions. This figure shows that genetic and environmental inputs determine the vulnerability to depression with corticosteroids and their receptors as critical mediators. Once the balance in MR/GR-mediated actions is disturbed, the individual loses the ability to maintain homeostasis if challenged, e.g. by experiencing inability to cope with an adverse life event (psychosocial trigger) (de Kloet, 1991; de Kloet *et al.*, 1998b, 1999). This leads to neuroendocrine dysregulation, impaired behavioural adaptation and possibly depression. In this scheme, drug action should be directed to restore the MR/GR-balance in order to facilitate behavioural adaptation.

Basal and stress-induced ACTH and corticosterone levels are increased in the deprived animal. The stress-hyporesponsive period therefore is maintained predominantly by maternal care. If aspects of maternal care are mimicked in the deprived animal the brain and adrenal components of the HPA axis are differentially restored. For instance, stroking the deprived pup three times with a warm wet artist's brush restored stress markers in the brain, while for recovery of the quiescent adrenal function additional feeding is required. Interestingly, these effects of maternal deprivation and their recovery depend on the time and duration of the maternal separation, but also on the gender and the strain of the animals used.

Maternal deprivation may be considered as a model for child neglect, which can be postulated as a form of child abuse. In animal models based on maternal deprivation it will be possible to assess the molecular and cellular changes. At least in a part of the population it will be possible to relate these early changes in the brain to vulnerability factors for stress-related disorders, such as depression.

CONCLUDING REMARKS

Many different neuronal cells are affected by corticosteroid hormones via MR and/or GR activation. These effects depend on cellular context, both for the occurrence at the genomic level, as well as for the physiological expression of the effects. They also depend on duration of the steroid signal – acute or chronic activation of GRs has dramatically different effects on neuronal function. Thirdly, as was shown for hippocampal physiology, but also for spatial behavioural tasks in rats, the effects of the steroids depend on how the two corticosteroid receptor types, MRs and GRs, become activated.

In this chapter we have discussed the implications of MR and GR co-expression in the same cells as is the case in the hippocampal neurons. In such cells the set-point of homeostatic control appears dependent on co-ordinated antagonistic MR- and GR-mediated actions. MRs operate in a *proactive* mode, maintain stability and are protective. On a higher level of complexity MR-mediated effects govern neuronal networks involved in interpretation of information and selection of the appropriate behavioural response to limit disturbance of homeostasis. In contrast, GR-mediated responses initiated after the stressful disturbance operate in a *reactive* mode with the aim to facilitate recovery and to restore homeostasis. In co-ordination MR- and GR-mediated actions in brain serve behavioural adaptation.

Once the balance in MR/GR-mediated actions is disturbed, the individual loses the ability to maintain homeostasis if challenged, e.g. by experiencing an adverse life event. (de Kloet, 1991; de Kloet *et al.*, 1998b, 1999) (Figure 3). This leads to neuroendocrine dysregulation and impaired behavioural adaptation. In surpassing a certain threshold, this may enhance the vulnerability to depression to which the individual is predisposed. In this line of reasoning an MR/GR imbalance may lead to impaired regulation of corticosteroid responsive gene expression with products that are expected to promote changes in neuronal processes underlying behavioural adaptation. Using gene expression profiling technology these corticosteroid responsive genes or '*candidate plasticity genes*' are being identified (Datson *et al.*, 1999). In our view, novel strategies for treatment of stress-related disorders should exploit these targets in the stress response system. The objective of one strategy is to restore the imbalance in MR/GR balance. Another approach could target directly the dysregulated gene products with a potential role to promote the restorative capacity still present in the diseased brain.

ACKNOWLEDGEMENTS

The support by Netherlands Foundation of Scientific Research and Organon NV (STIGO 014-80–005) is gratefully acknowledged. We would like to thank Dr J.G. Goekoop for helpful discussions.

REFERENCES

Albeck, D.S., McKittrick, C.R., Blanchard, D.C. *et al.* (1997). Chronic social stress alters levels of corticotropin releasing factor and arginine vasopressin mRNA in rat brain. *J Neurosci* **17**, 4895–4903.

Arana, G.W., Santos, A.B., Laraia, M.T. *et al.* (1995). Dexamethasone for the treatment of depression: a randomized, placebo-controlled, double-blind trial. *Am J Psychiatry* **152**, 265–267.

Artigas, F., Romero, L., de Montigny, C. and Blier, P. (1996). Acceleration of the effect of selected antidepressant drugs in major depression by 5HT1a antagonists. *Trends Neurosci* **19**, 378–383.

Barden, N., Reul, J.M. and Holsboer, F. (1995). Do antidepressants stabilize mood through actions on the hypothalamic–pituitary–adrenocortical system? *Trends Neurosci* **18**, 6–11.

Blier, P. and de Montigny, C. (1994). Current advances and trends in the treatment of depression. *Trends Pharmacol Sci* **15**, 220–226.

Bliss, T.V. and Collingridge, G.L. (1993). A synaptic model of memory: long-term potentiation in the hippocampus. *Nature* **361**, 31–39.

Bohus, B., Benus, R.F., Fokkema, D.S. *et al.* (1987). Neuroendocrine states and behavioral and physiological stress responses. *Prog Brain Res* **72**, 57–70.

Bradbury, M.J., Akana, S.F. and Dallman, M.F. (1994). Roles of Type I and II corticosteroid receptors in regulation of basal activity in the hypothalamo–pituitary–adrenal axis during the diurnal trough and the peak: evidence for a nonadditive effect of combined receptor occupation. *Endocrinology* **134**, 1286–1296.

Brady, L.S., Gold, P.W., Herkenham, M., Lynn, A.B. and Whitfield, Jr, H.J. (1992). The antidepressants fluoxetine, idazoxan and phenelzine alter corticotropin-releasing hormone and tyrosine hydroxylase mRNA levels in rat brain: therapeutic implications. *Brain Res* **14**, 117–125.

Budziszewska, B. and Lason, W. (1994). Pharmacological modulation of glucocorticoid and mineralocorticoid receptors in the rat central nervous system. *Pol J Pharmacol* **46**, 97–102.

Checkley, S. (1996). The neuroendocrinology of depression and chronic stress. *Br Med Bull* **52**, 597–617.

Chrousos, G.P. and Gold, P.W. (1992). The concept of stress and stress system disorders. *JAMA* **267**, 1244–1252.

Cleare, A.J., Murray, R.M. and O'Keane, V. (1996). Reduced prolactin and cortisol responses to D-fenfluramine in depressed compared to healthy matched control subjects. *Neuropsychopharmacology* **14**, 349–354.

Dallman, M.F., Levin, N., Cascio, C.S. *et al.* (1989). Pharmacological evidence that the inhibiton of diurnal adrenocorticotropin secretion by corticosteroids is mediated via type I corticosterone-preferring receptors. *Endocrinology* **124**, 2844–2850.

Dallman, M.F., Akana, S.F., Scribner, K.A. (1991). Stress, feedback and facilitation in the hypothalamo–pituitary–adrenal axis. *J Neuroendocrinology* **4**, 517–526.

Datson, N.A., van der Perk-de Jong, J., van den Berg, M.P., de Kloet, E.R. and Vreugdenhill, E. (1999). MicroSAGE: a modified procedure for serial analysis of gene expression in limited amounts of tissue. *Nucl Acid Res* **27**, 1300–1307.

De Goeij, D.C.E., Kvetnansky, R., Whitnall, M.H., Jezova, D. and Berkenbosch F. (1991). Repeated stress-induced activation of corticotropin-releasing factor neurones enhances vasopressin stores and colocalization with corticotropin-releasing factor in the median eminence of the rat. *Neuroendocrinology* **53**, 150–159.

de Kloet, E.R. (1991). Brain corticosteroid receptor balance and homeostatic control. *Front Neuroendocrinolo* **12**, 95–164.

de Kloet, E.R., de Kock, S., Schild, V. and Veldhuis, H.D. (1988a). Antiglucocorticoid RU 38486 attenuates retention of a behaviour and disinhibits the hypothalamic–pituitary adrenal axis at different brain sites. *Neuroendocrinology* **47**, 109–115.

de Kloet, E.R., Vreugdenhill, E., Oitzl, M.S. and Joels, M. (1998b). Brain corticosteroid receptor balance in health and disease. *Endocrinol Rev* **19**, 269–301.

de Kloet, E.R., Oitzl, M.S. and Joels, M. (1999). Stress and cognition: are corticosteroids good or bad guys? *Trends Neurosci* **22**, 422–426.

de Quervain, D.J.-F., Roozendaal, B. and McGaugh, J.L. (1998). Stress and glucocorticoids impair retrieval of long-term spatial memory. *Nature* **394**, 787–790.

Deuschle, M., Weber, B., Colla, M. *et al.* (1998). Mineralocorticoid receptor also modulates basal activity of hypothalamus–pituitary–adrenocortical system in humans. *Neuroendocrinol* **68**, 355–360.

Diamond, D.M., Bennett, M.C., Fleshner, M. and Rose, G.M. (1992). Inverted-U relationship between the level of peripheral corticosterone and the magnitude of hippocampal primed burst potentiation. *Hippocampus* **2**, 421–430.

Diamond, D.M., Fleshner, M. and Rose, G.M. (1994). Psychological stress repeatedly blocks hippocampal primed burst potentiation in behaving rats. *Behav Brain Res* **62**, 1–9.

Dinan, T.G., Lavelle, E., Cooney, J. *et al.* (1997). Dexamethasone augmentation in treatment-resistant depression. *Acta Psychiatr Scand* **95**, 58–61.

Dodt, C., Kern, W., Fehm, H.L. and Born, J. (1993). Antimineralocorticoid canrenoate enhances secretory activity of the hypothalamus–pituitary–adrenocortical (HPA) axis in humans. *Neuroendocrinology* **58**, 570–574.

Dorn, L.D., Burgess, E.S., Dubbert, B. *et al.* (1995). Psychopathology in patients with endogenous Cushing's syndrome: 'atypical' or melancholic features. *Clin Endocrinol* **43**, 433–442.

Eiring, A. and Sulser, F. (1997). Increased synaptic availability of norepinephrine following desipramine is not essential for increases in GR mRNA. *J Neural Transm* **104**, 1255–1258.

Frances, D., Diorio, J., Liu, D. and Meaney, M.J. (1999). Nongenomic transmission across generations of maternal behaviour and stress responses in the rat. *Science* **286**, 1155–1158.

Ghadirian, A.M., Engelsmann, F., Dhar, V. *et al.* (1995). The psychotropic effects of inhibitors of steroid biosynthesis in depressed patients refractory to treatment. *Biol Psychiatry* **37**, 369–375.

Gold, P.W. and Chrousos, G.P. (1998). The endocrinology of melancholic and atypical depression: relation to neurocircuitry and somatic consequences. *Proc Assoc Am Physic* **111**, 22–34.

Gray, J.A. and McNaughton, B. (1983). Comparison between the behavioural effects of septal and hippocampal lesions: a review. *Neurosci Biobehav Rev* **7**, 119–188.

Haller, J., Millar, S. and Kruk, M.R. (1998). Mineralocorticoid receptor blockade inhibits aggressive behavior in male rats. *Stress* **2**, 201–207.

Henry, J.P. and Stephens, P.M. (1976). *Stress, Health and the Social Environment. A Sociobiological Approach to Medicine.* Springer: New York.

Herman, J.P. and Cullinan, W.E. (1997). Neurocircuitry of stress: central control of the hypothalamo–pituitary–adrenocortical axis. *Trends Neurosci* **20**, 78–84.

Heuser, I.J., Yassouridis, A. and Holsboer, F. (1994). The combined dexamethasone/CRH test: a refined laboratory test for psychiatric disorders. *J Psychiatr Res* **28**, 341–356.

Holsboer, F. (1999). The rationale for corticotropin releasing hormone receptor (CRH-R) antagonists to treat depression and anxiety. *J Psychiatr Res* **33**, 181–214.

Holsboer, F. and Barden, N. (1996). Antidepressants and hypothalamic–pituitary–adrenocortical regulation. *Endocrinol Rev* **17**, 187–205.

Holsboer, F., Lauer, C.J., Schreiber, W. and Krieg, J.-C. (1995). Altered hypothalamic–pituitary–adrenocortical regulation in healthy subjects at high familial risk for affective disorders. *Neuroendocrinology* **62**, 340–347.

Joels, M. and de Kloet, E.R. (1992). Coordinative mineralocorticoid and glucocorticoid receptor-mediated control of responses to serotonin in rat hippocampus. *Neuroendocrinology* **55**, 344–350.

Joels, M. and de Kloet, E.R. (1994). Mineralocorticoid and glucocorticoid receptors in the brain. Implications for ion permeability and transmitter systems. *Progr Neurobiol* **43**, 1–36.

Joels, M. and de Kloet, E.R. (2000). Effects of glucocorticoids and norepinephrine on the excitability in the hippocampus. *Science* **245**, 1502–1505.

Karten, Y.J., Nair, S.M., van Essen, L., Sibug, R. and Joels, M. (1999). Long term exposure to high corticosterone levels attenuates serotonin responses in rat hippocampal CA1 neurones. *Proc Natl Acad Sci* **96**, 13456–13461.

Kendler, S., Karkowski, L.M. and Prescott, C.A. (1999). Causal relationship between stressful life events and the onset of major depression. *Am J Psychiatry* **156**, 837–841.

Korte, S.M., de Boer, S.F., de Kloet, E.R. and Bohus, B. (1995). Anxiolytic-like effects of selective mineralocorticoid and glucocorticoid antagonists of fear-enhanced behavior in the elevated plus-maze. *Psychoendocrinology* **20**, 385–394.

Korte, S.M., de Kloet, E.R., Buwalda, B., Bouman, S.D. and Bohus, B. (1996a). Antisense to the glucocorticoid receptor in hippocampal dentate gyrus reduces immobility in forced swim test. *Eur J Pharmacol* **301**, 19–25.

Korte, S.M., Korte-Bouws, G.A.H., Koob, G.F., de Kloet, E.R. and Bohus, B. (1996b). Mineralocorticoid and glucocorticoid receptor antagonists in animal models of anxiety. *Pharmacol Biochem Behav* **54**, 261–267.

Lamberts, S.W., Koper, J.W. and Jong, F.H. (1991). The endocrine effects of long-term treatment with mifepristone (RU 486). *J Clin Endocrinol Metab* **73**, 187–191.

Levine, S. (1967). Maternal and environmental influences on the adrenocortical response to stress in weaning rats. *Science* **156**, 258–260.

Loscertales, M., Rose, S.P. and Sandi, C. (1997). The corticosteroid synthesis inhibitors metyrapone and aminoglutethimide impair long-term memory for a passive avoidance task in day-old chicks. *Brain Res* **769**, 357–361.

Lupien, S.J., Gaudreau, S., Tchiteya, B.M., Maheu, F. *et al.* (1997). Stress-induced declarative memory impairment in healthy elderly subjects: relationship to cortisol reactivity. *J Clin Endocrinol Metab* **82**, 2070–2075.

Makino, S., Smith, M.A. and Gold, P.W. (1995). Increased expression of corticotropin-releasing hormone and vasopressin messenger ribonucleic acid (mRNA) in the hypothalamic paraventricular nucleus during repeated stress: association with reduction in glucocorticoid receptor mRNA levels. *Endocrinology* **136**, 3299–3309.

Margarinos, A.M., Deslandes, A. and McEwen, B.S. (1999). Effects of antidepressants and benzodiazepine treatments on the dendritic structure of CA3 pyramidal neurons after chronic stress. *Eur J Pharmacol* **371**, 113–122.

Meaney, M.J., Aitken, D.H., van Berkel, C., Bhatnagar, S. and Sapolsky, R.M. (1988). Effect of neonatal handling on age-related impairments associated with the hippocampus. *Science* **239**, 766–768.

Meijer, O.C. and de Kloet, E.R. (1998). Corticosterone and serotonergic neurotransmission in the hippocampus: functional implications of central corticosteroid receptor diversity. *Crit Rev Neurobiol* **12**, 1–20.

Meijer, O.C., Kortekaas, R., Oitzl, M.S. and de Kloet, E.R. (1998). Acute rise in corticosterone facilitates 5HT1A receptor-mediated behavioral responses. *Eur J Pharmacol* **351**, 7–14.

Meijer, O.C., Steenbergen, P.J. and de Kloet, E.R. (2000). Differential expression and regional distribution of steroid receptor coactivators SRC-1 and SRC-2 in brain and pituitary. *Endocrinology* **141**, 2192–2199.

Modell, S., Lauer, C.J., Schreiber, W. *et al.* (1998). Hormonal response patterns in the combined Dex-CRH test is stable over time in subjects at high familial risk for affective disorders. *Neuropsychopharmacology* **18**, 253–262.

Murphy, B.E.P. (1997). Antiglucocorticoid therapies in major depression: a review. *Psychoendocrinology* **22**, S125–S132.

Murphy, B.E.P., Filipini, D. and Ghadirian, A.M. (1993). Possible use of glucocorticoid receptor antagonists in the treatment of major depression: preliminary results using RU 486. *J Psychiatry Neurosci* **18**, 209–213.

Murphy, B.E.P., Ghadirian, A.M. and Dhar, V. (1998). Neuroendocrine responses to inhibitors of steroid biosynthesis in patients with major depression resistant to antidepressant therapy. *Can J Psychiatry* **43**, 279–286.

Newcomer, J.W., Slek, G., Melson, A.K. *et al.* (1999). Decreased memory performance in healthy humans induced by stress-level cortisol treatment. *Am J Psychiatry* **56**, 527–533.

Oitzl, M.S. and de Kloet, E.R. (1992). Selective corticosteroid antagonists modulate specific aspects of spatial orientation learning. *Behav Neurosc* **106**, 62–71.

Oitzl, M.S., Fluttert, M. and de Kloet, E.R. (1994). The effect of corticosterone on reactivity to spatial novelty is mediated by central mineralocorticoid receptors. *Eur J Neurosci* **6**, 1072–1079.

Oitzl, M.S., van Haarst, A.D., Sutanto, W. and de Kloet, E.R. (1995). Corticosterone, brain mineralocorticoid receptors (MRs) and the activity of the hypothalamic–pituitary–adrenal (HPA) axis: the Lewis rat as an example of increased central MR capacity and a hyporesponsive HPA axis. *Psychoendocrinology* **20**, 655–675.

Oitzl, M.S., Fluttert, M., Sutanto, W. and de Kloet, E.R. (1998). Continuous blockade of brain glucocorticoid receptors facilitates spatial learning and memory in rats. *Eur J Neurosci* **10**, 3759–3766.

Pariante, C.M., Pearce, B.D., Pisell, T.L., Owens, M.J. and Miller, A.H. (1997). Steroid-independent translocation of the glucocorticoid receptor by the antidepressant desipramine. *Mol Pharmacol* **52**, 571–581.

Peiffer, A., Veilleux, S. and Barden, N. (1991). Antidepressants and other centrally acting drugs regulate glucocorticoid receptor messenger RNA levels in rat brain. *Psychoneuroendocrinology* **16**, 505–515.

Pepin, M.C., Govindan, M.V. and Barden, N. (1992). Increased glucocorticoid receptor gene promoter activity after antidepressant treatment. *Mol Pharmacol* **41**, 1016–1022.

Przegalinski, E. and Budziszewska, B. (1993). The effect of long-term treatment with antidepressant drugs on the hippocampal mineralocorticoid and glucocorticoid receptors in rats. *Neurosci Lett* **161**, 215–218.

Przegalinski, E., Budziszewska, B., Siwanowicz, J. and Jaworska, L. (1993). The effect of repeated combined treatment with nifedipine and antidepressant drugs or electroconvulsive shock on the hippocampal corticosteroid receptors in rats. *Neuropharmacology* **32**, 1397–1400.

Purba, J.S., Hoogendijk, W.J., Hofman, M.A. and Swaab, D.F. (1996). Increased number of vasopressin- and oxytocin-expressing neurons in the paraventricular nucleus of the hypothalamus in depression. *Arch Gen Psychiatry* **53**, 137–143.

Ratka, A., Sutanto, W., Bloemers, M. and de Kloet, E.R. (1989). On the role of the brain type I and type II corticosteroid receptors in neuroendocrine regulation. *Neuroendocrinology* **50**, 117–123.

Reul, J.M., Probst, J.C., Skutella, T. *et al.* (1997) Increased stress-induced adrenocorticotropin response after long-term intracerebroventricular treatment of rats with antisense mineralocorticoid receptor oligodeoxynucleotides. *Neuroendocrinology* **65**, 189–199.

Ribeiro, S.C.M., Tandon, R., Grunhaus, L. and Greden, J.F. (1993). The DST as a predictor of outcome in depression: a meta-analysis. *Am J Psychiatry* **150**, 1618–1629.

Rots, N.Y., de Jong, J., Workel, J.O., Cools, A.R. and de Kloet, E.R. (1996). Neonatal maternally deprived rats have as adults elevated basal pituitary-adrenal activity and enhanced susceptibility to apomorphine. *J Neuroendocrinol* **8**, 501–506.

Sandi, C. and Rose, S.P. (1994). Corticosterone enhances long-term retention in one-day-old chicks trained in a weak passive avoidance learning paradigm. *Brain Res* **647**, 106–112.

Schulkin, J., Gold, P.W. and McEwen, B.S. (1998). Induction of corticotropin-releasing hormone gene expression by glucocorticoids: implication for understanding the states of fear and allostatic load. *Psychoneuroendocrinology* **23**, 219–243.

Seckl, J.R. and Fink, G. (1992). Antidepressants increase glucocorticoid and mineralocorticoid receptor mRNA expression in rat hippocampus. *Neuroendocrinology* **55**, 621–626.

Shors, T.J. and Dryver, E. (1994). Effect of stress and long-term potentiation (LTP) on subsequent LTP and the theta burst response in the dentate gyrus. *Brain Res* **666**, 232–238.

Spencer, R.L., Kim, P.J., Kalman, B.A. and Cole, M.A. (1998). Evidence for mineralocorticoid receptor facilitation of glucocorticoid receptor-dependent regulation of hypothalamic-pituitary-adrenal axis activity. *Endocrinology* **139**, 2718–2726.

Thakore, J.H. and Dinan, T.G. (1995). Cortisol synthesis inhibition: a new treatment strategy for the clinical and endocrine manifestations of depression. *Biol Psychiatry* **37**, 364–368.

Thase, M.E., Dube, S., Bowler, K. *et al.* (1996). Hypothalamic–pituitary–adrenocortical activity and response to cognitive behavior therapy in unmedicated, hospitalized depressed patients. *Am J Psychiatry* **153**, 886–891.

van Haarst, A.D., Oitzl, M.S., Workel, J.O. and de Kloet, E.R. (1996). Chronic brain glucocorticoid receptor blockade enhances the rise in circadian and stress-induced pituitary–adrenal activity. *Endocrinology* **137**, 4935–4943.

van Haarst, A.D., Oitzl, M.S. and de Kloet, E.R. (1997). Facilitation of feedback inhibition through blockade of glucocorticoid receptors in the hippocampus. *Neurochem Res* **22**, 1323–1328.

van Londen, L., Goekoop, J.G., van Kempen, G.J.M. *et al.* (1997). Plasma levels of arginine vasopressine elevated in patients with major depression. *Neuropsychopharmacology* **17**, 284–292.

van Oers, H.J., de Kloet, E.R., Whelan, T. and Levine, S. (1998). Maternal deprivation effect on the infant's neural stress markers is reversed by tactile stimulation and feeding but not by suppressing corticosterone. *J Neurosci* **18**, 10171–10179.

van Praag, H.M. (1996). Faulty cortisol/serotonin interplay. Psychopathological and biological characteristics of a new, hypothetical depression subtype (SeCA depression). *Psychiatry Res* **65**, 143–157.

Wolkowitz, O.M. and Reus, V.I. (1999). Treatment of depression with anti glucocorticoid drugs. *Psychosom Med* **61**, 698–711.

Workel, J.O. (1999). *Maternal Deprivation: Implications for Stress Cognition and Aging.* Leiden University.

Xu, L., Anwyl, R. and Rowan, M.J. (1997). Behavioural stress facilitates the induction of long-term depression in the hippocampus. *Nature* **387**, 497–500.

3

Stress, Monoamines and the Immune System

B.E. LEONARD

Pharmacology Department, National University of Ireland, Galway, Ireland

INTRODUCTION

The concept of depression as an immunological disease can be traced back to the observations of Galen in 200 AD who suggested that women of melancholic temperament were more susceptible to cancer than those of sanguine temperament. Numerous anecdotal reports have appeared in the medical literature since that time supporting the view that depression is associated with an impairment of immune function thereby predisposing the patient to infections and cancers. George Day, for example, cited unhappiness as a cause of lowered resistance in patients with tuberculosis (Day 1951). Such observations ultimately led to the seminal publication of Ader (1981) who helped to lay the scientific basis of psychoimmunology by reviewing the evidence for a complex interaction between the brain and the immune system and, more importantly, of the functional biodirectional communication that exists between the immune system and the central nervous system. This has led to the view that the nervous, endocrine and immune systems are so intimately linked that they should be regarded as a single network rather than three separate systems.

It is self-evident that psychological stress not only plays a vital role in precipitating major psychiatric illness in the vulnerable patient but also is responsible for compromising immune function as a result of the activation of the pituitary–adrenal axis. In the case of depression, a rise in the concentration of circulating cortisol would be expected to suppress many aspects of cellular immunity. This would explain the increased susceptibility of such patients to cancer and infections. However, while there is ample evidence that lymphocyte and natural killer cell activities are suppressed in the depressed patient (see Maes *et al.*, 1995), there is also convincing evidence that activa-

tion of macrophages occurs in these patients: a situation in which pro-inflammatory cytokines released by the activated macrophages play a key role
(Maes *et al.*, 1992; Leonard, 2000a). Such findings have led to the hypothesis
that the change in central monoamine function that has traditionally been
viewed as the cause of depression may occur as a consequence of an activation of the pituitary–adrenal axis that is caused by a rise in the concentration
of pro-inflammatory cytokines (see Connor and Leonard, 1998). The disturbance in the relationship between the central monoaminergic systems and the
immune and endocrine sytems as the cause of depression will form the basis
of this chapter. The evidence is summarized in Figure 1.

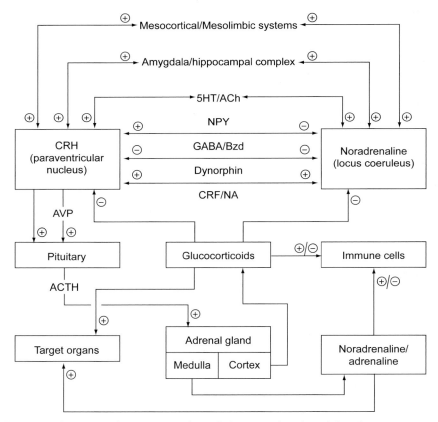

Figure 1. Diagrammatic representation of the central and peripheral components of
the stress system. (Modified with permission, from Chrousos and Gold, 1992). Key:
CRH, corticotrophin releasing hormone; NPY, neuropeptide Y; NA, noradrenaline;
AVP, arginine vasopression; ACTH, adrenocorticotrophic hormone; GABA–Bzd,
gamma aminobenzoic acid/benzodiazepine receptor complex; 5HT/ACh, serotonin/
acetylcholine; +, activation; –, inhibition.

STRESS AND DISORDERS OF THE IMMUNE SYSTEM

There are many definitions of stress but one of the most satisfactory may be attributed to Sklar and Anisman (1981) who defined it as the reactions of an organism to deleterious forces such as infections and other states that disturb normal homeostasis. The stimulus that causes such a disruption is termed the stressor. With such a broad definition it is essential to clarify the severity of the stressor, whether it is avoidable or unavoidable, of a physical or a psychological nature. The effect of the stressor will also depend on the age, gender and genetic composition of the subject. In addition, some types of stress will alter the general metabolism, for example exposure to heat or cold.

The impact of stress on the endocrine system is generally determined by assessing the plasma glucocorticoid concentrations. There is evidence that stress and the increase in plasma glucocorticoids are closely related (Owens and Nemeroff, 1991). The glucocorticoid release from the adrenal glands is partly dependent on the duration of the stress; acute stress is usually associated with a marked rise in glucocorticoid secretion, whereas following chronic stress, glucocorticoid secretion is often decreased (Owens and Nemeroff, 1991).

Stress activates both the hypothalamic–pituitary–adrenal (HPA) axis and the sympathetic nervous system and therefore it is not surprising to find that most acute stressors affect the immune response. Lymphocytes have adrenoceptors on their outer membranes which respond to the action of catecholamines that are released following an acute stressor. In addition, the secretion of glucocorticoids is commonly associated with the suppression of many aspects of cellular immunity. In animal studies, it has been shown that acute stressors such as social defeat or maternal separation suppress cellular immunity, while chronic stress such as overcrowding can suppress aspects of cellular and humoral immunity (Maier et al., 1994).

There is now ample clinical and experimental evidence to demonstrate that not all stressors produce identical changes in the endocrine and immune systems. Thus different stressors produce different degrees of endocrine and sympathetic activation (Mason, 1971). Coping strategies are also important in modifying the adverse impact of a stressor (Mormede et al., 1988). Thus, ultimately, the specific immune response involves a complex cascade of events in which the catecholamines, glucocorticoids, endorphins and other neuropeptides play vital roles (see Croiset et al., 1987).

The impact of stress on antibody synthesis depends on the temporal relationship between the antigen challenge and the time at which the stressor is applied. For example, a stressor will interfere with antibody synthesis only if it is applied near the time of the antibody exposure (Fleshner et al., 1995). Such a finding serves as a caution in extrapolating conclusions from studies in which the impact of stress on the immune system has been determined at only one time point. Furthermore, many immune changes are non-specific and reflect an intermediate aspect of the immune response (for example, the synthesis of interleukins or the proliferative response of T-cells to mitogens) rather than the end-point of the immune response that destroys virus infected cells, etc. It is apparent that the immune system contains a high degree of redundancy so that changes in a specific aspect of the immune cascade are not in themselves evidence of a significant change in the immune process (Cunnick *et al.*, 1991). Nevertheless, there is a growing literature to support the view that stressful life events predispose an individual to physical illness and while such correlations are relatively small, possibly accounting for 10% of the variance (Weisse, 1992), they are consistent across populations and following different types of adverse life events.

Stress, life events and altered immune response

Bereavement stress has been the subject of many studies. However, it is apparent that the risk of ill health following marital separation or divorce is greater than that occurring following bereavement (Kiecolt–Glaser *et al.*, 1987). Thus separated or divorced women showed defects in immune function in five of six immunological variables when compared with matched sample of married women. Somewhat similar findings were reported for separated and divorced men (Kiecolt–Glaser and Glaser, 1988).

Similarly, the effects of chronic stress on carers of patients with Alzheimer's disease have shown that such individuals have a high risk of depression (Crook and Miller, 1985) and impaired immunological function (Kiecolt–Glaser *et al.*, 1991). These, and other studies (for example, on people living in the vicinity of Three Mile Island, in the USA where an accident occurred at the nuclear power station (Davidson and Baum, 1986)) show that chronic stress does not necessarily result in adaptive changes in the immune system. This would not appear to be the situation in rodents, however, where experimental evidence shows that acute stress is largely immunosuppressive, whereas chronic stress is usually associated with adaptive changes (Cohen and Crnic, 1982).

Even relatively short-term stress can impair different aspects of the immune response. For example, examination stress in university students has been shown to decrease the activity of natural killer cells (NKCs) that normally protect against viral and carcinogen assults (Kiecolt–Glaser and Glaser, 1988). Interestingly, it was found that the application of relaxation techniques did not fully reverse the changes in cellular immunity caused by examination stress.

A major difficulty that occurs in predicting the effect of stress on the immune system arises because the same stressor may elicit different effects on different individuals. In addition, due to the wide variation in immune responses that normally occurs, small but physiologically important changes may be difficult to detect. Furthermore, selecting the immune parameters which accurately reflect the true status of an individual's immune defences is frequently difficult. Such factors make the interpretation of the effect of stress on the individual difficult.

INTERACTION BETWEEN THE BRAIN, IMMUNE AND ENDOCRINE SYSTEMS IN DEPRESSION

Changes in the central nervous system or endocrine systems inevitably are associated with changes in immune function and, conversely, changes in immune function directly or indirectly impact on the endocrine and central nervous systems (Leonard and Song, 1999). Such a close interrelationship between these three systems has a structural and functional basis. Thus noradrenergic and cholinergic terminals innervate both the thymus gland and bone marrow thereby directly influencing the development of immune cells. In addition, lymphocytes and monocytes contain adrenoceptors that directly respond to changes in the blood concentration of catecholamines and neuropeptides that are secreted in response to stress, Similarly, glucocorticoids secreted by the adrenals can directly modulate immune function by activating glucocorticoid receptors on immune cells. However, there is also abundant evidence that the immune system can modulate both central neurotransmitter and endocrine function. Thus some cytokines that are produced by immune cells in the periphery, and by microglia in the brain, are potent activators of the pituitary–adrenal axis. In addition, pro-inflammatory cytokines such as interleukins (IL) 1 and 6 and tumour necrosis factor alpha (TNFα) can modulate central neurotransmission indirectly by activating cyclo-oxygenase activity; this results in elevated prostaglandins of the E series which modulate neurotransmitter release (see Bost, 1988; Farrar, 1988; Connor and Leonard, 1998). Such 'cross-talk' between these three systems could account not only for the changes seen following the impact of an acute or chronic stressor but also for the changes that arise in depressed patients. These changes are reflected in a reduction in NKC activity, T-cell proliferation and neutrophil phagocytosis but also in the rise in the concentrations of positive acute phase proteins, immunoglobulins A and M and complement C3 and C4. Such changes in depression are largely a reflection of the increased release of IL-I, TNFα and interferon alpha (INFα) from activated macrophages; the antipro-inflammatory cytokines IL-4 and IL-10 are reduced in depression (see Maes *et al.*, 1992, 1995; Song *et al.*, 1994; Leonard and Song, 1999).

In addition to the functional changes in the immune system that are associated with depression, structural changes also occur. Thus the weights of the thymus gland and the spleen are decreased while that of the adrenals is increased both in depression and following chronic stress (Dohmus and Metz, 1991). The elevation of the glucocorticoid concentration that occurs under these conditions contributes to the atrophy of the thymus gland and to the secondary changes in cellular immunity. Secondary changes also occur in the brain of untreated (or inadequately treated) depressed patients which contribute to the psychopathology of the condition. Thus the enlargement of the cerebral ventricles and the shrinking of the hippocampus and other regions have been attributed to increased apoptosis (see Duman *et al.*, 1997) resulting from the chronic increase in glucocorticoids and possibly pro-inflammatory cytokines.

Such observations raise interesting questions. Glucocorticoids are known to be effective anti-inflammatory agents and would thereby be anticipated to suppppress pro-inflammatory mediators that would arise in stress or depression (Almawi *et al.*, 1996). However, it is well documented that glucocorticoids can act synergistically with the cytokines and strongly potentiate the effects of the pro-inflammatory IL-1 and IL-6 induction of acute phase proteins by the liver (Baumann and Gauldie, 1994). Furthermore, the expression of many cytokine receptors is strongly upregulated by glucocorticoids. These receptors include IL-1, 2, 4 and 6, INFγ and TNFα (Wiegers and Reul, 1998). This may help to explain why in depression there is both a hypersecretion of cortisol and an increase in the concentration of pro-inflammatory cytokines.

Following an acute stressor, the rise in the plasma cortisol concentration is usually attenuated due to the steroid inducing a negative feedback or the further release of corticotrophin releasing hormone (CRH) and adrenocorticotrophic hormone (ACTH) by the hypothalamus and anterior pituitary gland, respectively. However, in depression, or following chronic stress, the glucocorticoid receptors become subsensitive to the negative feedback mechanism and, as a consequence, glucocorticoid hypersecretion occurs. This situation is further accentuated by the activation of the hypothalamic–pituitary pathway by IL-1. The lack of suppression of macrophage activity by the increase in the circulating glucocorticoids could also arise as a consequence of the decreased sensitivity of the glucocorticoid receptor on these cells. The role that the glucocorticoids play in the aetiology of depression was formulated by Dinan (1994) and can now be extended to include the involvement of the pro-inflammatory cytokines.

The interrelationship between the cytokines and the glucocorticoids in pathological changes associated with depression is further exemplified by the increase in autoimmune diseases that frequently occur in the depressed patient. For example, there is evidence that some allergies involve inappropriate helper T-cell responses. While it is certainly true that exogenously applied glucocorticoids are effective in the treatment of many autoimmune diseases, it is also known that they may exacerbate the condition by inducing helper T-cells to secrete IL-4 and other cytokines (Blotta, 1997). As a consequence of this action, the synthesis of immunoglobulin E, a principal mediator of autoimmune dieases, is increased (Wu *et al.*, 1991). Thus an understanding of the complex interrelationship between the endocrine and immune systems may help explain why autoimmune diseases are often associated with depression.

IMMUNE–NEUROTRANSMITTER INTERACTIONS AND DEPRESSION

The amine hypothesis of depression, which postulates that the symptoms arise as a consequence of a primary defect in noradrenaline, serotonin and possibly dopamine, has been widely accepted for the past 30 years. As a consequence of improvements in methodology, emphasis has largely switched from studies of presynaptic mechanism governing the synthesis and release of the biogenic amines to changes in the function of postsynaptic receptors and their second messenger systems. This has resulted in an extension of the monoamine hypothesis to include amine receptor adaptation, and ultimately gene expression that signals the release of nerve growth factors that initiate new synaptic contacts (see Leonard, 2000b). The question therefore arises regarding the mechanism whereby pro-inflammatory cytokines impede central neurotransmission, and therefore contribute to the aetiology of depression.

There is substantial evidence to show that major depression is accompanied by an acute phase protein response (Song et al., 1994) and increased secretion of prostaglandins of the E series in the brain (Calabrese et al., 1986; McAdams and Leonard, 1992) and by an excessive secretion of pro-inflammatory cytokines (Maes et al., 1995). Such changes suggest that immune activation may play a crucial role in the pathogenesis of depression and provide the basis for the macrophage theory of depression (Smith, 1991). Thus inflammatory cytokine or bacterial cell wall lipopolysaccharide (LPS) administered to animals or to man result in sickness behaviour, many of the symptoms of which simulate those seen in major depression (Connor and Leonard, 1998). These behavioural changes are associated with an activation of the hypothalamic–pituitary–adrenal axis. The increase in the concentrations of IL-1 and IL-6 mediate the acute phase protein response in the liver (Song et al., 1994); these proteins reduce the plasma free tryptophan concentration and thereby affect the availability of the amine acid to the brain.

In addition to this indirect effect of the pro-inflammatory cytokines on the tryptophan pool in the brain (therefore leading to a reduction in the synthesis of serotonin), there is also evidence from in vitro studies that IL-1 activates the serotonin transporter directly (Ramamoorthy et al., 1995) thereby leading to an increased reuptake of the transmitter from the synaptic cleft. Receptors for IL-1 are widely distributed in the brain, including the serotonergic neurons (Cunningham and de Souza, 1996), and there is experimental evidence that the serotonergic cell bodies respond to IL-1 which is increased during an inflammatory process. Thus a reduction in the availabilty of tryptophan for the synthesis of serotonin caused by elevated acute phase proteins, and an enhanced reuptake of the transmitter from the synaptic cleft due to the direct action of IL-1, may directly contribute to the malfunctioning of the serotonergic system.

In addition to the modulation of central serotonergic function by IL-1, there is also experimental evidence that this cytokine can enhance the activity of cycloxygenase and thereby increase the synthesis of prostaglandins of the E series (PGEs). *In vitro*, PGE2 has been shown to activate monocytes, an important source of IL-1 in the periphery, and inhibit neutrophil phagocytosis at concentrations similar to those found in depressed patients (McAdams and Leonard, 1992); PGEs can reduce neurotransmitter release by reducing calcium mobility (Hedqvist, 1976). While it still remains to be shown that these changes occur *in vivo* in the brain of the depressed patient, it is known that antidepressants suppress pro-inflammatory cytokines (Xia *et al.*, 1996) and that different classes of antidepressant decrease the synthesis of PGEs (Manku *et al.*, 1977; Mtabaji *et al.*, 1977) The results of such studies suggest that the pro-inflammatory cytokines act as common mediators for the action of external (e.g. psychosocial) and internal (infections, toxins, etc.) stressors that are known to be important trigger factors for depression. Effective antidepressant treatment would therefore appear to be associated with a reduction in pro-inflammatory cytokines and PGEs as well as a normalization of central neurotransmitter function. The macrophage hypothesis of depression thus raises interesting questions regarding the mechanism whereby antidepressants act at the cellular level and the possibility that the changes in monoamines, that have so often been assumed to be the primary cause of the antidepressant response, may be secondary to changes in the immune–endocrine systems.

REGULATION OF BRAIN IL-1 DURING STRESS AND ITS RELEVANCE TO THE BIOLOGY OF DEPRESSION

Dysregulation of the HPA axis is widely accepted as the key element in the biology of major depression (Nemeroff *et al.*, 1984; Gold *et al.*, 1996). As there is experimental evidence to show that stress-induced IL-1 β gene expression in the brain is regulated by endogenous adrenal steroids (Licinio and Wong, 1999), it may be speculated that the symptoms of major depression might be affected by the balance between the activation of the HPA axis and the synthesis of IL-1. This led Licinio and Wong (1999) to propose that, in major depression, the stress-related increase in IL-1 would stimulate the HPA axis which would, as a consequence, suppress IL-1 synthesis. The reduction in IL-1 would then lead to a reduced stimulation of the HPA axis thereby resulting in an increase in IL-1 synthesis and a continuation of the cycle (Figure 2).

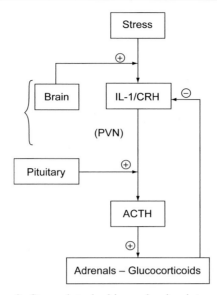

Figure 2. Stress–interleukin–endocrine interactions.

This constant interplay between IL-1 and the glucocorticoids might help to explain why most patients with major depression do not present with overt clinical features of either endocrine or immune disease. However, it does not account for the down-regulation of central glucocorticoid receptors that characterizes many patients with major depression (Dinan, 1994). This event has been explained by the adaptive mechanism that arises in response to the chronic over-activation of the glucocorticoid receptors which reflects a chronic hypersecretion of glucocorticoids in these patients. Furthermore, the medical consequences of untreated major depression (such as decreased bone mineral density (Michelson *et al.*, 1996), increased coronary artery disease (Glassman and Shapiro, 1998) and neurodegeneration (Skeline *et al.*, 1996) support the hypothesis that a prolonged activation of the HPA axis and the pro-inflammatory cytokine pathway could also play a causal role in the physical ill health of these patients. Experimental studies also support such views (Nguyen *et al.*, 1988). Thus the IL-1 induced stimulation of the nucleus coeruleus, the main noradrenergic cell body region in the brain activated by stress, is attenuated by the administration of the IL-1 receptor antagonist (IL-1 ra). Furthermore, experimental studies have shown that chronic antidepressant treatments cause a marked elevation in the concentration of IL-1 ra in the hypothalamus (Suzuki *et al.*, 1996). Such experimental findings, if relevant to the clinical situation in depressed patients, could provide evidence of a new mechanism of action of antidepressants whereby the impact of stress as a major trigger factor for depression is attenuated.

It is often forgotten that the only Nobel Prize ever awarded to a psychiatrist was to Wagner Jauregge in 1927 for his research on the beneficial effect of immune activation in the treatment of schizophrenia with malaria. Despite this, an understanding of the role that the mediators of the immune response play in the biology of mental disorders is still in its infancy. However, there is increasing evidence that cytokines acting in the brain, particularly IL-1 and related pro-inflammatory mediators, play a role in major depression and that these actions are terminated by chronic antidepressant treatment.

Such a conclusion is not unreasonable in view of the fact that these cytokines are known to adversely affect food intake, body weight, sleep pattern, memory, cognition, body temperature and neuroendocrine regulation in a manner that qualitatively resembles the changes seen in patients with major depression. Such is the persuasive evidence in favour of the view that depression is a neuroimmune–endocrine disease and that effective treatment brings about the normalization of these dysfunctional endocrine and immune systems.

CONCLUSIONS

The concept that changes in the immune and endocrine systems determine many of the biological changes associated with stress and are ultimately connected to the cause of major depression dates back many decades even though the precise mechanism linking the immune, endocrine and neurotransmitter systems with behaviour is a relatively recent discovery. It is interesting to note for example that Sigmund Freud was aware of the possible role that the endocrine system played in the pathogenesis of the neuroses when he wrote: 'From a clinical standpoint the neuroses must necessarily be put alongside the intoxications and such disorders as Graves disease. These are conditions arising from an excess or a relative lack of certain highly active substances, whether produced inside the body or introduced into it from the outside. In short, they are disturbances of the chemistry of the body, toxic conditions' (Freud, 1923).

However, despite the advances that have been made in psychoneuroimmunoendocrinology in recent years, there are many open questions regarding the relationship between the immune and endocrine systems and the impact of stress in the aetiology of depression. Many of these points have been critically considered by Leonard and Song (1999) and may be illustrated by the following.

The variation in an immune parameter between patients and their controls may be statistically signficant but still within the normal range for immune function. It would appear that there is a high degree of physiological redundancy in many aspects of the immune response. While there is evidence that the incidence of cancer and autoimmune disease is higher in patients with major depression than in a control population, it is also evident that the increased mortality rate in such patients is due to suicide or accidents rather than related to a disorganized immune system (Martin *et al.*, 1985). Furthermore, it is evident that both stressful and non-stressful environmental events can profoundly affect the immune system. However, the degree to which a stressor can cause immunosuppression is influenced by the perception of the stressful event. From experimental studies it is known that the immune system can be classically conditioned (Ader and Cohen, 1991); animals can learn to immunosuppress or immunoenhance different aspects of cellular immunity (Dark *et al.*, 1987), but such conditioning is rarely taken into consideration in clinical studies. With regard to the impact of glucocorticoids on the immune system, it is known that these steroids exert paradoxical effects on cytokine expression and cytokine regulated biological responses. However, an understanding of these complex interrelationships is hampered by the fragmented information obtained from studies in which only the immune changes have been determined. Thus a comprehensive approach, involving changes in specific cytokines as well as the glucocorticoids and other endocrine markers, is essential if any meaningful data are to be determined.

Despite these limitations, there are exciting developments relating to the interactions between the immune and endocrine systems and the brain in patients subject to chronic stress and depression. In future, research into the basic physiological processes that underlie these interactions, and their relevance to the development and outcome of psychiatric illness will be particularly pertinent. In the meantime, a clearer understanding of the cytokines, their receptors and the various neuromodulators and neurotransmitters may help in the development of novel psychotropic drugs.

REFERENCES

Ader, R. (Ed.) (1981). *Psychoneuroimmunology*. Academic Press, New York.
Ader, R. and Cohen, N. (1991). Conditioning the immune system. *Neth J Med* **39**, 263–276.
Almawi, W.Y., Beyuhum, H.N., Rahme, A.A. and Rider, M.J. (1996). Regulation of cytokine and cytokine receptor expression by glucocorticoids. *J Leucocyte Biol* **60**, 5563–5572.
Baumann, H. and Gauldie, J. (1994). The acute phase response. *Immunol Today* **15**, 74–80.
Blotta, M.H. (1997). Corticosteroids inhibit IL-12 production in human monocytes and enhance their capacity to induce IL-4 synthesis in CD4+ lymphocytes. *J Immunol* **158**, 5589–5595.
Bost, K.L. (1988). Hormone and neuropeptide receptors on mononuclear leucocytes. *Prog Allergy* **43**, 68–83.

Calabrese, J.H., Skwerer, R.G., Banra, B. *et al.* (1986). Depression, immunocompetence and prostaglandins of the E scries. *Psychiatr Res* **17**, 44–47.

Chrousos, G.P. and Gold, P.W. (1992). The concepts of stress and stress system disorders: overview of physical and behavioural homeostasis. *JAMA* **267**, 1244–1252.

Cohen, J.J. and Crnic, L.S. (1982). Glucocorticoids, stress and the immune response. In: Webb D.R. (Ed.), *Immunopharmacology and the Regulation of Leucocyte Function*. Marcel Dekker, New York, pp. 61–83.

Connor, T.J. and Leonard, B.E. (1998). Depression, stress and immunological activation: the role of cytokines in depressive disorders. *Life Sci* **62**, 583–606.

Croiset, G., Heijnen, C.J., Veldhuis, H.D., de Wied, D. and Ballieux, R.E. (1987). Modulation of the immune response by emotional stress. *Life Sci* **40**, 775–782.

Crook, T.H. and Miller, NW. (1985). The challenge of Alzheimer's disease. *Am Psychol* **40**, 1245–1250.

Cunnick, J.E., Lysle, D.T., Aronfield, A. and Rabin, B.S. (1991). Stressor induced changes in mitogenic activity are not associated with decreased IL-2 production or changes in lymphocyte subsets. *Clin Immunol Immunopathol* **60**, 419–429.

Cunningham, E.T. and de Souza, E.B. (1996). Interleukin 1 receptors in the brain and endocrine tissue. *Immunol Today* **14**, 171–176.

Dark, K., Peeke, H.V.S., Eliman, G. and Salfi, M. (1987). Behaviourally conditioned histamine release. *Ann NY Acad Sci* **496**, 578–582.

Davidson, R.A. and Baum, A. (1986). Chronic stress and post traumatic stress disorder. *J Consult Clin Psychol* **54**, 303–308.

Day, G. (1951). Cited by Solomon, G.F. and Amkran, T.A.A. (1981). *Ann Rev Microbiol* **35**, 155–184.

Dinan, T.G. (1994). Glucocorticoids and the genesis of depressive illness – a psychobiological model. *Br J Psychiatry* **164**, 365–371.

Dohmus, J.E. and Metz, A. (1991). Stress mechanism of immunosuppresslon. *Vet lmmunol Immunopathol* **30**, 89–109.

Duman, R.S., Henninger, G.R. and Nessler, E.J. (1997). A molecular and cellular theory of depression. *Arch Gen Psychiatry* **54**, 597–606.

Farrar, W.O. (1988). Evidence for the common expression of neuroendocrine hormones and cytokines in the immune and central nervous system. *Brain Behav Immunity* **2**, 322–327.

Fleshner, M., Bellgrau, D., Watkins, L.R., Laudenslager, M.L. and Maier, S.F. (1995). Stress induced reduction in the rat mixed lymphocyte reaction is due to macrophages and not to changes in T cell phenotypes. *J Neuroimmunol* **56**, 45–52.

Freud, S. (1923). The resistances to psychoanalysis. In: Strachey, J.(Ed.), *The Complete Psychological Works of Sigmund Freud, Vol. 19*, Hogarth Press, London, pp. 214–215.

Glassman, A.H. and Shapiro, P.A. (1998). Depression and the course of coronary artery disease. *Am J Psychiatry* **155**, 4–11.

Gold, P.W., Wong, M.L., Chrousos, G.P. and Licinio, J. (1996). Stress system abnormalities in melancholic and atypical depression: molecular pathophysiological and therapeutic implications. *Mol Psychiatry* **1**, 257–264.

Hedqvist, P. (1976). Effects of prostaglandins on autonomic neurotransmission. In: Karin, S.M.M. (Ed.), *Prostaglandins, Physiological, Pharmacological and Pathological Aspects*, MTP Press, Manchester, pp. 37–12.

Kiecolt–Glaser, J.K. and Glaser, R. (1988). Methodological issues in behavioural immunology research in humans. *Brain Behav Immunol* **2**, 67–78.

Kiecolt–Glaser, J.K., Fisher, L.K., Ogrocki, P. *et al.* (1987). Marital quality, marital disruption and immune function. *Psychosom Med* **49**, 13–34.

Kiecolt–Glaser, J.K., Dura, J.R., Speicher, C.E., Tarsk, O.J. and Glaser, R. (1991). Spousal caregivers of dementia victims: longitudinal changes in immunity and health. *Psychosom Med* **53**, 345–362.

Leonard, B.E. (2000a). Stress, depression and the activation of the immune system. *World J Biol Psychiatry* **1**, 17–25.

Leonard, B.E. (2000b). Clinical implications of mechanisms of action of antidepressants. *Adv Psychiatr Treat* **6**, 178–186.

Leonard, B.E. and Song, C. (1999). Stress, depression and the role of cytokines. In: Dantzer, R. (Ed.), *Cytokines, Stress and Depression*, Kluwer Academic Plenum, New York, pp. 251–265.

Licinio, J. and Wong, M.L. (1999). The role of inflammatory mediators in the biology of major depression: central nervous system cytokines modulate the biological substrate of depressive symptoms, regulate stress-response systems and contribute to neurotoxicity and neuroprotection. *Mol Psychiatry* **4**, 317–327.

McAdams, C. and Leonard, B.E. (1992). Effect of prostaglandin E2 and thromboxane A2 on monocyte and neutrophil phagocytes *in vitro*. *Med Sci Res* **20**, 673–674.

Maes, M., Planken, V.D. and Stevens, W.J. (1992). Leucocytosis, monocytosis and neutrophilia: of severe depression. *J Psychiatr Res* **261**, 125–134.

Maes, M., Smith, R. and Scharpe, S. (1995). The monocyte T lymphocyte hypothesis of major depression. *Psychoneuroendocrinology* **20**, 111–116.

Maier, S.F., Watkins, L.R. and Fleshner, M. (1994). Psychoneuroimmunology – the interface between behaviour, brain and immunity. *Am J Psychiatry* **49**, 1004–1017.

Manku, M.S., Myabaji, P.P. and Horrobin, D.F. (1977). Effects of prostaglandins on baseline pressure and responses to noradrenaline in a rat mesenteric artery preparation: PGE 1 as an antagonist of PGE2. *Prostaglandins* **3**, 701–707.

Martin, R.C., Cloninger, R., Guze, S. and Clayton, P. (1985). Mortality in a follow-up to 500 pychiatric outpatients in total mortality. 2. Cause specific mortality. *Arch Gen Psychiatry* **42**, 47–54, 58–66.

Mason, J.W. (1971). A re-evaluation of the concept of non-specificity in stress theory. *J Psychiatr Res* **8**, 123–140.

Michelson, D., Stratakis, S., Hill, L. *et al.* (1996). Bone mineral density in women with depression. *New Engl J Med* **355**, 1176–1181.

Mormede, P., Dantze, R., Michael, B., Kelly, K. and Le Maoal, M. (1988). Influence of stressor predictability and behaviour control on lymphocyte reactivity, antibody response and neuroendocrine activation in rats. *Physiol Behav* **43**, 577–503.

Mtabaji, J.P., Manku, M.S. and Horrobin, D.F. (1977). Actions of the tricyclic antidepressant clomipramine on responses to pressor agents. Interactions with prostaglandin E2. *Prostaglandins* **14**, 125–132.

Nemeroff, C.B., Wilderlov, E., Bisette, G. *et al.* (1984). Elevated concentrations of CSF corticotrophin releasing factor-like immunoreactivity in depressed patients. *Science* **226**, 1342–1344.

Nguyen, K.T., Deak, T., Owens, S.M. *et al.* (1988). Exposure to acute stress induces brain interleukin beta protein in the rat. *J Neurosci* **18**, 2239–2246.

Owens, M.J. and Nemeroff, C.B. (1991). Physiology and pharmacology of corticotropin releasing factor. *Pharmacol Res* **43**, 425–473.

Ramamoorthy, S., Ramamoorthy, J.D., Pradoaol, P. *et al.* (1995). Regulation of the human serotonin transporter by interleukin-1 beta. *Biochem Biophys Res Comm* **216**, 560–567.

Skeline, Y.I., Wang, P.W., Gado, M.H. *et al.* (1996). Hippocampal atrophy in recurrent major depression. *Proc Natl Acad Sci USA* **93**, 3908–3913.

Sklar, L.S. and Anisman, H. (1981). Stress and cancer. *Psychol Bull* **89**, 369–406.

Smith, R.S. (1991). The macrophage theory of depression. *Med Hypoth* **35**, 298–306.

Song, C., Dinan, T.G. and Leonard, B.E. (1994). Changes in immunoglobulin, complement and acute phase protein concentrations in depressed patients and normal controls. *J Affect Disord* **30**, 283–288.

Suzuki, E., Shintani, F., Kanba, S. *et al.* (1996). Induction of interleukin-1 beta and interleukin-1 receptor antagonist in RNA by chronic treatment with various psychotropics in widespread area of rat brain. *Neurosci Lett* **215**, 201–204.

Weisse, C.S. (1992). Depression and immunocompetence: a review of the literature. *Psychol Bull* **111**, 475–487.

Wiegers, G.J. and Reul, J.M. (1998). Induction of cytokine receptors by glucocorticoids: functional and pathological significance. *Trends Pharmacol Sci* **19**, 317–321.

Wu, C.Y., Fargeas, C., Nakajima, T. and Delespesse, G. (1991). Glucocorticoids suppress the production of interleukin 4 by human lymphocytes. *Eur J Immunol* **10**, 2645–2647.

Xia, Z., De Piere, J.W. and Nassberger, L. (1996). TCAs inhibit IL-6, IL-1 and TNF release in human blood monocytes and IL-2 and interferon in T-cells. *Immunopharmacology* **34**, 27–37.

4

Epidemiology of the Relationship Between Depression and Physical Illness

PER BJÖRNTORP

Department of Heart and Lung Diseases, Sahlgren's University Hospital, University of Göteborg, Sweden

INTRODUCTION

Major depression and suicide are associated with a considerable elevation of the risk of developing physical illness. In fact, estimates have suggested that as a predictor of myocardial infarction, depression is of the same order of magnitude as established somatic risk factors such as dyslipidaemia. Clinicians and researchers in biomedical areas tend to underestimate, or are not aware of, this risk of developing physical illness. With the high prevalence of depression, or related panic and anxiety syndromes, this pathway to serious somatic disease probably contributes significantly to premature mortality. A substantial volume of literature is now available documenting such relationships.

There are a large number of physical illnesses related to depression. Attention will be given here to the field of diseases with background factors such as dysregulation of glucose and lipid metabolism as well as in haemodynamic systems, involving cardiovascular disease (CVD), and type 2 diabetes mellitus, and their established somatic risk factors in prospective epidemiological studies. Potential mechanisms for associations between depression and these physical illnesses and their risk factors will then be discussed.

THE RELATIONSHIP BETWEEN DEPRESSION AND CVD

This problem must be divided into events occurring after a myocardial infarction (MI) and the prediction of MI by established depression, occurring before an MI. There are numerous reports that subjects suffering from an MI are frequently depressed. Compared with euthymics, those with depression have a worse prognosis after MI (Cassem and Hackett, 1971). It is not surprising that disease in general, particularly disease as serious as MI, is followed by a reactive depression. However, in some instances a major melancholic depression develops, and this cannot be considered to be a functional, natural consequence of heart disease. It is important that this is not ignored by the responsible cardiologist, because it is amenable to effective treatment, which might also improve the prognosis of the heart disease (for review, see Carney et al.,1997).

Another question is whether or not depression precedes heart disease. To resolve this problem, prospective studies are needed. Several studies indicate that repeated depressive periods have occurred before an MI (Anda et al., 1993; Ford et al., 1994), although this is not always the case (Goldberg et al., 1979; Vogt et al., 1994). Most of these studies are, however, confounded by the fact that established, somatic risk factors apart from smoking have not been accounted for. Thus, an analysis of the impact of depression alone is not possible. Furthermore, treatment of depression with for example tricyclic antidepressants may have increased the risk of heart disease. It is a dilemma in psychiatry that panic disorder and anxiety are frequently mixed with depressive symptoms, and that the combination of these conditions which are highly interrelated might have an impact on physical ill-health.

A recent careful prospective study illustrates these points particularly well (Pratt et al., 1996). A randomized population was followed prospectively over 13 years. Sixty-four subjects had an MI during the observation period, and were free of heart problems before the time of observation. Dysphoria and a major depressive episode increased the risk of developing MI with odds ratios of 2.07, and 4.54, respectively; i.e. elevated risks compared with those patients with dyslipidaemia or hypertension. Treatment with tricyclic antidpressants or benzodiazepines did not account for these findings. A history of diabetes, hypertension, cigarette smoking and alcohol consumption was observed, and data suggested that such factors were not confounding the relationship between depression and the development of MI. Since the incidence of depression decreases with age and the incidence of MI shows the opposite effect, age was adjusted for with remaining significant associations between depression and MI. Interestingly, male gender and divorce increased the risk.

The strength of this study is its prospective design in a randomized population. The weakness is, however, that it is based on self-reported data, which opens up the risk for misclassification, and, in addition, makes the exclusion of conventional somatic risk factors uncertain. Apparently, no information was available on, for example, insulin resistance, obesity and dyslipidaemia, which are powerful risk factors for MI.

As discussed above, the single impact of depression on MI has apparently not been tested in rigorous statistical treatments, where somatic risk factors such as hypertension, dyslipidaemia, insulin resistance, abdominal obesity and thrombogenetic factors have been taken into account. However, this might not be an appropriate way to approach this problem. Depression and other psychiatric diseases are localized to the brain, and there must be some connection between these diseases and the rest of the body in order to precipitate physical illness, in this case MI. It may well be that this connection is operating via the generation of somatic risk factors, which in turn lead to heart disease and other physical illnesses. There is also the possibilty that risk factors, for example severe obesity, could lead to depression. In addition, depression could act in parallel with risk factors to precipitate physical disease. This is illustrated in Figure 1. An approach to this problem would be to examine depressive symptoms in relation to such somatic risk factors, and search for potential mechanistic links, preferrably in prospective studies in randomly selected population cohorts. This will be discussed in a later section.

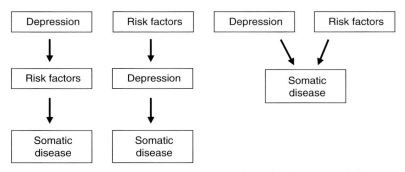

Figure 1. The relationship between depression, risk factors and disease.

THE RELATIONSHIP BETWEEN DEPRESSION AND TYPE 2 DIABETES MELLITUS

As is the case with MI, depression is frequently present in patients with diabetes mellitus (Koranyi, 1979; Lilliker, 1980). The cause and effect relationships are probably even more complex than in MI because not only awareness of the disease itself, but also hypoglycaemia and hyperglycaemia may affect mood and induce depressive traits. In addition diabetic complications have been observed to be associated with depression. There are, however, indications that depressive states are more common in diabetes than in other diseases with comparable physical and psychological suffering (Fris and Nanjundappa, 1986; Tun et al., 1987; Weyerer et al., 1989).

The interesting question from the point of view of pathogenesis is whether or not depression precedes the development of clinically manifest diabetes or its precursor states, impaired glucose tolerance and insulin resistance. This requires prospective studies to be resolved, and such studies are sparse in the literature. A study by Eaton *et al.* (1996) examined this problem prospectively in a total of 3481 household-residing adults who were followed up for 13 years. At this time 72% of survivors were available for self-report of the onset of diabetes during the observation period. The cumulative incidence of diabetes was 5.2%, comprising 89 cases. Major depressive symptoms or other forms of psychiatric disorder at the start of the study predicted the onset of diabetes with a risk ratio of 2.23. This prediction was independent of age, race, sex, socioeconomic status, education, use of health services, other psychiatric disorders and body weight. Milder forms of depressive symptoms did not, however, show such relationships with diabetes.

This study is well conducted and informative. Uncertainties remain, however, in the self-reported data. Undetected type 2 diabetes is a common problem and has been estimated to account for around 50% of clinically manifest diabetes (Harris, 1993). Another difficulty is that certain symptoms such as fatigue occur in both depression and in the early phases of diabetes, perhaps resulting in reports at the start of the observation period which have been misjudged as depression but were in fact early signs of diabetes, diagnosed during the observation time. Assuming that early phases of diabetes are proportional to clinically manifest diabetes, which seems reasonable, then the fact that impaired glucose tolerance and insulin resistance were not diagnosed would not prevent the conclusion that depression increases the risk for the development of diabetes.

Again, as in the case of MI, the linking mechanism between depressive symptoms and the periphery is not known, but of great interest. Type 2 diabetes is precipitated by a combination of insensitivity to the effects of insulin (insulin resistance) and an inability of the pancreatic insulin-producing beta cells to compensate for insulin resistance by increasing insulin secretion. The latter is considered to be mainly due to genetic factors, while insulin resistance is highly dependent on environmental factors. Obesity is the most common promoter of insulin resistance, but was not involved in the study referred to (Eaton *et al.*, 1996). Another important regulator is physical inactivity, which is followed by insulin insensitivity in muscles, the major site of systemic insulin resistance in prediabetic conditions (De Fronzo, 1987). Physical inactivity is difficult to estimate quantitatively, and was not recorded in the study discussed. However, long-term physical inactivity is frequently associated with obesity, and obesity was not a confounder in the study.

From this attempt to further analyse the prospective study by Eaton *et al.* (1996) it seems that additional factors than those included in the study must be examined in the relationship between depression and diabetes. Although the possibility that common genetic factors are associated with both depression and diabetes, the latter by influence on insulin secretion and/or insulin resistance, cannot be discounted, this seems to be a rather far-fetched idea. It seems more likely that depression is associated with signals to the periphery which are responsible for the induction of insulin resistance. Such possibilities will be discussed in a later section.

NEUROENDOCRINE ABNORMALITIES IN DEPRESSION

An established neuroendocrine abnormality in depression is the hyperactivity of the hypothalamic–pituitary–adrenal (HPA) axis. This results in hypercortisolaemia. Furthermore, the locus coeruleus–norepinephrine system, regulating outflow from the sympathetic nervous system, also shows elevated activity. As a consequence of the HPA axis activation, gonadal and growth hormone axes become inhibited (for review, see Gold and Chrousos, 1999). Proximal centres are involved such as those for regulation of emotional memory (amygdala), cognitive centres (hippocampus), dopaminergic reward centres as well as cortical modulation of the hypothalamic neuroendocrine functions (Gold and Chrousos, 1999).

The feedback regulation of the HPA axis is often deranged, as is indicated by the dexamethasone suppression test (Carrol et al., 1981). This feedback is regulated via glucocorticoid receptors (GRs), which when forming a hormone–receptor complex brake the activity of the HPA axis. With longstanding depression this blunted feedback is followed by severe damage of cognitive function and substance loss in the hippocampus area, visible by imaging techniques as lacunae (McEwen, 1998).

These abnormalities will be followed by multiple changes in peripheral hormonal concentrations as well as in the autonomic nervous system activities. These in turn will initiate disturbances in carbohydrate and lipid metabolism as well as in blood pressure regulation, generating risk factors for both MI and type 2 diabetes. This will be reviewed in the following section.

Cortisol

Cortisol has well known effects on the regulation of insulin sensitivity, and induces insulin resistance in several tissues, including muscle, liver and adipose tissue. The mechanisms for muscular insulin resistance are established and include effects on both the glucose transport system and the insulin receptor (McMahon et al., 1988). Since muscle is the major regulator of systemic insulin sensitivity, such cortisol-induced insulin resistance will result in insensitivity to insulin when measured as total body glucose regulation. Cortisol increases hepatic glucose production and therefore tends to elevate blood glucose, particulary in the fasting state (McMahon et al., 1988).

The effects on adipose tissue are of no direct consequence for systemic glucose uptake or insulin resistance, because total glucose uptake in adipose tissue is only a small fraction of total body glucose assimilation. Instead, cortisol exerts powerful effects on the mobilization of free fatty acids (FFAs) through several mechanisms. Firstly, cortisol displays a permissive effect on the catecholamine stimulation of triglyceride breakdown (lipolysis). Second, the sensitive inhibitory effect of insulin on the lipolytic activity is blunted. Third, glucose uptake is inhibited, which makes the re-esterification of FFAs in adipose tissue inefficient, because this process requires glucose. Together, these mechanisms will be followed by a pronounced outflow of FFAs from adipose tissue and elevated passive uptake in other tissues (for review, see Björntorp, 1996). This in turn will be followed by insulin resistance through blockage of several key steps in glucose metabolism, and worsen the insulin resistance created by cortisol itself. In fact evidence suggests that the major effect of cortisol on insulin resistance is mediated via FFAs (Guillaume-Gentil et al., 1993). This is summarized in Table 1.

Table 1. The effects of cortisol on insulin sensitivity.

Muscle	Receptor function inhibited	Glucose transport inhibited	
Liver	Glucose production enhanced		
Adipose tissue	Lipolysis enhanced	Insulin control inhibited	Glucose transport inhibited

Net effect on adipose tissue: free fatty acid outflow increased, which creates insulin resistance in muscle and liver.

Insulin resistance is an independent risk factor for both MI (Lapidus et al., 1984) and the most powerful precursor of type 2 diabetes (Haffner et al., 1990). The compensatory rise in insulin secretion is followed by dyslipidaemia (elevated low density and low high density lipoprotein cholesterol as well as elevated triglycerides) via mechanisms that are involved in both production and removal of these lipids (Reaven, 1995). It has also been suggested that the hyperinsulinaemia is involved in the pathogenesis of hypertension, although this is less well documented, and, as will be seen, is probably a consequence of central sympathetic nervous system activity. Nevertheless, insulin resistance, created by cortisol, generates several of the well-known risk factors for MI and is an immediate precursor to insulin secretion breakdown and type 2 diabetes.

Interestingly, cortisol elevation is also followed by centralization of body fat stores, creating abdominal, central or visceral obesity. This is seen dramatically clearly in Cushing's syndrome and disappears with successful treatment (Lönn et al, 1994). The mechanisms for this event are also known. Cortisol in the presence of insulin is a powerful stimulator of the major

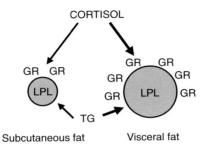

Figure 2. The effects of cortisol on lipid uptake in adipose tissue. Cortisol binds to glucocorticoid receptors (GRs) in adipose tissue and increases the expression of the main regulator of lipid (TG, triglyceride) uptake in adipose tissue, lipoprotein lipase (LPL). Lipid uptake will be higher in visceral than subcutaneous adipose tissue because of a higher density of GR.

controlling enzyme for lipid uptake in adipocytes, lipoprotein lipase. Since GRs are particularly dense in intra-abdominal adipose tissue, the lipid accumulating effects of lipoprotein lipase activity will be particularly marked in this adipose tissue region (Figure 2). Elevated internal fat mass can thus be considered to be a conveniently noticeable index of long-term cortisol effects, but other hormones are also involved, as well as gender and genetic factors, which will be reviewed in subsequent sections.

Sex steroid and growth hormones

Other prominent hormonal abnormalities in depression are diminished secretion of sex steroids and growth hormone, which is probably a consequence of elevated HPA axis activity (Chrousos and Gold, 1992). These hormonal abnormalities also have profound effects on peripheral metabolic events, often in combination by facilitating each other's effects. The sex steroid hormones are important for maintaining insulin sensitivity in muscles, and deficiency is followed by decreased activity of the regulatory steps in glucose metabolism, notably the insulin-sensitive enzymes responsible for glycogen synthesis. In other words, sex steroid hormones have opposite effects to those of cortisol, and a relative deficiency of these hormones will be followed by insulin resistance, particularly with concomitant increase of cortisol secretion. These interpretations of results from cellular and molecular studies are in excellent agreement with observations that deficiencies of these hormones are associated with insulin resistance, and that substitution is followed by near or full normalization in both animal and human intervention studies (for review, see Björntorp, 1993).

Diminished secretions of sex steroids and growth hormone are also followed by visceral fat accumulation. Again, intervention studies are followed by clear diminution of visceral fat mass (Björntorp, 1996). This is summarized in Table 2 and shown schematically in Figure 3.

Table 2. The effects of indicated hormones on visceral fat accumulation.

		Net effect
Cortisol	LPL activated, lipid mobilization inhibited	Mass elevated
Sex steroids and growth hormones	LPL inhibited, lipid mobilization stimulated	Mass diminished

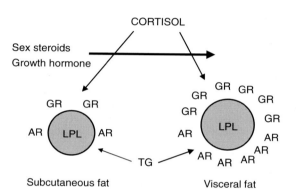

Figure 3. The interaction between cortisol and sex steroids and growth hormone in the uptake of lipids in adipose tissue. The cortisol effects (see Fig. 2) are counteracted by sex steroid hormones in concert with growth hormone by cellular effects which are opposite to those of cortisol. Sex steroid hormone receptors (AR) have, like glucocorticoid receptors (GR), higher density in visceral than subcutaneous adipose tissue. Therefore sex steroid and growth hormone effects will be more pronounced in visceral depots.

The sympathetic nervous system

Among a multitude of other functions the sympathetic nervous system regulates the central haemodynamic system and blood pressure. Elevated central activity of this system, as seen in depression, would thus be expected to raise blood pressure. This is also the mechanism by which primary hypertension is thought to be initiated in the early hyperkinetic states (Folkow, 1987). The multiple interconnections between the centres for HPA axis and sympathetic nervous system regulation probably have the consequence that these centres are activated simultaneously (Chrousos and Gold, 1992), and this may be the reason why both these centres are aroused in depression.

The sympathetic nervous system is a major regulator of fat mobilization from human adipose tissue. Cortisol exerts 'permissive' effects, i.e. it amplifies the triggering effects of catecholamines to hydrolyse adipose tissue triglycerides into fatty acids and glycerol. These products of hydrolysis will then circulate and the FFAs exert marked inhibitory effects on insulin sensitivity in various tissues, notably muscles, creating systemic insulin resistance, as briefly reviewed above. This means that increased activity of the sympathetic nervous system will be followed by insulin resistance via elevated circulating FFAs. This is amplified by elevated cortisol and by enlarged adipose tissue, particularly when central depots are enlarged, because these tissues are particularly sensitive to the lipid mobilization effects of catecholamines. These phenomena probably explain the markedly elevated levels of circulating FFAs in abdominal obesity, and probably contribute to the insulin resistance seen in that condition (for review and references, see Björntorp, 1996).

Summary

The multiple neuroendocrine disturbances in depression are followed by perturbations of peripheral hormonal secretions and elevation of the activity of the sympathethic nervous system. These include cortisol, which is elevated, and the sex steroids and growth hormone, which are abnormally low. This is followed by mechanisms which create insulin resistance and, secondarily, dyslipidaemia by both increasing lipoprotein synthesis in the liver and inhibiting peripheral lipid uptake. Furthermore, visceral body fat accumulates. Finally, blood pressure is elevated, which is likely to be an effect of the accompanying activation of the sympathetic nervous system. These are all powerful risk factors for both CVD and type 2 diabetes. It may therefore be considered that the association between depression and CVD and type 2 diabetes is mediated via this generation of established risk factors by the neuroendocrine–endocrine perturbations. This is summarized in Figure 4.

RECENT POPULATION STUDIES OF THE RELATIONSHIP BETWEEN DEPRESSION AND CENTRALIZATION OF BODY FAT

The problem of associations between depression and physical illness may be approached by studies in the general population. The advantage of this method is that a non-selected population can be examined for putative associations between various potential disease-generating factors, including depression and related conditions, and the subsequent development of disease. We have performed several such studies, which will be reviewed in the following section.

In an earlier study, depressive symptoms were related to the waist–hip circumference ratio (WHR) (Lapidus et al., 1989). The WHR is an estimation of central adipose tissue mass. The reason for selecting the WHR was that

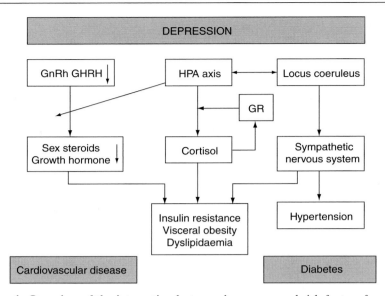

Figure 4. Overview of the interaction between hormones and risk factors for somatic disease and the neuroendocrine and autonomic arousal in depression. The activity of the HPA axis, controlled by glucocorticoid receptors (GR) is facilitated, and inhibits the gonadal and growth hormone axes (GnRH, gonadotrophin releasing hormone; GHRH, growth hormone releasing hormone). This results in elevated cortisol and diminished sex steroid and growth hormone secretions. In concert, these peripheral endocrine perturbations will induce insulin resistance by the mechanisms summarized in Table 1, and visceral fat accumulation, by the mechanisms summarized in Table 2 and Figs 2 and 3. Dyslipidaemia (elevated low and very low density lipoproteins and low high density lipoproteins) is generated from the hyperinsulinaemia created by insulin resistance. The sympathetic nervous system activity from locus coeruleus is activated in parallel with the HPA axis centres, which results in elevated blood pressure and mobilization of free fatty acids, which amplify insulin resistance. The net result will be generation of several, powerful risk factors for cardiovascular disease and type 2 diabetes mellitus.

this had turned out to be an unusually powerful risk predictor for MI and related diseases, type 2 diabetes and stroke, in prospective studies in both men and women (for review, see Björntorp, 1993). We then found, first in women, that the WHR was associated with several depressive traits, including reports of self-perceived equivalents to depression, consumption of antidepressants and anxiolytics, and certain types of sleep disturbances (Lapidus et al., 1989). This was confirmed in other studies (Wing et al., 1991), and was also found in subsequent studies in both men and women (Rosmond et al., 1996a), and is consequently a robust, reproducible phenomenon. These psychiatric traits were frequently followed by other phenomena such as psychosocial and socioeconomic handicaps (living alone, divorce, poor education, physical types of work with low salaries, unemployment, early retirement, problems at work when employed, etc.). The psychosocial observations had some gender bias, men apparently showing stronger associations than women with anthropometric variables (Rosmond *et al.*, 1996b; Rosmond and Björntorp, 1999). Furthermore, high alcohol consumption and tobacco smoking were also often found to be associated problems.

The factors in this cluster of phenomena are strongly interrelated. It may be considered that the primary, triggering factor might be any one of those mentioned, resulting in the development of the other phenomena. For example, depressive or anxiety traits could be followed by increased alcohol consumption as well as psychosocial and socioeconomic handicaps. Alternatively, alcohol, psychosocial or socioeconomic problems are likely to precipitate depressive moods. In the populations we have studied, a rough estimation of the prevalence of depressive symptoms is in the order of 10%, in accordance with other reports of a high prevalence of this condition (Weissman and Olfson, 1995). It is thus apparent that depression might frequently be a primary factor in a presumed chain of events, leading to the other problems mentioned. Depressive equivalents and their neuroendocrine and autonomic consequences, generating risk factors as described above, are probably therefore a prevalent route towards MI and diabetes.

Relationships between depression, the WHR and neuroendocrine perturbations in population studies

Having seen these associations, originally with the WHR, we started to examine potential mechanisms. Centralization of body fat, or central visceral obesity, is seen dramatically clearly in Cushing's syndrome, where elevated cortisol secretion is the cause of the disease. Furthermore, the associations between an elevated WHR and depression and anxiety symptoms, and the frequently elevated cortisol secretion in these conditions, made us direct our attention to explanatory mechanisms in the regulation of cortisol secretion.

The regulation of cortisol secretion by the HPA axis occurs by a balance between central, facilitating factors and the feedback control, exerted by GRs in the central nervous system, notably in the hippocampus area. Examination of these loci in humans is usually performed with methods aimed at diagnosing severe perturbations such as Cushing's syndrome or melancholic depression. They include determinations of cortisol in the circulation and excretion in the urine, as well as inhibitory tests of the feedback regulation, usually performed in hospital settings. Although useful for the purposes mentioned, milder, functional forms of HPA axis regulatory errors might not be discernable by such methods. For example, the unfamiliar milieu of a hospital or a laboratory, as well as venous puncture probably disrupt or exaggerate limited regulatory perturbations of the system, which are active in the everyday life of examined probands. Therefore, other approaches must be selected.

Cortisol in saliva has frequently been used recently for such purposes (Kirschbaum and Hellhammer, 1989). The advantages include non-invasive sampling, the convenience of using such methods during everyday life except sleep, and the fact that the free, active fraction of circulating cortisol is measured. Saliva cortisol is apparently independent of saliva flow, and correlates strongly with circulating, free cortisol (Kirschbaum and Hellhammer, 1989).

The utility of this method is illustrated by a recent report where normal subjects delivered saliva samples at several randomly selected time points over a day, reporting the concomitantly perceived stress factors. The results showed striking, 'dose-dependent' correlations between, for example, current, previous and anticipated stress as well as current mood (Smyth *et al.*, 1998). These results demonstrate not only the usefulness of cortisol concentrations in saliva, but also the sensitivtiy of the regulating system.

We have recently used this method in population samples of middle-aged men or women, selected from population registers, and born in the same year (men 1944, women 1956). These results have been described and reviewed in detail recently, and readers are referred to these publications for details and references (Rosmond *et al.*, 1998, 2000; Björntorp, 1999; Björntorp *et al.*, 1999). These findings are summarized here, focusing on depressive symptoms and related factors.

Functional characteristics of the HPA axis were determined in repeated saliva cortisols, collected by the probands over an ordinary working day. Among the variables measured were the shape of the diurnal curve, including morning and evening values, the response to a standardized lunch and to perceived stress. A low dose (0.5 mg) dexamethasone suppression test (DST) was also performed at home.

The normal diurnal curve of cortisol, with high morning and low evening cortisols was found in a majority of the men. Stress-related cortisol was elevated in about one-third of subjects. These men showed positive correlations with abdominal distribution of body fat, insulin, glucose, plasma lipids and blood pressure. This cluster of risk factors for MI and type 2 diabetes is now frequently called the 'Metabolic syndrome'. With the background reviewed in previous sections, we believe that the elevated cortisol secretion is responsible for the risk factor pattern. In just under 10% of the men sampled, a pathological HPA axis function was found with low morning values and a general picture of a low plasticity of the regulation. This type of cortisol secretion has previously been found in several conditions with severe 'life events', chronic pain, 'vital exhaustion' due to apparently irreversible poor environment, and has been labelled a 'burn out' (McEwen, 1998). The DST was frequently mildly inefficient with the low dose of dexamethasone used. In these men associations to abdominal obesity and the metabolic syndrome were particularly strong. This is, however, unlikely to be a consequence of cortisol secretion, because total cortisol secretion was about 75% lower than in the normal men.

In this group with an apparent 'burn-out' of the HPA axis function, we also found consistent decreases of the secretion of sex steroids and growth hormone. With the background of the function of these hormones on insulin resistance and visceral fat accumulation, briefly reviewed above, we have suggested the possibility that deficiencies of these hormones may be responsible. Furthermore, there was consistent evidence that this condition is followed by elevated activity of the central sympathetic nervous system, which will probably be followed by elevated blood pressure and worsening of the metabolic risk factors by mechanisms outlined above.

The regulatory feedback system seems to be mildly perturbed, particularly in the condition of the severely disturbed function of the HPA axis.

In the population of women a moderate hyperandrogenicity (< 3–4 nmol/l of testosterone) is prominently associated with somatic disease risk factors. Such hyperandrogenicity is found in about 25% of the women, and is a powerful risk factor for the development of type 2 diabetes and other prevalent diseases (Björntorp, 1993). These androgens are probably of adrenal origin because they are secreted in parallel with other steroids which originate exclusively in the adrenals, such as dihydroepiandrosterone sulphate and cortisol. Such secretion is also associated with symptoms of depression as well as socioeconomic problems and low educational status suggesting that environmental stress is involved (Baghaei et al., 2000).

In summary, associations with centralization of body fat stores were found in two groups of men, one with elevated stress-related cortisol and another with a 'burned-out' function of the HPA axis, associated with low sex steroid and growth hormone secretions as well as an elevated activity of the sympathetic nervous system. Reasonably likely mechanisms for these statistical associations between endocrine and autonomic nervous system perturbations on the one hand, and the central accumulation of body fat and risk factor pattern for MI and type 2 diabetes have been provided. In women a moderate hyperadrogenicity is tightly coupled to such phenomena.

In these studies we have again seen the statistical associations between depressive moods, often combined with symptoms of anxiety, on the one hand, and, on the other, not only centralization of body fat but also perturbations of the regulation of the HPA axis. In women, hyperandrogenicity is associated with depressive traits (Baghaei et al., 2000) . It should be noticed that the degree of depression seldom reaches the degree of manifest disease as indicated by the Beck Depression Inventory, the Hamilton or the Montgomery–Asberg Depression Rating Scales (Ahlberg et al., 2001). Nevertheless, these 'subclinical' symptoms appear to be associated with a disrupted HPA axis regulation, which testifies to the usefulness of salivary cortisol analyses.

CENTRAL INTEGRATION OF NEUROENDOCRINE PERTUBATIONS IN DEPRESSION WITH ASSOCIATED RISK FACTORS FOR PHYSICAL ILLNESS

There are numerous interactions between neuroendocrine and autonomic regulatory centres (Chrousos and Gold, 1992). Among those that we see in our population studies, the increased actvity of the HPA axis regulation is probably responsible for the inhibition of gonadal and growth hormone axes. Furthermore, results of studies indicate that there are close interactions between the hypothalamic centres for HPA axis regulation and the centres for regulation of the autonomic nervous system. One consequence of this is that one axis is usually not activated without concomitant activation of the other. Furthermore, when the HPA axis fails and is reaching a 'burn-out' condition, the regulatory centres of the sympathetic nervous system seem to be activated, perhaps as a compensation to maintain homeostatic or allostatic conditions. We believe that what we are seeing in our population studies are consequences of these interactions. Depression, or usually a subclinical equivalent, is apparently an integrated part of this picture in accordance with the summary of the neuroendocrine perturbations in the hyperarousal condition of depression (Gold and Chrousos, 1999).

Gold and Chrousos (1999) also describe a condition of atypical depression with hypersomnia, lethargy, fatigue and relative apathy, which is associated with hypofunction of central neuroendocrine centres. If such subjects are present in our populations they would be expected to be found in the group of low cortisol secretion, where, however, the sympathetic nervous system activity on average seems to be elevated.

The sleep disturbances we see are of interest in relation to this discussion. They might be part of depressive symptoms or due to other factors such as shift work. Sleep deprivation has recently been found to be associated with elevated activity in both the HPA axis and the sympathetic nervous system, with associated early signs of metabolic disturbances (Spiegel *et al.*, 1999). Whatever the reason for sleep disturbances in our population studies, this factor alone seems to have a profound effect on both neuroendocrine and metabolic regulation.

STUDIES IN MELANCHOLIC DEPRESSION

Although prospective data indicate that depression precedes MI and type 2 diabetes, studies on the associations with the risk factors for physical illness, discussed here, have seldom been performed in patients with melancholic depression as primary inclusion criterion. A recent study has described an elevated mass of intra-abdominal, visceral adipose tissue in patients with melancholic depression (Thakore *et al.*, 1997). With the background reviewed above, it seems likely that this statistical association is indeed due to the perturbed neuroendocrine functions of such patients, directing storage fat preferentially to central depots.

We have recently completed a study where this problem was addressed. Fifty-nine middle-aged men with moderate obesity with a varying degree of centralization of body fat were studied with a number of detailed anthropometric, endocrine, metabolic and haemodynamic variables. They were also examined with the Hamilton Depression and Anxiety Rating Scales, the Montgomery–Asberg Depression Rating Scale and the Beck Depression Inventory. Although measurements with these scales showed highly varying results among the men, none could be classified as established melancholic depression. The men with centralization of body fat (abdominal obesity) had clearly higher values in all the depression and anxiety scales utilized, and they also showed mild signs of HPA axis perturbations. In these men there were also several perturbations in metabolic variables, particularly those indicating insulin resistance and glucose intolerance (Ahlberg et al., 2001). These results suggest the rather remarkable possibility that even minor degrees of depressive and anxiety traits with mild neuroendocrine abnormalities are associated with abdominal obesity and other risk factors for type 2 diabetes mellitus and MI. These statistical relationships may be causally connected by the mechanisms reviewed above. Such risk factors might be more prevalent and powerful when depression and/or anxiety are more pronounced, such as in melancholic depression.

THERAPEUTIC CONSIDERATIONS

There is thus considerable evidence that the neuroendocrine–autonomic system perturbations in depression might be the triggers for the generation of risk factors for somatic disease, whereby such illnesses may be precipitated. This suggests that correcting these perturbations would be followed by improvements in the risk factor pattern and therefore less prevalence of the somatic diseases.

Successful treatment of depression is usually followed by correction of the neuroendocrine and autonomic nervous system abnormalities, as evidenced for example by a normalization of the dexamethasone suppression test. However, studies of the possibility of improving conventional risk factors for MI and diabetes do not seem to have been performed.

With the background described above, we have started to examine this possibility in an exploratory pilot study. A group of about 20 men selected for abdominal obesity and associated metabolic and haemodynamic risk factors, but without depressive symptoms were studied. They were given citalopram for 6 months. This is a serotonin reuptake inhibitor and an efficient antidepressant drug without effects on energy intake regulation. The latter is important, because a body weight decrease during treatment would be expected to be a severely confounding factor, changing neuroendocrine factors by presumably other mechanisms than those of interest to this study. After treatment, there was evidence of diminished sympathetic nervous system activity. Morning cortisol levels were abnormally low at the outset which was interpreted as meaning that the regulation of the HPA axis was abnormal in analogy with the findings in the population studies (see above). After treatment morning cortisol levels were higher and approached those of normal controls. This occurred without elevation of total cortisol secretion; in fact, there was a tendency to lower total cortisol secretion. We have interpreted this to mean that the HPA axis regulation began to normalize.

Taken together, these results indicate that the neuroendocrine and autonomic systems reacted upon treatment in the same manner as in patients with depression, where abnormalities of these regulations are frequent, and where normalization occurs with antidepressant treatment. Concomitantly, glucose tolerance improved and there was some evidence for an increased sensitivity to insulin, in other words an apparent early improvement of somatic risk factors for somatic disease. (Ljung *et al.*, 2000). These results indicate that intervention at a central level may be followed by improvement of disease risk factors, and encourage further studies along the same lines.

It seems particularly interesting that these men did not have pathological scores on several depression scales (Beck, Hamilton, Montgomery-Asberg), and the scores did not change after treatment. This finding might indicate that a potential improvement of neuroendocrine, autonomic output and of risk factors for somatic disease is independent of the mental state of depression. In addition, to lend support to the pathogenetic pathways for physical illness in depression and in abdominal obesity, as reviewed above, these findings may open completely novel avenues for therapy of prevalent somatic disease. We are therefore now embarking on a larger study of a similar design.

CONCLUSIONS

There is an established connection with physical illness of different kinds in depressive states. The risk of depression appears to be of the same magnitude as that of established somatic risk factors for MI and type 2 diabetes, such as dyslipidaemia and hypertension. It is therefore important to try to understand the mechanisms of the statistical relationships between depression and physical illness.

In this review it is suggested, based on the results of clinical, statistical, intervention and cellular studies, often based on randomly selected populations, that the mechanistic factors in operation are the established neuroendocrine arousal seen in depression, which via peripheral endocrine and autonomic nervous system perturbations generate risk factors for MI and type 2 diabetes. Observations in population and case-control type of studies suggest that this may be the case even in mild, subclinical symptoms of depression. It is anticipated that this would be more pronounced in clinically manifest melancholic depression, and information is now beginning to appear to suggest that this is indeed a possibility. It is also anticipated that therapeutic strategies for depression, which normalize the neuroendocrine perturbations, would also diminish risk factors for physical illness, and therefore diminish risk of serious somatic disease. Further studies in this area are of interest not least because of the potential for therapeutic selection and developments.

REFERENCES

Ahlberg, A.-C., Ljung, T., Rosmond, R et al. (2001). Mood disturbance and anthropometric measurements in men. *Psychiatry Res* in press.

Anda, R., Williamson, D., Jones, D. et al. (1993). Depressed affect, hopelessness, and the risk of ischemic heart disease in a cohort of US adults. *Epidemiology* **4**, 285–294.

Baghaei, F., Rosmond, R., Westberg, L. et al. (2000). Androgens and disease predictors in women. (submitted).

Björntorp, P. (1993). Visceral obesity: a 'civilization syndrome'. *Obes Res* **1**, 206–222.

Björntorp, P. (1996). Review: the regulation of adipose tissue distribution in humans. *Int J Obes* **20**, 291–302.

Björntorp, P. (1999). Neuroendocrine perturbations as a cause of insulin resistance. *Diabet Metab Res Rev* **15**, 1–15.

Björntorp, P., Holm, G. and Rosmond, R. (1999). Hypothalamic arousal, insulin resistance and type 2 diabetes mellitus. *Diabet Med* **16**, 1–11.

Björntorp, P., Holm, G., Rosmond, R. and Folkow, B. (2000). Hypertension and the metabolic syndrome: closely related central origin? *Blood Press* **9**, 71–82.

Carney, R.M., Freedland, K.E., Sheline, Y.I. and Weiss, E.S. (1997). Depression and coronary heart disease: A review for cardiologists. *Clin Cardiol* **20**, 196–200.

Carrol, B.J., Feinberg, M., Greden, J.F. et al. (1981). A specific laboratory test for the diagnosis of melancholia. *Arch Gen Psychiatry* **38**, 15–22.

Cassem, H. and Hackett, T.P. (1971). Psychiatric consultations in a coronary care unit. *Ann Int Med* **75**, 9–14.

Chrousos, G.P. and Gold, P.W. (1992). The concept of stress and stress-related disorders. Overview of physical and behavioral homeostasis. *JAMA* **267**,1244–1252.

De Fronzo, R.A. (1987). The triumvirate: beta-cell, muscle, liver. A collusion responsible for NIDDM. Lilly lecture. *Proc Natl Acad Sci* **75**, 667–687.

Eaton, W.W., Armenian, H., Gallo, J., Pratt, L. and Ford, D.E. (1996). Depression and risk for onset of type II diabetes. A prospective population-based study. *Diabet Care* **19**, 1097–1102.

Folkow, B. (1987). Stress, hypothalamic function and neuroendocrine consequences. *Acta Med Scand* **723**, 61–69.

Ford, D.E., Mead, L.A., Chang, P.P., Levine, D.M. and Klag, M.J. (1994). Depression predicts cardiovascular disease in men: the precursors study. *Circulation* **90** (suppl. I), I-614.

Fris, R. and Nanjundappa, G. (1986). Diabetes, depression and employment status. *Soc Sci Med* **23**, 471–475.

Gold, P.W. and Chrousos, G.P. (1999). The endocrinology of melancholic and atypical depression: relation to neurocircuitry and somatic consequences. *Proc Assoc Amer Physicians* **111**, 22–34.

Goldberg, E.L., Comstock, G.W. and Hornstra, R.K. (1979). Depressed mood and subsequent physical illness. *Am J Psychiatry* **136**, 530–534.

Guillaume-Gentil, C., Assimacopoulos-Jeanneau, I.F. and Jeanrenaud, B. (1993). Involvement of non-esterified fatty acid oxidation in glucocorticoid-induced peripheral insulin resistance *in vivo* in rats. *Diabetologia* **36**, 899–906.

Haffner, S.M., Stern, M.P., Mitchell, P.D., Hazuda, P.D. and Patterson, J.K. (1990). Incidence of diabetes type II in Mexican Americans predicted by fasting insulin and glucose levels, obesity and body fat distribution. *Diabetes* **39**, 283–288.

Harris, M. (1993). Undiagnosed NIDDM: clinical and public health issues. *Diabet Care* **16**, 642–652.

Kirschbaum, C. and Hellhammer, D.H. (1989). Salivary cortisol in psychoneuroendocrine research: an overview. *Neuropsychobiology* **22**, 150–169.

Koranyi, E.K. (1979). Morbidity and rate of undiagnosed physical illnesses in a psychiatric clinic population. *Arch Gen Psychiatry* **36**, 414–419.

Lapidus, L., Bengtsson, C., Larsson, B. *et al.* (1984). Distribution of adipose tissue and risk of cardiovascular disease and death: 12 year follow-up of participants in the population study of women in Gothenburg, Sweden. *Br Med J* **289**,1257–1261.

Lapidus, L., Bengtsson, C., Hällström, T. and Björntorp, P. (1989). Obesity, adipose tissue distribution and health in women: results from a population study in Gothenburg, Sweden. *Appetite* **12**, 25–35.

Lilliker, S.L. (1980). Prevalence of diabetes in a manic-depressive population. *Psychiatry* **21**, 270–275.

Ljung, T., Ahlberg, A.C., Holm, G. *et al.* (2000). Treatment of abdominally obese men with a serotonin reuptake inhibitor (submitted).

Lönn, L., Kvist, H., Ernest, I. and Sjöström, L. (1994). Changes in body composition and adipose tissue distribution after treatment of women with Cushing's syndrome. *Metabolism* **43**, 1517–1522.

McEwen, B.S. (1998). Protective and damaging effects of stress mediators. *New Engl J Med* **338**, 171–179.

McMahon, M., Gerich, J. and Rizza, R. (1988). Effects of glucocorticoids on glucose metabolism. *Diabet Metab Rev* **52**, 17–30.

Pratt, L.A., Ford, D.E., Crum, R.M. *et al.* (1996). Depression, psychotropic medication, and risk of myocardial infarction. Prospective data from the Baltimore ECA folow-up. *Circulation* **94**, 3123–3129.

Reaven, G.M. (1995). Pathophysiology of insulin resistance in human disease. *Physiol Rev* **75**, 473–486.

Rosmond, R. and Björntorp, P. (1998). Psychiatric ill-health of women and its relationship to obesity and body fat distribution. *Obes Res* **6**, 338–345.

Rosmond, R. and Björntorp, P. (1999). Psychosocial and socio-economic factors in women and their relationship to obesity and regional body fat distribution. *Int J Obes Relat Metab Disord* **23**, 138–145.

Rosmond, R., Lapidus, L. and Björntorp, P. (1996a). Mental distress, obesity and body fat distribution in middle-aged men. *Obes Res* **4**, 245–252.

Rosmond, R., Lapidus, L. and Björntorp, P. (1996b). The influence of occupational and social factors on obesity and body fat distribution in middle-aged men. *Int J Obes Relat Metab Disord* **20**, 599–607.

Rosmond, R., Dallman, M.F. and Björntorp, P. (1998). Stress-related cortisol secretion in men:relationships with abdominal obesity and endocrine, metabolic and hemodynamic abnormalities. *J Clin Endocrinol Metab* **83**,1853–1859.

Rosmond. R, Holm, G. and Björntorp, P. (2000). Food-induced cortisol secretion in men in relation to anthropometric, metabolic and haemodynamic variables. *Int J Obes Rel Metab Disord* **24,** 416–422.

Smyth, J., Ockenfels, M.C., Porter, L. *et al.* (1998). Stressors and mood measured on a momentary basis are associated with salivary cortisol secretion. *Psychoneuroendocrinology* **23**, 353–370.

Spiegel, K., Leproult, R. and Van Cauter, E. (1999). Impact of sleep on metabolic and endocrine function. *Lancet* **354**, 1435–1439.

Thakore, J.H., Richards, P.J., Reznek, R.H., Martin, A. and Dinan, T.G. (1997). Increased intra-abdominal fat mass in patients with major depressive illness as measured by computed tomography. *Biol Psychiatry* **41**, 1140–1142.

Tun, P.A., Perlmuter, L.C., Russo, P. and Nathan, D.M. (1987). Memory self-assessment and performance in aged diabetics and non-diabetics. *Exp Aging Res* **13**, 151–157.

Vogt, T., Pope, C., Mullooly, J. and Hollis, J. (1994). Mental health status as a predictor of morbidity and mortality: a 15–year follow-up of members of a health maintenance organization. *Am J Public Health* **84**, 227–231.

Weissman, M.M. and Olfson, M. (1995). Depression in women: implications for health care research. *Science* **269**, 799–801.

Weyerer, S., Hewer, W., Pfeifer-Kurda, M. and Dilling, H. (1989). Psychiatric disorders and diabetes – results from a community study. *J Psychosom Res* **33**, 633–640.

Wing, R.R., Matthews, K.A., Kuller, L.H., Mellahn, E.N. and Plantinga, P. (1991). Waist to hip ratio in middle-aged women. Associations with behavioral and psychosocial factors and with changes in cardiovascular risk factors. *Arterioscl Thromb* **11**, 1250–1257.

5

Psychiatric Illness and the Metabolic Syndrome

JONATHAN MANN[a] and JOGIN H. THAKORE[b]

*[a]Department of Psychiatry, Royal South Hants Hospital, Southampton, UK
and [b]St Vincent's Hospital Dublin, Ireland*

INTRODUCTION

The link between psychiatric and physical illness is well recognized and may take many forms. An important example clinically is the fact that a primary psychiatric condition may mimic a physical illness, and vice versa. For example, patients with panic disorder may present with complaints of difficulty in breathing or chest pain. Alternatively, patients with an acute confusional state may present with prominent psychotic symptoms.

However, psychiatric and medical illnesses are not mutually exclusive and patients may suffer from both simultaneously. Indeed it has been stated that 'there are no psychiatric patients – only medical patients with varying degrees of psychopathology' (Schiffer *et al.*, 1988). With this in mind there has been considerable interest regarding the degree of comorbidity between these medical conditions, although, in general, research has concentrated on the prevalence of psychiatric illness in patients with established medical diseases. A classic example is the high incidence of depression in patients with Cushing's syndrome (Kelly, 1996).

The high prevalence of psychopathology in certain medical illnesses may be due to a number of causes. For example, it may be due to a psychologically mediated response to the diagnosis of a serious medical illness. Alternatively, it may be related to biological factors, either in sharing some underlying aetiological mechanism, or as a result of complications of the physical disease. Whatever the reason, this issue is of clinical importance as some types of psychiatric illness may adversely influence the outcome of certain medical disorders. This can be demonstrated by the finding that patients who experience a major depressive episode after a myocardial infarction carry a poorer prognosis (Carney *et al.*, 1997).

A more controversial point of view is the possibility that psychiatric disorders may actually predispose an individual to the development of certain medical diseases. If this were the case then psychiatric patients should have a greater comorbidity than expected with some types of medical illnesses, and suffer increased mortality (and morbidity) as a result. This chapter will focus on the 'functional' psychiatric illnesses, depression and its association with features of the metabolic syndrome (diabetes, hypertension and dyslipidaemias). It is vital to exclude organic brain syndromes (delirium and dementia) from this discussion as it is well established that both are strongly associated with high degrees of medical comorbidity.

PSYCHIATRIC ILLNESS, PHYSICAL DISEASE AND EARLY DEATH

Patients suffering with severe mental illness have a reduced life expectancy. A good example of this fact is provided by Tsuang et al. (1980) who concentrated on the mortality rates among affective disorders and schizophrenia. They studied a sample of 225 depressive, 100 manic and 200 schizophrenic patients collected from 3800 consecutive admissions to the Iowa Psychiatric Hospital between 1934 and 1944. For a comparison group they used 160 surgical patients who had undergone relatively minor procedures. The groups were followed up over the next 30–40 years, and in 1974, 97% of the sample was accounted for. From the group of psychiatric patients traced at the end of the follow-up period, 53% were dead. The groups were analysed with respect to gender, age and diagnosis. The survival times of each major psychiatric diagnosis were examined individually. The depressive patients' survival time was shortened by 15–22 years for females, and by 11–18 years for males. The female manic patients' survival time was reduced by 14 years, although the male manic patients showed no differences. Both male and female schizophrenic patients had a life-span reduction of about 10 years. These results are interesting as they provide estimates of 'real time' reduction in life expectancy in patients who suffer with serious mental illness. Unfortunately, the causes of death were not closely examined in this study, although, as would be expected, high rates from unnatural causes (suicide) were noted.

The premature death of psychiatric patients is not wholly due to suicide, but can also be a result of natural death. Koranyi (1977) demonstrated this by studying a sample of 2070 psychiatric outpatients in Canada over a three-year period. At the end of the follow up period 28 fatalities were noted. This was twice that found in the general population. Thirteen patients from this group of 28 died from natural causes as assessed by autopsy reports and coroners' death certificates. The average age of these 13 patients was 56.2 years, about 20 years younger than the national average at the time. Due to the small subsample size, the cause of death and its relationship to specific psychiatric diagnoses in individual subjects could not be accurately assessed. In addition, it is worth noting that this study was conducted on outpatients whose psychiatric histories were not made explicit. This may be of importance as patients with higher degrees of inpatient care may differ from an outpatient group in a number of ways including severity of illness and treatment regimes, and may therefore have different rates of death from natural causes.

In a study investigating the severity and degree of comorbid physical health problems in living psychiatric patients, Maguire and Granville-Grossman (1968) conducted a retrospective case note study in which they scrutinized the inpatient records of 200 consecutive admissions to a psychiatric unit in a general hospital. They categorized the patients according to gender and diagnosis, and also noted the presence of physical illness, which was graded as 'severe' or 'less severe'. A rating of severe was recorded if the physical illness was considered to be 'at least of comparable importance to the psychiatric illness, to cause considerable disability to the patient and to require investigation and treatment'. Overall they found that one-third (67) of the sample had a physical illness, two-thirds of which (47) were graded as severe. Of further interest is the fact that half of the patients diagnosed as having a physical illness were not aware of its presence before admission, suggesting that 'silent' medical problems may remain undetected in this patient group. In their analysis of the data they found that gender did not influence the overall distribution of disease. However, age was important and, as might be expected, rates of physical illness increased particularly in those aged over 60. Predictably, a diagnosis of organic 'mental reactions' was strongly associated with physical illness, with nine out of 15 (60%) patients showing concurrent physical disease, underscoring the fact that it is important to differentiate this group from those with 'functional' psychiatric disorder. There were no significant differences between the other diagnostic categories, which included schizophrenia, severe affective disorder, other functional psychoses, moderate affective disorder, other neuroses and personality disorder, thus representing a broad range of psychiatric problems. However, when reviewing the data provided in the original paper with respect to functional serious mental illness, there is an important point to be made. Out of 54 subjects with severe affective disorder, 20 with depression are recorded as having a physical illness, 15 of which are rated as severe. In addition, out of 41 patients with moderate affective disorders, 13 with depression are recorded as having a physical illness, of which seven are rated as severe. From a further 27 schizophrenic subjects, five were stated to have a physical illness, of which two were severe. The individual ages of patients are not provided and therefore the effect of this important variable cannot be controlled for in re-examining the data. However, this study, despite its case record approach, which is likely to underestimate any association between psychiatric and physical disease, predicts that about one-third of psychiatric patients will have comorbid medical problems.

Importantly, and not stressed by the original authors, this overall figure seems to apply more to 'functional' psychiatric illness such as affective disorders and schizophrenia, than to organic mental conditions. Although the diagnostic categories contain relatively small numbers, this study is useful as it provides a rough estimate of the order of magnitude (and severity) of physical health problems found in general psychiatric patients. Unfortunately, a major weakness of the above studies is that they do not demonstrate any particular association between various categories of physical and mental disorder. This is a crucial point, because if the possible relationship between psychiatric and physical illness is to be of clinical importance it is vital to consider two questions. First, are any particular medical disorders implicated? Secondly, are the medical disorders significant and potentially responsible for a natural premature death? Bearing these questions in mind the chapter will concentrate on the relationship between psychiatric illnesses and cardiovascular disease.

The possibility that a positive association might exist between cardiovascular disease and psychiatric illness has long been suspected. A review of the studies examining this relationship was undertaken by Hayward (1995), and draws attention to the methodological weaknesses in many of the research methods and concludes that the overall evidence is unconvincing. However, several recent papers have brought the topic to the foreground again. A large review paper by Harris and Barraclough (1997) concluded that psychiatric patients suffer with increased morbidity and mortality as a result of medical problems. Although a specific association between depression and circulatory disease was not made, one was made with bipolar affective illness. Furthermore, since that review was published, other important studies have supported an association between affective disorders and cardiovascular disease. Everson et al. (1998) followed up a community sample of 6676 subjects for 25 years and found that those with depressive symptoms at baseline suffered an increased risk of developing cardiovascular disease, and in particular cerebrovascular accidents. Another study investigated and followed up 1190 male medical students. After 40 years follow-up the cumulative incidence of depression was 12%, and was associated with a significantly increased risk of coronary heart disease and myocardial infarction (Ford et al., 1998). Furthermore, as part of the Normative Ageing Study, Sesso et al. (1998) followed up 1305 male subjects over a seven-year period and found that coronary heart disease was positively associated with symptomatic depression. The fact that depression appears to predispose to cardiovascular disease has received increasing amounts of interest recently and was addressed briefly in an editorial in the BMJ (Dinan, 1999).

Further robust scientific research is needed to establish whether the connection between psychiatric illness and cardiovascular disease is indeed causative. However, if this is the case, as the above recent studies seem to suggest, then consideration should also be given to the possible pathophysiological mechanisms responsible for this link. To put it more simply: How do psychiatric disorders cause cardiovascular disease?

THE METABOLIC SYNDROME

It is well established that certain physiological (e.g. hypertension) and metabolic abnormalities (e.g. diabetes and hypercholesterolaemia) predispose to cardiovascular disease (Ostfeld, 1980). These states may all exist independently, although they are commonly present simultaneously in the same individual, and over the last decade have been collectively referred to as the 'metabolic syndrome'. The metabolic syndrome is also known by a number of pseudonyms including 'syndrome X' (Reaven, 1988), 'metabolic syndrome X' and Insulin Resistance Syndrome. Each contains a common triad of core factors: hypertension, type 2 diabetes mellitus and abnormal lipid profiles. When considering diabetes it is useful to think of glucose utilization in more general terms, and therefore physiological parameters such as hyperinsulinaemia, which reflects insulin resistance and some degree of glucose intolerance, should also be included. Other factors have also been associated with the metabolic syndrome, and include increased plasminogen activator inhibitor 1 levels and changes in plasma thromboxane levels, both of which alter fibrinolysis and may increase the risk of arteriosclerosis (Hughes et al., 1998).

The presence of aspects of the metabolic syndrome in an individual is a powerful predictor of cardiovascular disease, and though the underlying cause of the metabolic syndrome is not yet known, it is well established that obese individuals are prone to the development of its core features (Wannamethee et al., 1998). The importance of this association is demonstrated by the fact that obese subjects suffer increased morbidity and mortality as a result of cardiovascular disease (Rexrode et al., 1996). In obese subjects, it appears that those with a more centralized pattern of fat storage (referred to as abdominal obesity) suffer greater adverse physical health consequences than those with a more peripheral pattern (Freedman, 1995). This last point may be particularly important with respect to psychiatric disorders and will be examined in more detail later.

When considering the relationship between obesity and the metabolic syndrome it is reasonable to concentrate on energy balance (and degrees of adiposity) in general, rather than each aspect of the syndrome individually. This is because each factor of the metabolic syndrome may be derived from a different biochemical pathway, and can be considered collectively as 'spokes on a wheel rather than links on a chain' (Hopkins et al., 1996). The central role played by increased adiposity (i.e. the hub of the wheel) in the development of aspects of the metabolic syndrome is underscored by the fact that reducing the weight (fat content) of obese individuals may reduce blood pressure and improve glucose tolerance. Further consideration of the possible mechanisms by which individual features of the metabolic syndrome are produced are beyond the scope of this chapter and the interested reader should consult the article by Hopkins *et al.* (1996). Assuming that increased adiposity is central to the formation of multiple aspects of the metabolic syndrome, it is important to examine the concept of energy balance in more detail.

Energy balance

A comprehensive discussion of energy balance in general is not necessary, but the consideration of some of the more pertinent aspects, with regard to the main theme of this chapter, is required.

Energy balance refers to a complex physiological mechanism by which the body regulates energy intake and energy expenditure in an attempt to maintain a constant body weight. Energy intake is provided by food in the form of protein, carbohydrate and fat. Energy expenditure occurs as a result of metabolic processes within the body and physical activity, the latter being the main component. A positive energy balance refers to situations where energy intake is greater than energy output, with the excess energy subsequently being stored in the body as adipose tissue. Under normal conditions the body strives to maintain a constant weight, as demonstrated experimentally by Liebel *et al.* (1995) who examined the effects of changes in weight, induced by manipulating diet, on energy expenditure in humans. An increase in weight was associated with an increase in energy expenditure, with the opposite applying to weight loss. The compensatory changes in energy expenditure resulted in individuals returning to their original body weight. This pattern of events will be recognized by obese individuals who have successfully completed weight loss programmes, only to rapidly put the weight back on again afterwards. This may indicate that under normal conditions individuals may have a 'set' body weight, which resists and then corrects any changes imposed by behavioural techniques such as changes in diet or levels of exercise, unless these behavioural techniques are maintained.

Eating (energy intake) and physical activity (energy expenditure) occupy key roles in the equation of energy balance, and should be seen as representing the observable aspects of the final pathway of a complex internal regulatory system. The exact nature of this system is not known but is thought to involve complex interactions between a number of sub-systems including central neural networks, the autonomic nervous system and neuroendocrine components.

Certain parts of the brain, in particular the hypothalamus, have long been known to influence eating behaviour. Experiments on rodents in which the hypothalamus has been electrically stimulated produced marked changes in feeding behaviour. Stimulation of the lateral aspect of the hypothalamus has been shown to result in excess eating, leading to obesity, whereas stimulation of the medial aspect has been shown to lead to a reduction in food intake. In humans the hypothalamus is also thought to be the site of a complex central nervous system involved in the regulation of feeding behaviour and the integration of central and peripheral signals.

Within the central nervous system several neuropeptides exert major effects upon energy balance. Neuropeptide Y (NPY) is a transmitter that is expressed widely throughout the brain. NPY axons project from the arcuate nucleus to the paraventricular nucleus (PVN) within the hypothalamus. Central NPY administration leads to an increase in energy intake, which is coupled with a decrease in energy expenditure (Sainsbury et al., 1996). A subsequent positive energy balance may ensue resulting in a state of excess lipid storage. Corticotrophin-releasing hormone (CRH) which is synthesized in the PVN also acts centrally, with opposite effects to that of NPY, and causes a reduction in food intake. It should also be noted that CRH acts on the anterior pituitary gland to promote the secretion of adrenocorticotrophic hormone (ACTH), which in turn promotes the release of glucocorticoids from the adrenal glands. A state of glucocorticoid excess is associated with increased adiposity as demonstrated in patients with Cushing's syndrome (Yoshida et al., 1991; Wajchenberg et al., 1995). The effect of the glucocorticoids on energy balance is significant and will be considered in more detail later.

The activities of NPY and CRH are regulated by a number of factors, including leptin, which is a protein secreted predominantly by adipose tissue, and thought to act as a satiety factor at the hypothalamus. The plasma levels of leptin reflect total body adiposity and are the product of the ob (obesity) gene. In mice with mutations of the ob gene (ob/ob), severe obesity occurs as a result of a failure to secrete leptin. On the other hand, mice with a mutation of the db gene (db/db) also become obese, because of a mutation of the leptin receptor, which induces a state of 'leptin resistance'. Studies in humans have revealed higher levels of leptin in the plasma of obese subjects compared with that found in lean subjects, and also that leptin concentrations increase as body fat increases (Considine et al., 1996). This implies that some types of obesity in humans may be associated with reduced leptin receptor sensitivity. Leptin levels change with alterations in body weight, and though the correlation is positive, the changes in leptin are of a much greater magnitude. For example, an increase in body weight of 10% results in a 300% increase in serum leptin levels (Kolaczynski et al., 1996). Leptin levels are also influenced by acute changes in calorie intake, and a single day of massive overfeeding leads to an increase in leptin, whereas fasting leads to a dramatic decrease. Therefore, plasma leptin levels are influenced by factors other than total adiposity.

Leptin has been shown to attenuate neuropeptide Y induced feeding in *ob/ob* mice. In addition, leptin appears to cause an increase in the levels of CRH, which might serve to amplify its effect on reducing energy intake. Furthermore, leptin has been shown to increase the activity of the sympathetic nervous system, which may increase the resting metabolic rate and lead to further weight reduction by stimulating lipolysis of formed fat stores. Glucocorticoids influence the functions of leptin, and a deficiency of cortisol enhances the ability of leptin to promote weight loss. On the other hand, an excess of circulating cortisol is associated with an increase in the level of leptin, which may be mediated by the increased adiposity associated with states of hypercortisolism.

In addition to the biological variables described above other important factors involved in the regulation of energy balance include peripheral signals such as insulin and glucose. The circulating levels of insulin, like leptin, correlate with total body adiposity, with obese individuals showing hyperinsulinaemia. A raised level of plasma insulin is an indicator of impaired glucose tolerance and, as suggested earlier, should be considered a core feature of the metabolic syndrome. Further similarities between insulin and leptin include having receptors in the key areas of the hypothalamus, which when stimulated result in a decrease in food intake with subsequent weight loss.

All of the above signals, and possibly many others, interact to control feeding behaviour and energy expenditure, thus regulating body weight and adiposity. However, the equilibrium of the system may be disturbed by a large number of factors, both external (behaviour) and internal (illness). Therefore changes in diet and/or levels of physical activity, or of parts of the internal regulatory system may result in changes in weight. An increase in weight reflects increased adiposity and enhances the risk of developing aspects of the metabolic syndrome. Although the degree of adiposity in general is important, the site of any excess lipid storage must also be considered. Individuals with a more centralized (abdominal) pattern of obesity are more prone to developing features of the metabolic syndrome than those with a peripheral pattern. The former group of subjects can be subdivided further and those with a more visceral (intra-abdominal), as opposed to subcutaneous, pattern of abdominal fat distribution are particularly prone to the development of core features of the metabolic syndrome. Therefore the regulation of adipose tissue itself, particularly with respect to visceral fat, is of interest and relevant to this discussion.

Regulation of adipose tissue and distribution of body fat

As with energy balance the regulation of adipose tissue storage is complex and influenced by many factors (Björntorp, 1996). At the level of the adipocyte two enzymes are of particular importance. Lipoprotein lipase (LPL) converts free fatty acids (FFAs) in the plasma into triglycerides (TGs) which are then stored in the fat mass. Hormone sensitive lipase (HSL) has the opposite effect and converts stored TGs into FFAs, which are then released into the circulation. The activities of both of these enzymes are influenced by circulating hormones and the sympathetic nervous system, the net result of which leads to differences in the patterns of body fat distribution, which is perhaps demonstrated most effectively by the differences noted between males and females.

As described above fat can be seen as being deposited peripherally and centrally. Peripheral fat storage refers to areas such as the buttocks, hips and thighs, referred to as gynoid (female) obesity, whereas central storage refers to the abdomen, and is referred to as android (male) obesity (Vague, 1956). The collection of adipose tissue situated in the peripheral or subcutaneous regions may be easily visible to the naked eye, and is what we commonly refer to in describing cases of phenotypic obesity. Fat around the abdomen can be stored in the subcutaneous compartment, or more deeply around the visceral organs. Obese subjects who have excess deposits of subcutaneous adipose tissue may also have increased amounts of visceral fat, but this is not always the case. For example, Japanese Sumo wrestlers have massive amounts of subcutaneous and peripheral fat, but very little amounts of visceral fat (Karam, 1996). It is therefore possible to speculate that the opposite scenario may exist where individuals have excess visceral fat but are not phenotypically obese. This is of clinical importance as visceral fat is independently associated with health risks similar to those of generalized obesity (Reaven, 1988).

Abdominal obesity can be measured indirectly by calculating the waist–hip ratio (WHR), or directly using imaging techniques such as computed tomography and magnetic resonance imaging. A waist–hip ratio gives an estimate of the ratio between central and peripheral fat storage, and the greater the WHR, the greater the risk of developing aspects of the metabolic syndrome (Bray, 1987). By using direct imaging methods, such as computerized tomography, one can more accurately measure the actual amount and pattern of distribution of abdominal fat present.

It is of interest that patients with Cushing's syndrome, and excess circulating plasma cortisol, have been consistently shown to preferentially promote the collection of excess adipose tissue within the visceral area. Not surprisingly, patients with Cushing's syndrome are also very prone to the development of the core features of the metabolic syndrome (Friedman et al., 1996). Therefore, with respect to visceral obesity it is reasonable to place particular emphasis on the role played by glucocorticoids. Cortisol has been shown to act on adipose tissue directly and increases and decreases the activity of LPL (Ottoson et al., 1995) and HSL (Samra et al., 1998), respectively, the net effect being the promotion of fat storage. This applies particularly to the intra-abdominal fat depot which has a glucocorticoid receptor density of up to four times that of subcutaneous fat (Pederson et al., 1994). Since overactivity of the HPA axis and hypercortisolaemia is associated with depression (Dinan, 1994) and to a lesser extent schizophrenia (Lammers *et al.*, 1995) it is possible that these conditions are also associated with an increased abdominal distribution of fat storage. Because of the health risks implied with this association it is important to examine whether the major psychiatric disorders are associated with any abnormalities of energy balance and/or fat distribution.

ENERGY BALANCE AND PSYCHIATRIC ILLNESS

Changes in biological features such as appetite and activity levels occur commonly in psychiatric illness. These may be most striking during acute severe episodes of affective disorders or schizophrenia. However, patients with serious mental disorders may continue to experience more chronic subtle changes in their behaviour. This may particularly apply to patients with schizophrenia who may suffer from profound negative symptoms, and to patients suffering with chronic depression. Both states may lead to a reduced level of energy expenditure and promote the onset of weight gain and obesity. The impact that these behavioural changes might have on energy balance, and fat distribution, is of importance when considering the relationship between depression and the metabolic syndrome.

Typical episodes of major depression are often associated with a marked reduction in physical activity, though weight loss occurs presumably as a result of a greater reduction in appetite and calorie intake. Although a loss of weight during a depressive episode would be expected to reduce the risk of developing features of the metabolic syndrome, this does not take into account the necessary longitudinal view of disease processes. It is important to note that there may be differences in examining the acute and long-term effects of a depressive disorder. The intensity, duration and frequency of depressive episodes may also be of major importance.

Patients with melancholic depression have been shown to have increased CSF levels of CRH (Banki *et al.*, 1992) and decreased levels of neuropeptide Y (Gjerris *et al.*, 1992). Both of these factors may act at the hypothalamus to reduce food intake. Despite the reduction in calorie intake and weight loss associated with depressive episodes, the levels of plasma leptin have been reported to be normal in depressed patients (Deuschle *et al.*, 1996). From our current understanding of the functions of leptin we would expect to find that a reduction in calorie intake, with associated weight loss, would result in a decrease in leptin levels. The reason for this discrepancy is not yet clear, but may indicate that the hypercortisolism often present during episodes of major depression enhances the secretion of leptin and counteracts the effect of the weight loss (Antonijevic *et al.*, 1998). It is also worth noting that in rodents leptin appears to promote the release of CRH (Van Dijk *et al.*, 1999), and therefore its failure to decrease in depressed humans despite weight loss might contribute to HPA system overactivity.

The changes that may take place in important regulatory neuropeptides in more chronic, or recurrent, states of depression have not been closely examined. The most consistently demonstrated neuroendocrine abnormality associated with major depression of the melancholic subtype is overactivity of the hypothalamic–pituitary–adrenal (HPA) axis, resulting in hypercortisolism (Dinan, 1994). As stated earlier, hypercortisolism, as seen in patients with Cushing's syndrome, is associated with the impairment of the actions of leptin, and may result in excess lipid storage. It is therefore possible that the excess cortisol circulating at times of major depressive episodes may predispose to lipid accumulation, particularly in the intra abdominal area. In addition, a subgroup of patients with major depressive disorder also demonstrate a persistent mild hyperactivity of the HPA axis, and as a result this group of patients might, in the long term, be particularly vulnerable to increased visceral fat accumulation. A further speculative point of interest is that the unresponsiveness of leptin to a loss of weight may also apply to an increase of weight/adiposity, thereby robbing the body, to some degree, of its powerful internal regulatory system.

BODY FAT DISTRIBUTION AND PSYCHIATRIC ILLNESS

An interest in the relationship between body shape and psychiatric illness is certainly not a new idea. The changes in body shape (and energy balance) that accompany the eating disorders, and in particular anorexia nervosa, have long been recognized and are useful in establishing diagnosis. However, when considering major 'functional' psychiatric illness in general there has been little interest until relatively recently. With the growing body of literature regarding the health consequences of obesity in general, and visceral fat in particular, psychiatric patients have received some attention.

In general, obesity, including abdominal obesity, is more prevalent in the chronically mentally ill compared with the general population (Wallace and Tennant, 1998; Sharpe and Hill, 1998). Because of the possible differences between major diagnostic categories it is important to examine each mental disorder separately.

A number of studies have examined the relationship between depression and any associated changes in the pattern of body fat distribution. Rosmond et al. (1996) studied 1040 middle-aged Swedish men and concluded that depressive traits were independently associated with an increase in the WHR. Wing et al. (1991) found the same association to apply to premenopausal female subjects. Of further interest is that Lloyd et al. (1996) have demonstrated some longitudinal evidence for a positive correlation between changes in depressive symptomatology and the value of the WHR.

As stated earlier the WHR provides an estimate of the ratio between the degrees of central and peripheral fat storage, and is an indirect measurement.

The only study to date to have specifically measured the amount of abdominal fat, by direct methods, in patients with established depressive illnesses was conducted by Thakore *et al.* (1997). They used a single slice computerized tomography (CT) scan at the level of the fourth lumbar vertebra to measure the amount and pattern of distribution of abdominal fat in six female patients suffering with melancholic depression. They found that the depressed subjects had twice the amount of visceral fat compared with that found in the six matched controls. This study provides some important direct evidence of an increase in intra-abdominal fat associated with a current depressive disorder, though needs replication on a larger, more longitudinal scale. For a more extensive discussion of the relationship between melancholic depression and increased levels of intra-abdominal fat the reader is referred to a review article written by the authors (Mann and Thakore, 1999).

PSYCHIATRIC ILLNESS AND FEATURES OF THE METABOLIC SYNDROME

Examination of the postulated relationship between the metabolic syndrome and psychiatric illness can be approached in a structured manner. This section will look at some of the individual factors that make up the metabolic syndrome and try to establish whether they are associated with the major depression.

Diabetes

There is a lot of research literature regarding the prevalence of depression in patients with established diabetes. A review by Gavard *et al.* (1993) concluded that while studies often show a higher than expected rate of depression in diabetic patients, this is partly offset by methodological problems, and overall the specific association with diabetes relative to other medical illnesses is not proven. They do state however that depression has an overall negative effect on diabetes management, probably due to the fact that depressed diabetic patients may not comply with treatment as effectively as wished. Similarly, Marcus *et al.* (1992) found that current depressive symptoms did not alter glycaemic control in 66 obese patients with type 2 diabetes, but noted that subjects with a history of major depression were less likely to complete the 52 week diabetes management behavioural programme. In agreement with this fact Lustman *et al.* (1997) have demonstrated that major depression was responsible for worsening glycaemic control in a five-year follow up study of 25 patients with established diabetes.

Does the presence of major depression increase the likelihood of developing type 2 diabetes mellitus? This important point has been addressed by Eaton et al. (1996) who conducted a 13-year follow-up study of a community sample in Baltimore, USA. In 1981 a total of 3481 subjects agreed to participate, and those with diabetes were subsequently excluded. At the end of the follow-up period in 1994, there were 89 new cases of diabetes among a population at risk sample of 1715. A history of depression was assessed by means of a self-report questionnaire. They found that the presence of major depression, but not of milder forms of depression, predicted the onset of diabetes. This relationship was not weakened by controlling for age, sex, race, social status, education, other psychiatric disorders or body weight. In addition, Kawakami et al. (1999) conducted a similar study in Japan and followed 2764 male subjects over an eight-year period. They found that subjects with moderate or severe levels of depression, as measured by the Zung Self-Rating depression scale, were just over twice as likely to be diagnosed as suffering with type 2 diabetes at the end of the follow-up period as those who were not depressed. Although these studies have some methodological weaknesses, in particular with respect to the self-report assessment of depression, the large sample sizes and longitudinal design encourage serious consideration of their conclusions.

Other studies have investigated the glucose utilization of individuals with major depression in closer detail by means of an oral glucose tolerance test (OGTT). Winokur et al. (1988) administered a five–hour OGTT to 28 depressive subjects and 21 control subjects and measured the responses of serum glucose, insulin and glucagon. The depressed patients showed significantly greater basal glucose levels, and also had greater cumulative glucose responses than the control group. In addition, the depressive patients also had a larger cumulative insulin response, indicating some degree of insulin resistance. The glucagon responses between the two groups did not differ. A similar response using the intravenous glucose tolerance test has also been observed (Wright et al., 1978). Another way of testing insulin resistance is by examining the response of plasma glucose to insulin administration. Menna-Perper et al. (1984) compared the responses to insulin infusion among three groups of subjects: major depression, dysthymic disorder and normal controls. In support of the above evidence they found that the rate of change in glucose levels in patients with major depression was significantly less than the other groups tested, again indicating some degree of insulin resistance.

The above studies suggest that certain groups of patients suffering with depression may have some degree of insulin resistance and glucose intolerance. The important question of whether or not glucose utilization returns to normal with successful treatment has recently been addressed by Okamura et al. (1999). In accordance with the above data they found that depressed subjects exhibited features of glucose intolerance. Successful treatment of the current depressive state using antidepressant medication restored normal glucose tolerance. Although their study used a very small sample of three subjects, it is of significance that the changes in glucose utilization, as measured by the oral glucose tolerance test, were not related to changes in body weight or diet. In addition, glycaemic control as measured by glycated haemoglobin in type 2 diabetes mellitus patients with superimposed major depression has been shown to improve with treatment of the comorbid depression. Importantly, this effect was independent of any changes in the subjects self-monitoring of blood glucose or weight changes. This suggests that depression itself may worsen glycaemic control by a mechanism that is as yet unidentified. It seems possible to speculate further, that if depression can worsen glycaemic control in an established type 2 diabetes patient, then perhaps by interacting with other risk factors (such as mild obesity) a state of type 2 diabetes might be induced.

Hypertension

A recent large epidemiological study by Jonas *et al.* (1997) examined whether depression acts as an independent risk factor for hypertension. They followed a normotensive, mixed race and sex population of 2992 subjects for a period of between 7 and 16 years. Baseline recordings included levels of anxiety and depression. The main outcome measure was hypertension, either treated at some point during the study (treated hypertension), or noted at the end of the follow-up period (incident hypertension). The results were statistically adjusted for known hypertension risk factors and stratified by race and age. For whites aged 25–44 depression was an independent predictor of treated hypertension. For whites aged 45–64, depression remained an independent predictor of both treated and incident hypertension. In blacks, depression was an independent predictor of both treated and incident hypertension across the entire 25–64 age range. Although the frequency and type of depressive episodes are not known, the results of this study indicate that depression is associated with this aspect of the metabolic syndrome. It also highlights the fact that different populations may be more at risk than others.

The prevalence of hypertension in depressed inpatients with concurrent hyperactivity of the HPA axis has also been examined. Pfohl *et al.* (1991) investigated whether or not depressed patients with an abnormal dexamethasone suppression test (DST) exhibited the classic physiological stigmata of Cushing's syndrome. Of 230 subjects they found that hypertension was significantly more frequent amongst DST non-suppressors than it was amongst normal suppressors. Age, gender, body weight and the use of antihypertensive medication did not account for this difference. This is of interest as it raises the possibility that the hyperactive HPA axis observed in depression is related to the development of high blood pressure. However, this study did not examine the effects of treatment, and therefore the relationship between the HPA axis and hypertension in these depressed subjects cannot be regarded as causative.

Lipid profiles

Abnormal lipid states, and in particular increased low density lipoprotein (LDL) cholesterol and reduced high density lipoprotein (HDL) cholesterol are strongly associated with the development of cardiovascular disease.

Some abnormalities of lipid profiles have been found in depressed patients, with lower levels of HDL cholesterol being demonstrated (Horsten *et al.*, 1997). However, there is no clear evidence that LDL cholesterol is increased. Increased levels of LDL triglyceride have also been reported, and though this may predispose to cardiovascular disease, the effect is not as strong as that associated with increased levels of LDL cholesterol. It must be noted however that patients suffering with depression have also been found to have reduced levels of plasma cholesterol.

Clotting abnormalities

High levels of thromboxane A_2 and B_2 have been reported in patients with major depression, and appear to be associated with excess HPA activity (Piccirillo *et al.*, 1994). In addition, Musselman *et al.* (1996) have shown that platelets of depressives show higher baseline and responsive activation. Both of these factors may increase the risk of arteriosclerotic disease.

CONCLUSIONS

Patients who suffer from major psychiatric disorders have a reduced life expectancy partly due to natural causes. Cardiovascular disease seems to be a good candidate for the premature death experienced by some patients, and may be mediated by an association between psychiatric illness and the metabolic syndrome. The relationship between psychiatric disease and the metabolic syndrome may be as a result of HPA overactivity predisposing to an increased visceral adipose tissue collection.

If the association is correct then there are some important considerations. For example, psychiatric patients suffering from severe mental disorders may need to be screened more carefully for 'silent' medical problems. In addition, general medical patients might also need closer monitoring for, and the appropriate treatment of, any comorbid psychiatric disorders.

Overall, a more comprehensive and holistic approach to the care of patients suffering from severe mental disorders may be required. This would hopefully lead to enhanced general care, for as we are already aware, 'there are no psychiatric patients. . .only medical patients with varying degrees of psychopathology' (Schiffer *et al.*, 1988).

REFERENCES

Antonijevic, I.A., Murck, H., Frieboes, R.M. *et al.* (1998). Elevated nocturnal profiles of serum leptin in patients with depression. *J Psychiatr Res* **32**, 403–410.

Banki, C.M., Karmacsi, L., Bissette, G. and Nemeroff, C.B. (1992). Cerebrospinal fluid neuropeptides in mood disorder and dementia. *J Affect Disord* **25**, 39–45.

Björntorp, P. (1996). The regulation of adipose tissue distribution in humans. *Int J Obes* **20**, 291–302.

Bray, G.A. (1987). Overweight is risking fate. Definition, classification, prevalence, and risks. *Ann NY Acad Sci* **499**, 14–28.

Carney, R.M., Freedland, K.E., Sheline, Y.I. and Weiss, E.S. (1997). Depression and coronary heart disease. A review for cardiologists. *Clin Cardiol* **20**, 196–200.

Considine, R.V., Sinha, M.K., Heiman, M.L. *et al.* (1996). Serum immunoreactive-leptin concentration in normal weight and obese humans. *New Engl J Med* **334**, 292–295.

Deuschle, M., Blum, W.F., Englaro, P. *et al.* (1996). Plasma leptin in depressed and healthy controls. *Hum Metabol Res* **28**, 714–717.

Dinan, T.G. (1994). Glucocorticoids and the genesis of depressive illness. A psychobiological model. *Br J Psychiatry* **164**, 365–371.

Dinan, T.G. (1999). The physical consequences of depressive illness (editorial). *Br Med J* **318**, 826.

Eaton, W.W., Armenian, H., Gallo, J., Pratt, L. and Ford, D.E. (1996). Depression and risk for onset of type 2 diabetes: A prospective population based study. *Diabet Care* **19**, 1097–1102.

Everson, S.A., Roberts, R.E, Goldberg, D.E and Kaplan, G.A. (1998). Depressive symptoms and increased risk of stroke mortality over a 29 year period. *Arch Intern Med* **158**, 1133–1138.

Ford, D.E., Mead, C.A., Chang, P.P. *et al.* (1998). Depression is a risk factor for coronary artery disease in men. The precursors study. *Arch Int Med* **158**, 1422–1426.

Freedman, D.S. (1995). The importance of body fat distribution in early life. *Am J Med Sci* **310**, (Suppl 1), 72–76.

Friedman, T.C., Mastorakos, G., Newman, T.D. *et al.* (1996). Carbohydrate and lipid metabolism in endogenous hypercortisolism: shared features with metabolic syndrome X and non insulin dependent diabetes. *Endocrinol J* **43**, 645–655.

Gavard, J.A., Lustman, P.J. and Clouse, R.E. (1993). Prevalence of depression in adults with diabetes. An epidemiological evaluation. *Diabet Care* **16**, 1167–1178.

Gjerris, A., Widerlov, E, Werdelin, L. and Ekma, R. (1992). Cerebrospinal fluid concentrations of neuropeptide Y in depressed patients and in controls. *J Psychiatry Neurosci* **17**, 23–27.

Hagg, S., Joelsson, L., Mycorindal, T. *et al.* (1998). Prevalence of diabetes and impaired glucose tolerance in patients treated with clozapine compared with patients treated with conventional depot neuroleptic medications. *J Clin Psychiatry* **59**, 294–299.

Harris, C.E. and Barraclough, B. (1997). Excess mortality of mental disorder. *Br J Psychiatry* **173**, 11–53.

Hayward, C. (1995). Psychiatric illness and cardiovascular disease risk. *Epidemiol Rev* **17**, 129–138.

Hopkins, P.N., Hunt, S.C., Wu, L.L., Williams, G.H. and Williams, R.R. (1996). Hypertension, dyslipidaemia and insulin resistance:links on a chain or spokes on a wheel? *Curr Opin Lipidol* **7**, 241–253.

Horsten, M., Wamala, S.P., Vingerhoets, A. and Orth-Gomer, K. (1997). Depressive symptoms, social support, and lipid profile in healthy middle aged women. *Psychosom Med* **59**, 521–528.

Hughes, K., Choo, M., Kuperan, P., Ong, C.N. and Aw T.C. (1998). Cardiovascular risk factors in non insulin dependent diabetics compared to non diabetic controls: a population based survey among Asians in Singapore. *Atherosclerosis* **136**, 25–31.

Jonas, B.S., Franks, P. and Ingram, D.D. (1997). Are symptoms of anxiety and depression risk factors for hypertension? Longitudinal evidence for the NH and nutrition exam survey 1 epidemiological follow up study. *Arch Fam Med* **6**, 43–49.

Karam, J.H. (1996). Reversible insulin resistance in non-insulin dependent diabetes mellitus. *Horm Metab Res* **28**, 440–444

Kawakami, N., Takatsuka, N., Shimizu, H. and Ishibashi, H. (1999). Depressive symptoms and occurrence of type 2 diabetes among Japanese men. *Diabet Care* **22**, 1071–1076.

Kelly, W.F. (1996). Psychiatric aspects of Cushing's syndrome. *Q J Med* **89**, 543–551.

Kolaczynski, J.W., Considine, R.V., Ohannesian, J. *et al.* (1996). Responses of leptin to short term fasting and refeeding in humans:a link with keteogenesis but not ketones themselves. *Diabetes* **45**, 1511–1515.

Koranyi, E.K. (1977). Fatalities in 2070 psychiatric outpatients. *Arch Gen Psychiatry* **34**, 1137–1142.

Lammers, C.H., Garcia-Borregeuro, D., Schmider, J., Gotthardt, U., Dettling, M., Holsboer, F. and Heuser, I.J. (1995). Combined dexamethasone/ corticotropin-releasing hormone test in patients with schizophrenia and in normal controls: II. *Biol Psychiatry* **38**, 803–807.

Liebel, L., Rosenbaum, M. and Hirsch, J. (1995). Changes in energy expenditure resulting from altered body weight. *New Engl J Med* **332**, 621–628.

Lloyd, C.E., Wing, R.R. and Orchard, T.J. (1996). Waist to hip ratio and psychosocial factors in adults with adults with insulin dependent diabetes mellitus: the Pittsburgh Epidemiology of Diabetes Complications study. *Metabolism* **45**, 268–272.

Lustman, P.J., Griffith, L.S., Freedland, K.E. and Clouse, R.E. (1997). The course of major depression in diabetes. *Gen Hosp Psychiatry* **19**, 138–143.

Maguire, G.P. and Granville-Grossman, K.L. (1968). Physical illness in psychiatric patients. *Br J Psychiatry* **114**, 1365–1369.

Mann, J.N. and Thakore, J.H. (1999). Melancholic depression and abdominal fat distribution: a mini-review. *Stress* **3**, 1–15

Marcus, M.D., Wing, R.R., Guane, J., Blair, E.H. and Jawaad, A. (1992). Lifetime prevalence of major depression and its effect on treatment outcome in obese type 2 diabetic patients. *Diabet Care* **15**, 253–255.

Menna-Perper, M., Rochford, J., Meuller, P.S. *et al.* (1984). Differential response of plasma glucose, amino acids and non-esterified fatty acids to insulin in depressed patients. *Psychoneuroendocrinology* **9**, 161–171.

Musselman, D.L., Tomer, T., Manatunga, A.K. *et al.* (1996). Exaggerated platelet reactivity in major depression. *Am J Psychiatry* **153**, 1313–1317.

Okamura, F., Tashiro, A., Utsumi, A. *et al.* (1999). Insulin resistance in patients with depression and its changes in the clinical course of depression: a report on 3 cases using the minimal model analysis. *Int Med* **38**, 257–260.

Ostfeld, A.M. (1980). A review of stroke epidemiology. *Epidemiol Rev* **2**, 136–152.

Ottoson, M., Marin, P., Karason, K., Elander, A. and Björntorp, P. (1995). Blockade of the glucocorticoid receptor with RU 486: effects in vitro and in vivo on human adipose tissue lipoprotein lipase activity. *Obes Res* **3**, 233–240.

Pederson, S.B., Jonler, M. and Richelsen, B. (1994). Characterization of regional and gender differences in glucocorticoid receptors and lipoprotein lipase activity in human adipose tissue. *J Clin Endocrinol Metab* **78**, 1354–1359.

Piccirillo, G., Fimognari, F.L., Infantino, V. *et al.* (1994). High plasma concentrations of cortisol and thromboxane B2 in patients with depression. *Am J Med Sci* **307**, 228–232.

Pfohl, B., Rederer, M., Loryell, W. and Stangl, D. (1991). Association between post-dexamethasone cortisol level and blood pressure in depressed patients. *J Nerv Ment Dis* **179**, 44–47.

Reaven, G.M. (1988). The role of insulin resistance in human disease. *Diabetes* **37**, 1595–1607.

Rexrode, K.M., Manson, J.E. and Hennekens, C.H. (1996). Obesity and cardiovascular disease. *Curr Opin Cardiol* **11**, 490–495.

Rosmond, R., Lapidus, L., Marin, P. and Björntop, P. (1996). Mental distress, obesity and body fat distribution in middle aged men. *Obes Res* **4**, 245–252.

Sainsbury, A., Cusin, I., Doyle, P., Rohner-Jeanren, F. and Rohner-Jeanren, B. (1996). Intracerebroventricular administration of NPY to normal rats increases ob gene expression in white adipose tissue. *Diabetalogia* **39**, 353–356.

Samra, J.S., Clark, M.L., Humphries, S.M., McDonald, I.A., Bannister, P.A. and Frayn, K.N. (1998). Effects of physiological hypercortisolaemia on the regulation of lipolysis in subcutaneous adipose tissue. *J Clin Endocrinol Metab* **83**, 626–631.

Sesso, H.D., Kawachi, I., Vokonas, P.S. and Sparrow. D. (1998). Depression and the risk of coronary heart disease in the Normative Ageing Study. *Am J Cardiol* **82**, 851–856.

Schiffer, R.B., Klein, R.F. and Sider, R.C. (1988). *The Medical Evaluation of Psychiatric Patients*. Plenum, New York, p. 28.

Sharpe, J.K and Hill, A.P. (1998). Anthropometry and adiposity in a group of people with chronic mental illness. *Aust NZ J Psychiatry* **32**, 77–81.

Thakore, J.H., Richards, P.J., Reznek, R.H., Martin, A. and Dinan, T.G. (1997). Increased intra-abdominal fat deposition in patients with major depressive illness as measured by computed tomography. *Biol Psychiatry* **41**, 1140–1142.

Tsuang, M.T., Woolson, R.F. and Fleming, J.A. (1980). Premature deaths in schizophrenia and affective disorders. An analysis of survival curves and variables affecting the shortened survival. *Arch Gen Psychiatry* **37**, 979–983.

Vague, J. (1956). The degree of masculine differentiation of obesities: A factor determining predisposition to diabetes, gout and uric calculous disease. *Am J Clin Nutr* **4**, 20–34.

Van Dijk, G., Seeley, R.J., Thiele, T.E. *et al.* (1999). Metabolic, gastrointestinal and CNS neuropeptide effects of brain leptin administration in the rat. *Am J Physiol* **276**, R1425–R1437.

Wallace, B. and Tennant, C. (1998). Nutrition and obesity in the chronic mentally ill. *Aust NZ J Psychiatry* **32**, 82–85.

Wajchenberg, B.L., Bosco, A., Marone, M.M. *et al.* (1995). Estimation of body fat and lean tissue distribution by dual energy X-ray absorptiometry and abdominal body fat evaluation by computed tomography in Cushing's disease. *J Clin Endocrinol Metab* **80**, 2791–2794.

Wannamethee, S.G., Shaper, A.G., Durrington, P.N. and Perry, I.J. (1998). Hypertension, serum insulin, obesity and the metabolic syndrome. *J Hum Hypertens* **12**, 735–741.

Wing, R.R., Matthews, K.A., Kuller, L.H., Meilahn, E.N. and Plantinga, P. (1991). Waist to hip ratio in middle aged women. Association with behavioural and psychosocial factors and with changes in cardiovascular risk factors. *Arteriosclerot Thrombosis* **11**, 1250–1257.

Winokur, A., Maislin, G., Phillips, J.L. and Amsterdam, J.D. (1988). Insulin resistance after oral glucose tolerance testing in patients with major depression. *Am J Psychiatry* **145**, 325–330.

Wright, J.H., Jacism, J.J., Radin, N.S. and Bell, R.A. (1978). Glucose metabolism in unipolar depression. *Br J Psychiatry* **132**, 386–393.

Yoshida, S., Inadera, H., Ishikawa, Y. *et al.* (1991). Endocrine disorders and body fat distribution. *Int J Obes* **15** (suppl. 2), 37–40.

6

Depression and Osteoporosis: Association or Causal Relationship?

GIOVANNI CIZZA[a], ALEJANDRO AYALA[a], MARIANNE DALEY[c], PHILIP W. GOLD[a] and GEORGE P. CHROUSOS[b]

[a]Clinical Neuroendocrinology Branch, NIMH, [b]Pediatric and Reproductive Endocrinology Branch, NICHD, Bethesda, MD, and Merck Research Laboratories, Rahway, NJ, USA

INTRODUCTION

Hippocrates was among the first to hypothesize an association between mental and physical illness. The idea that melancholia was caused by 'excess black bile' was based on the premise that mental illness resulted from imbalances of the four dominant body humours (blood, phlegm, yellow bile and black bile), a concept accepted and propagated by Plato and Aristotle. In the Renaissance, Paracelsus introduced the idea that psychiatric illnesses are not caused by supernatural forces but are a consequence of 'natural' maladaptations to the environment. Robert Burton integrated these ideas in his famous text, *The Anatomy of Melancholia*.

During the 20th century, neuroscience and psychobiology became increasingly popular areas of research. Within the last decade, a growing body of evidence has accumulated which suggests that some endocrine correlates of depression, such as hypercortisolism, might be responsible for some of the somatic derangements frequently observed in depressive patients (Chrousos and Gold, 1998). Currently, researchers are intensively investigating not only the biological bases of mental illness, but also the putative somatic consequences of these disorders.

Depression is a common disorder, affecting 5–9% of women, and 1–2% of men (Robbins *et al.*, 1984). This disorder carries a considerable risk of morbidity and is associated with a two- to three-fold increase in all-cause, non-suicide-related mortality, especially in men (Zheng *et al.*, 1997). In addition to their psychological manifestations, depressed subjects exhibit changes in body composition characterized by a decrease of their lean body mass and increased central adiposity, alterations in haemostasis and endothelial functions, which together increase their risk of cardiovascular events. Depression is also associated with changes in the inflammatory response which may predispose to pathologies associated with dysregulation of the immune response, such as periodontitis and other diseases (Genco, 1999).

Another area where depression may play a role is in the pathogenesis of osteoporosis, a serious disease that develops slowly and silently over many years and results in fractures and associated health care costs (Ravn *et al.*, 1999a). We recently reported that young and middle-aged premenopausal women with depression had low bone mineral density, a factor that may predispose them to osteoporosis and fractures later in life (Michelson *et al.*, 1996). The scope of this chapter is to examine the association between depression and osteoporosis, two common medical conditions. We will then discuss the endocrine factors potentially responsible for the bone loss observed in endocrine abnormalities, such as hypercortisolism, hypogonadism, and growth hormone deficiency, which may also be responsible for the bone loss that is associated with depression.

DEPRESSION AND OSTEOPOROSIS

Review of existing studies

Several studies have examined the association between major depression and osteoporosis (Table 1).

In one study, the density of the trabecular bone, assessed by single-energy quantitative computerized tomography (CT) at the level of the lumbar spine, was approximately 15% lower in 80 depressed men and women older than 40 years – with an average age of 62 years for women and 58 years for men as compared with 57 non-depressed men and women (Schweiger *et al.*, 1994). Risk factors for bone loss, such as smoking, lifetime history of excessive or inadequate levels of exercise, or history of oestrogen treatment in women did not yield an additional effect, suggesting an effect of depression *per se* on bone loss. However, at study entry, neither age of onset nor total duration of depression correlated with bone loss. A follow-up study recently published by the same group on 18 depressed men and women and 21 comparison subjects from the originally reported series, indicated that bone loss over 24 months or more was significantly greater in depressed subjects than in comparison subjects. Interestingly, bone loss was more severe in depressed men than in depressed women (Schweiger *et al.*, 2000).

Another study was conducted where bone mineral density was measured at the spine, hip, and radius in 24 premenopausal women, average age 41 years, with past or current major depression and 24 control women matched for age, body mass index, menopausal state and race; depressed women had significantly lower bone mineral density (Michelson *et al.*, 1996). Specifically, bone mineral density was 6.5% lower at the spine, 13.6% lower at the femoral neck and at Ward triangle, and 10.8% lower at the trochanter; no differences were observed at the radius. In 10 of the 24 depressed women, bone mineral density was in the osteoporotic range (greater than 2 SD below the expected peak density), and eight of these women were 44 years old or younger. In contrast, no normal women had a deficit of similar magnitude. This suggests that in these relatively young women the lifetime risk of osteoporotic fracture related to depression is substantial. However, as recruitment in this study was not population-based, it is not possible to extrapolate what the actual prevalence of low bone mineral density in depressed women of that age would be.

The bone loss observed in depressed women in that study could be due to decreased bone formation, increased bone resorption, or both. Serum osteocalcin, a marker of bone formation, was approximately 20% lower in depressed women, suggesting a decrease in osteoblastic activity. Urinary deoxypyridinoline crosslinks excretion, a marker of osteoclastic activity, was also approximately 30% lower in this group. However, the urinary excretion of *N*-telopeptide, another marker of bone resorption, was not altered. Finally, depressed women had higher urinary free cortisol excretion than controls, although these levels in many of the patients were within the normal range.

A prospective, cohort study conducted at five different centres in the USA in more than 9000 white women older than 65 years, examined the association between depression, bone mineral density, falls and risk of fractures (Whooley *et al.*, 1999). Depression was evaluated by the Geriatric Depression Score, a 15-item validated checklist of symptoms designed to detect depression in the elderly. Bone mineral density was measured at the lumbar spine and hip by dual-energy X-ray absorptiometry (DEXA), incident vertebral fractures documented by comparing lateral spine films between baseline and follow-up visits, and self-reported falls were collected at follow-up visits. The prevalence of depression in this cohort of elderly women was 6.3%. Women with depression were more likely to fall (70% v. 59%) and had a greater incidence of vertebral (11% v. 5%) and non-vertebral (28% v. 21%) fractures, than women without depression. The greater incidence of fractures observed in depressed women was not clearly associated with a lower bone mineral density as, overall, there were no significant differences in mean spine and hip bone mineral density between women with and women without depression. However, in *post-hoc* analyses, a significant interaction between depression, bone mineral density, and body mass index was detected. In the subgroup of women in the highest tertile of body mass index (greater than 27.6), women with depression had a 4.6% lower spine bone mineral density, and a 2.6% lower hip bone mineral density than women without depression.

Table 1. Summary of reports on depression and osteoporosis.

Study	Authors	Subjects	Measurements	Study design/ setting	Evaluation of depression	Findings
1	Schweiger et al., 1994	80 depressed men and women, 57 controls	Spine BMD by CT	Cross-sectional	DSM-IIIR	15% lower spine BMD in depressed subjects
2	Schweiger et al., 2000	18 depressed, 21 controls	Spine BMD by CT	Longitudinal	DSM-IIIR	Greater bone loss over time in depressed subjects, greater bone loss in depressed men than in depressed women
3	Michelson et al., 1996	24 depressed women 24 control women	BMD at various sites, endocrine measurements	Cross-sectional	DSM-IIIR	Lower BMD in depressed women (6.5%, spine 13.6%, femoral neck, 13.6%, Ward's triangle, 10.8%, trochanter)
4	Whooley et al., 1999	7414 elderly women	Spine and hip BMD, falls, fractures	Prospective cohort	Geriatric depression scale	Greater incidence of falls but no differences in spine BMD between depressed and non-depressed women

5	Halbriech et al., 1995	33 women and 35 men with various mental disorders, 21 depressed subjects	Spine and hip BMD, endocrine measurements	Inpatient psychiatric clinic	DSM-IIIR	Low BMD in depressed subjects, especially depressed men; inverse correlation between plasma cortisol and BMD
6	Coelho et al., 1999	102 women randomly selected	Spine and hip BMD	Cross-sectional, epidemiological, population-based	Beck Depression Inventory / Hopkins Symptom Checklist-90	Higher levels of depressive symptoms and depression in women with osteoporosis
7	Reginster et al., 1999	121 healthy postmenopausal women	Spine and hip BMD	Cross-sectional outpatient clinic for osteoporosis	General Health Questionnaire	No association between depressive symptoms and BMD
8	Liu et al., 1998	8239 cases, age 66 or older	Hip fractures	Case-control study	Use of antidepressants	Greater incidence of falls and hip fractures in women with depression
9	Granek et al., 1987	184 'fallers' older than 65 living in long-term care, 184 controls	Odds of falling by drugs and medical conditions	Case-control study	Use of antidepressants	Depression and osteoarthritis are associated with increased risk of falling
10	Yaffe et al., 1999	8333 older women not on oestrogens	Calcaneal and hip BMD at baseline and follow-up	Prospective cohort, community dwelling	Geriatric depression scale – shortened, Cognitive evaluations	Correlation between cognition and BMD, adjustment for depression did not affect the correlation

Low rather than high body mass index is usually associated with low bone mineral density (Ravn *et al.*, 1999b); therefore, the finding of decreased bone mineral density in the subgroup of overweight or obese women is interesting and will be discussed below. The higher number of fractures observed in depressed women might have been explained in part by the greater propensity to fall observed in this group, although the reasons for this propensity were not clear. Adjustment for use of antidepressants or sedatives/hypnotics did not influence the association between depression and fracture. The authors suggested that falls in depressed women seemed to be related to unknown factors, such as poor adjustment to old age or others. They also speculated that the association between depression and osteoporosis might be limited to younger women and/or to more severe and long-lasting cases of depression. This study underscored the importance of depression as a risk factor for osteoporotic fractures, but did not find a clear association between bone mineral density and depression in elderly women.

In a series of male ($N = 35$) and female ($N = 33$) psychiatric inpatients (mean age 39±12 years; range 20–66 years of age) consecutively admitted for depression or other mental conditions, such as schizophrenia, mania, schizoaffective disorder, and adjustment disorders, depressed subjects had a significantly lower bone mineral density than age- and gender-matched controls (Halbreich *et al.*, 1995). In men there was a positive correlation between bone mineral density and testosterone whereas no correlation was observed in women between oestradiol plasma levels and bone mineral density at any site. In depressed subjects of both genders there was a negative correlation between plasma cortisol and bone mineral density. Finally, bone mineral density losses were worse in depressed men than in depressed women.

In a community study, women with osteoporosis had significantly higher levels of depressive symptomatology independent of other risk factors for osteoporosis, such as age or body mass index (Coelho *et al.*, 1999). In this study 102 Portuguese white women, aged 40–80 years, were selected by random digital dialing. General evaluations included clinical and reproductive history, medication use, physical activity, and dietary history. Depressive symptoms were evaluated by the Beck Depression Inventory, and a total score greater than 9, comprising cases of mild to severe depression, was used as the cut-off to define depression; in addition the Hopkins Symptom Checklist, a scale aimed at evaluating psychological distress, was administered. Bone mineral density was measured at the lumbar spine and femur by dual energy X-ray absorptiometry, and osteoporosis defined as a bone mineral density of less than 2.5 standard deviations below the young adult reference range at any of the measured sites. The prevalence of osteoporosis in this sample was 47%. When compared with the 54 women with normal bone mineral density, the 48 women with osteoporosis presented with a higher number of depressive episodes. The overall prevalence of depression in this random sample of women was surprisingly high at 65%, and depression was significantly more common in osteoporotic (77%), than in non-osteoporotic (54%), women. Specifically, the odds ratio favouring osteoporosis in depressed women was 2.9 (95% CI: 1.0–7.6). Osteoporotic women also had significantly higher mean values of the Beck Depression Inventory, even after adjusting for age and body mass index. No differences were found in the mean general well-being scores, suggesting that in these asymptomatic women with a densitometric diagnosis of osteoporosis, depression was not a consequence of pain or physical distress.

Depressive symptomatology, apart from depression itself, does not seem to be an independent risk factor for osteoporosis in postmenopausal women (Reginster *et al.*, 1999). Depressive symptoms, as assessed by the General Health Questionnaire (GHQ), an index of future vulnerability to depression, were not associated with changes in bone mineral density at the hip or spine in 121 postmenopausal women, 44–77 years old, spontaneously attending a screening visit for osteoporosis. This would suggest that osteoporosis is not associated with a depressive trait but with depression itself.

Psychotropic medications, falls and fractures

The use of certain classes of drugs, such as antidepressants and sedatives/hypnotics has been associated with a greater incidence of falls and fractures, especially in the elderly. Medications can increase the risk of falling by various mechanisms, such as inducing orthostatic hypotension and syncope, dizziness, vertigo, blurred vision, ataxia, sedation and other non-specific mechanisms. However, it is not clear whether the drugs prescribed for depression or the depression itself is the major contributor to falling and resultant fractures.

A case-control study, conducted in Canada, investigated the risk of hip fractures associated with the use of two widely used classes of antidepressants, tricyclics (TCAs) and selective serotonin-reuptake inhibitors (SSRIs) (Liu *et al.*, 1998). Patients were 66 years or older, and had been discharged from an acute care hospital with a hip fracture. Each patient was matched to five controls by age and gender. Comorbidity and risk of falls in the previous 3 years were determined by hospital records. 8239 cases were identified; 77.5% were women, and 39.8% were older than 85 years. Depression was approximately three times more common in patients who experienced hip fractures than in those who did not: 14.9% of the patients and 5.7% of the controls carried a diagnosis of depression. Of the cases, 6.6% had been exposed to SSRIs, 2.6% to secondary TCAs, and 9.0% to tertiary TCAs. Users of antidepressants had a greater risk of hip fractures than non-users. There was a consistent association between time of exposure and risk, i.e. current users had a higher risk than former users. After adjusting for confounding variables, the risk of hip fractures associated with current use of antidepressants was still greater, 2.4 for SSRIs, 2.2 for secondary amine TCAs, and 1.5 for tertiary amine TCAs. However, no relation between dose of antidepressants and risk of hip fracture was observed. This study suggested that in elderly people there is an association between hip fracture and the use of antidepressants. As no measurements of bone mineral density were obtained, it is unclear whether this finding reflected an association between osteoporosis and depression and, if so, whether osteoporosis would have been caused by depression or whether depression was the result of a debilitating fracture.

Another case-control study was conducted to ascertain the incidence of falls and correlating factors in residents of a long-term facility who were older than 65 years (Granek et al., 1987). A significant association between falls and medications was found and, in general, this association was related more to the drug prescribed than to the underlying condition for which the drug was prescribed. In addition, the use of three or more drugs increased the risk of falling. However, only two of the 12 diagnostic categories, depression and osteoarthritis, were consistently associated, across different therapeutic classes, with an increased risk of falling, suggesting an independent effect of these two medical conditions.

Psychotropic medications and bone mineral density

In addition to potentially impairing arousal and balance and thus increasing the risk of falls, many of the drugs prescribed in depression have potential effects on calcium metabolism and, possibly, bone mineral density. The contribution of these factors to the fractures that result from falls associated with use of these medications is however unclear.

Lithium carbonate, a drug used for bipolar and unipolar affective disorders or other mental conditions, may potentially affect bone mineral density by potentiating calcium-induced inhibition of parathyroid hormone (PTH) secretion via an intracellular post-calcium receptor mechanism, changing the set point of PTH secretion. Use of this drug has also been associated with secondary hyperparathyroidism. In a small, cross-sectional, study spine and hip bone mineral density were normal and no changes in calcium or PTH plasma levels were observed in 23 patients (5 men, 18 women) on lithium (average use 0.6–9.9 years) for various affective disorders. This suggests that there is no clear negative effect of lithium carbonate on bone mineral density in this population (Cohen et al., 1998). The only abnormality reported was an increase in the urinary excretion of hydroxyproline, suggesting an increased bone turnover.

Thyroid hormones have known negative effects on bone mineral density. Endocrinological studies have shown that thyroid stimulating hormone (TSH)-suppressive thyroxine treatment is associated with decreased bone mineral density. This hormone, and also triiodothyronine, are sometimes used in doses sufficient to suppress TSH as an adjunct treatment to antidepressive therapy in patients with major depression or rapid-cycling bipolar disorders. A small, cross-sectional study evaluated bone mineral density in 10 (nine premenopausal and one postmenopausal) women with bipolar disorder treated with thyroxine for a minimum of 18 months (82±83 months; mean±SD) (Gyulai et al., 1997). In this small series of patients, use of thyroxine was not associated with decreased bone mineral density at any site. This suggests that use of neither lithium nor thyroid hormone appears to be associated with decreased bone mineral density in a psychiatric setting.

Oestrogen levels are known for their effects in women on mood, cognitive function, and bone loss. In a study to test the hypothesis that there may be an association between bone mineral density and cognitive function, two markers of cumulative oestrogen exposure, calcaneal and hip bone mineral density were measured in 8333 non-demented women 65 years or older (Yaffe et al., 1999). Cognitive tests included a modified Mini-Mental State Exam, Trails B, and the Digit Symbol; prevalence of depression was measured by the Depression Scale–Shortened. Women with osteoporosis and fractures had poorer cognitive function and greater risk of cognitive deterioration. However, adjustment for depression score did not affect the association between bone mineral density and cognition in this sample of elderly women. This suggests that the association observed in younger women between depression and osteoporosis may be lost at an older age.

Psychiatric conditions and osteoporosis

Decreased bone mineral density has been reported in subjects affected by mental conditions other than depression, including anorexia nervosa and schizophrenia. This poses a question of specificity of the association between depression and osteoporosis, as psychiatric conditions share several risk factors of bone loss, including use of psychotropic medications, nutritional deficiencies or other lifestyle factors such as alcohol and drug abuse, smoking, excessive or inadequate physical activity.

Anorexia nervosa is a chronic illness that affects 1% of adolescent females, has high morbidity, and may be fatal in 10–15% of cases. Women with anorexia nervosa do not attain peak bone mass, have low bone mineral density and are, therefore, at high risk for osteoporotic fractures. The pathophysiology of low bone mass in anorexic women is multifactorial in nature and may include oestrogen deficiency, glucocorticoid excess, hyperprolactinaemia, reduced insulin growth factor-1 (IGF-1) levels, secondary hyperparathyroidism due to low calcium intake and vitamin D deficiency, protein-energy malnutrition, and intense exercise. Cortical bone in anorexic women is not easily regained upon improvement of body weight, and bone mineral density remains low several years after recovery (Rigotti et al., 1991). Oral contraceptives seem to exert some protection in terms of bone mass at the spine, but not at the hip.

The bone loss that is associated with anorexia nervosa shares several clinical features and pathogenetic mechanisms with depression-related osteoporosis. These include a greater prevalence in women and several common endocrine mechanisms, including hypogonadism and increased activity of the hypothalamic pituitary adrenal axis (Chrousos and Gold, 1992). However, bone loss in anorexia nervosa is more severe than in depression, which may be due both to the earlier age of onset in this condition that does not allow full achievement of bone peak mass and to the marked malnutrition of the former group of patients.

Bone loss in schizophrenic patients seems to be mainly due to 'non-specific' factors (Abraham et al., 1995). These include hyperprolactinaemia secondary to the use of neuroleptics, psychogenic polydipsia and negative life factors such as alcoholism, dietary deficiencies, immobility and lack of sunshine.

GLUCOCORTICOID-INDUCED OSTEOPOROSIS

Osteoporosis is a known consequence of chronic steroid use. The mechanism of bone loss in glucocorticoid-induced osteoporosis is probably similar to that observed in endogenous Cushing's syndrome and has relevance to depression-related osteoporosis. Thus, it is important to review the clinical features of bone loss in both forms of hypercortisolism.

Endogenous Cushing's syndrome

Harvey Cushing first recognized that endogenous hypercorticolism (Cushing's syndrome) caused osteoporosis. Hypercortisolism-induced bone loss seems to be caused primarily by decreased bone formation; the relative contribution of increased bone resorption is currently not known. The bone loss is more marked in trabecular than in cortical bone, and frequently leads to fractures at various sites (Hermus et al., 1995). The degree of bone loss correlates with the severity and the duration of Cushing's syndrome, rather than the underlying cause of Cushing's syndrome, including the factitious form of the condition, provided the condition is sufficiently severe (Cizza et al., 1996). This bone loss is only partially reversible once the disease is cured and the process may take many years. The recovery of the bone is better in younger than in older patients.

In a series of 20 patients with Cushing's syndrome, the majority had osteoporosis associated with their condition, and similar bone loss was observed at the spine and femoral neck (Hermus et al., 1995). No improvements in bone mineral density were observed up to 6 months after curative surgery. From 6 months onward bone mineral density increased; however, in most patients it did not reach normal values, even at the last measurement (follow-up duration 18–60 months). As early as 3 months after curative surgery, osteocalcin levels increased, suggesting an activation of osteoblastic activity. Interestingly, in women with depression bone loss was more accentuated at the hip than at the spine compared with the bone loss observed in Cushing's syndrome (Michelson *et al.*, 1996).

Endogenous hypercortisolism is particularly deleterious to the bone during the period of bone accretion, as indicated by a longitudinal study conducted in two identical twin girls, one of whom was diagnosed at 14 years of age with an ACTH-secreting pituitary adenoma (Leong *et al.*, 1996). The affected twin had very low bone mineral density (–3.2 SD at the lumbar spine), as well as decreased osteocalcin and pyrimidine crosslink levels. Surgical cure led to an increase in bone formation, as indicated by increased osteocalcin levels. However, more than 2 years after surgery, bone mineral density, although markedly improved in the affected twin, was still low (–1.9 SD). In addition, the final height of the affected twin was 21 cm less than that of her identical twin. The affected twin had delayed puberty associated with suppressed gonadotrophin and oestradiol secretion, and changes in body composition such as a decrease in lean mass and an increase in fat mass.

Bone loss in Cushing's syndrome can be restored by specific anti-osteoporotic treatments. Treatment with alendronate, a potent bisphosphonate that inhibits bone resorption, improved bone mineral density at the spine and hip in patients with active Cushing's syndrome (Di Somma *et al.*, 1998). In a prospective, open-label, uncontrolled study, 39 consecutive patients with Cushing's syndrome (18 women, 21 men; 29–51 years old) underwent selective adenomectomy. Cured patients ($N = 21$) were randomly allocated to treatment with alendronate 10 mg daily or no treatment; non-cured patients ($N = 18$) were randomly allocated to either ketoconazole (200–600 mg) ($N = 8$), an inhibitor of the adrenal steroidogenesis, or to ketoconazole plus alendronate 10 mg/day ($N = 10$). At study entry, bone mineral density was lower at the spine and hip in all Cushing's patients than in age- and body mass index-matched healthy comparison subjects. Nine patients with Cushing's syndrome were osteoporotic and 20 patients were osteopenic. Treatment with alendronate for 12 months increased bone mineral density both in patients with cured disease and in patients with active disease by approximately 1.7% and 2.4% at the spine, and 1.2% and 1.8% at the hip, respectively. No improvements in bone mineral density were observed in the patients with active disease who received only ketoconazole.

Exogenous Cushing's syndrome

Bone loss is often observed in patients that receive long-term pharmacological therapy with glucocorticoids for various reasons. A 48-week, randomized, double-blind, placebo-controlled study of alendronate in 477 men and women, 17–83 years of age, receiving glucocorticoid therapy for various underlying diseases, was published recently (Saag *et al.*, 1998). Patients requiring long-term (at least one year) use of 7.5 mg or more of prednisone or its equivalent, were followed for 48 weeks after randomization to daily placebo or three different doses (2.5, 5, or 10 mg) of daily alendronate. In addition, all patients received 800–1000 mg of elemental calcium, and 250–500 IU of vitamin D daily. At baseline, a substantial proportion of patients, 32%, had osteoporosis and approximately 16% of subjects had incident vertebral fractures. Treatment with alendronate significantly increased bone mineral density in this population; mean bone mineral density at the lumbar spine increased after 48 weeks of treatment by $2.9\pm0.3\%$ in the alendronate 10 mg group and decreased by $0.4\pm0.3\%$ in the placebo group.

In a study with a smaller number of subjects with glucocorticoid-induced osteoporosis, another bisphosphonate, etidronate was employed (Adachi *et al.*, 1997). Oral etidronate was given to 141 men and women for a total period of 12 months intermittently (400 mg/day for 14 days), followed by calcium (500 mg/day for 76 days) for four cycles. Spine and hip bone mineral density did not change after 52 weeks of treatment in etidronate-treated subjects, whereas they declined in the placebo group. Finally, there was an 85% decrease in the population of postmenopausal women with new vertebral fractures in the etidronate group.

Elevated cortisol levels may affect calcium metabolism by various mechanisms: decreased calcium absorption, increased calcium excretion, or transient hypocalcaemia, all of which may trigger secondary hyperparathyroidism. The conversion of vitamin D to its more active metabolites is also affected, which may result in further impairment of intestinal calcium absorption. Calcium and vitamin D are an effective preventive treatment of glucocorticoid-induced osteoporosis. 103 patients starting corticosteroid therapy were randomly assigned to receive calcium 1000 mg/day and either calcitriol (0.5–1 g/day orally) plus salmon calcitonin (400 IU/day intranasally), or calcitriol plus a placebo nasal spray, or double placebo for one year (Sambrook *et al.*, 1993). Calcitriol with or without calcitonin prevented more bone loss from the lumbar spine than calcium alone. However, bone loss at the femoral neck and distal radius was not significantly affected by any treatment.

Finally, it is worth noting that the rate of bone loss in placebo-treated patients in some clinical trials of glucocorticoid-induced osteoporosis was somewhat less severe than what would have been expected based upon the clinical course of bone loss in endogenous hypercortisolism. Potential explanatory factors may include a 'clinical trial' effect, as calcium and vitamin D supplementation are usually administered in controlled trials together with the study drug, as well as some other unexplained factors, possibly related to a true placebo effect. This may be particularly relevant to depression, as controlled clinical trials conducted in depressed subjects are often characterized by a greater placebo effect than that observed in other groups of patients.

POTENTIAL MECHANISMS OF BONE LOSS IN DEPRESSION

As discussed previously, one of the mechanisms by which bone loss occurs in depression is hypercortisolism. This, as well as other mechanisms, appear to be the result of a dysregulation of the corticotrophin-releasing hormone (CRH) system, and hence the HPA axis. This dysregulation, in addition to bone loss may also be responsible for the other somatic consequences of depression, including insulin resistance and complications of accelerated atherosclerosis (Figure 1). As this topic has been reviewed recently, a brief summary as well as some critical comments will be included here (Chrousos and Gold, 1992).

Depression-induced CRH hypersecretion and hypercortisolism lead to inhibition of the reproductive axis and hypogonadism. The latter is an established

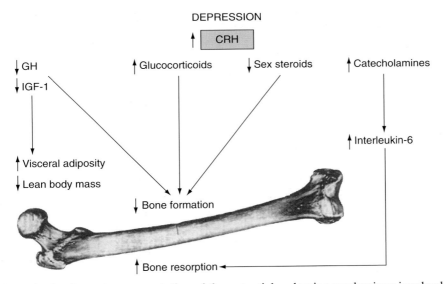

Figure 1. A schematic representation of the potential endocrine mechanisms involved in the bone loss that is associated with depression. Depression is associated with an hypersecretion of corticotrophin-releasing hormone (CRH) and of the hypothalamic–pituitary–adrenal (HPA) axis. Increased cortisol, decreased growth hormone (GH) and IGF-1, and decreased sex steroids result in decreased bone formation. Increased catecholamine levels stimulate the production of IL-6, a potent bone-resorption factor. The concurrent effect of increased bone formation and decreased bone resorption results in net bone loss and, eventually, osteoporosis and fractures in depressed subjects. In addition, decreased GH, increased cortisol, and decreased sex steroids are a risk factor for accumulation of visceral adipose tissue and decreased lean body mass. Similarly, subjects with Cushing's syndrome who have elevated cortisol levels and decreased GH and sex steroids, have characteristically increased visceral adiposity and a loss in lean body mass.

risk factor for bone loss in both genders. In addition, CRH hypersecretion and hypercortisolism cause decreased activity of the growth hormone/IGF-1 axis, an important stimulator of bone formation. Increased sympathetic activity, a corollary of CRH hypersecretion, is associated with increased interleukin-6 (IL-6) secretion. In depression, a dysfunction of several inflammatory mediators has been reported, and IL-6 may be implicated in the long-term medical consequences of major depression, including cardiovascular disease and osteoporosis (Licinio and Wong, 1999). Indeed, this cytokine, a major mediator of bone resorption, is elevated in depressed subjects, especially at an older age, in cross-sectional studies (Dentino et al., 1999).

Finally, both major depression and osteoporosis are likely to be associated with multiple genes. Recently it was proposed that genes involved in the regulation of phospholipids may be associated with both conditions (Horrobin and Bennett, 1999). Whether depression and osteoporosis share a common genetic predisposition, mediated by a common genetic set-up, remains to be determined.

CONCLUSIONS

The studies summarized are important because for the first time they covered the existence of a strong association between depression and osteoporosis. It is, however, important to note some of their limitations; most studies were cross-sectional in design and, as such, could only establish the existence of an association, rather than a causal link, between depression and osteoporosis. Different instruments were used to make the diagnosis of depression and to assess its severity. This factor may have contributed to the wide range of prevalence of depression reported and to some of the divergent results on the comorbidity of depression and osteoporosis. In several studies, actively depressed subjects were pooled together with subjects who only carried a history of depression. Retrospective evaluation of history of depression has limited reliability when it is based solely upon subject recollection, a factor that may have introduced a bias. Finally, many studies were small and the populations studied heterogeneous. In summary, according to the literature reviewed, there seems to be an undisputed association between depression and osteoporosis; however, this association was reported only at a younger, but not at an older, age, and mostly in women.

Although the influence of ageing on the hypothalamic–pituitary–adrenal axis is controversial, there is a consensus for progressively decreasing sensitivity to glucocorticoid negative feedback in elderly healthy subjects (Pavlov et al., 1986). The interactive net effect of ageing and repeated episodes of depression over a lifetime is not known. We hypothesize that in elderly subjects, depression does not always trigger hypercortisolism, and/or that with ageing, a different phenotype of depression, atypical depression, associated with hypocortisolism rather than with hypercortisolism, becomes more prevalent. Compatible with this hypothesis is the finding that ageing in the rat is associated with decreased activity and responsiveness of the HPA axis, which is mediated at the level of the hypothalamus and higher nervous structures (Cizza *et al.*, 1994).

The nature of the relation between depression and osteoporosis is known only in part. Summarized here is a list of questions that should be posed in future studies to determine whether there is a causal link between depression and osteoporosis and, if so, whether bone loss occurs only when a patient is actively depressed, as compared with when she or he is in clinical remission. In addition, it should be established whether successful treatment of depression has an impact on bone loss. Furthermore, the exact prevalence of osteoporosis in depressed subjects should be determined, and the subgroups of depressed subjects at higher risk for osteoporosis should be identified. More research is needed to understand the putative role of depression in osteoporosis in men, a condition poorly understood, and labeled as 'idiopathic' in approximately one-third of subjects. At a mechanistic level, it will be crucial to understand the specific role of the endocrine and paracrine factors responsible for bone loss in depression and the relative contribution of decreased bone formation and increased bone resorption to bone loss in depression. Such knowledge should guide therapeutic interventions aimed at restoring bone loss and preventing fractures. More genetic research is needed to establish how much of the individual variance in bone mass is due to hereditary factors and to identify which gene(s) are involved. Only prospective, long-term studies with sufficient statistical power will be able to answer some of these questions, and allow insight into the natural history of bone loss in depression, which remains largely unknown.

In conclusion, there is enough evidence to claim that depression is a risk factor for osteoporosis and, possibly, bone fractures. Therefore, the clinical work-up of subjects with idiopathic osteopaenia and osteoporosis should include an evaluation for depression, especially if there are no other obvious causes for the low bone mineral density, or if the subject is a premenopausal woman or a young or middle aged man. Conversely, a history of non-traumatic fractures in a depressed subject should alert the physician to the possibility of undiagnosed osteoporosis.

REFERENCES

Abraham, G., Friedman, R.H., Verhese, C. and de Leon, J. (1995). Osteoporosis and schizophrenia: can we limit known risk factors? *Biol Psychiatry* **38**, 131–132.

Adachi, J.D., Bensen, W.G., Brown, J. *et al.* (1997). Intermittent etidronate therapy to prevent corticosteroid-induced osteoporosis. *New Engl J Med* **337**, 382–387.

Chrousos G.P. and Gold P.W. (1992). The concept of stress and stress system disorders. *JAMA* **267**, 1244–1252.

Chrousos, G.P. and Gold, P.W. (1998). A healthy body in a healthy mind and vice versa: the damaging power of 'uncontrollable' stress. *J Clin Endocrinol Metab* **83**, 1842–1845.

Cizza, G., Calogero, A.E., Brady, L.S. *et al.* (1994). Male 344 Fischer rats show a progressive central impairment of the hypothalamic-pituitary-adrenal axis with advancing age. *Endocrinology* **134**, 1611–1620.

Cizza, G,. Nieman, L., Doppman, J. *et al.* (1996). Factitious Cushing's syndrome. *J Clin Endocrinol Metab* **81**, 3573–3577.

Coelho, R., Silva, C., Maja, A., Prata, J. and Barros, H. (1999). Bone mineral density and depression: a community study in women. *J Psychosom Res* **46**, 29–35.

Cohen, O., Rais, T., Lepkifker, E. and Vered, I. (1998). Lithium carbonate therapy is not a risk factor for osteoporosis. *Horm Metab Res* **30**, 594–597.

Dentino, A.N., Pieper, C.F., Rao, M.K. *et al.* (1999). Association of interleukin-6 and other biological variables with depression in older people living in the community. *J Am Geriat Soc* **47**, 6–11.

Di Somma, C., Colao, A., Pivonello, R. *et al.* (1998). Effectiveness of chronic treatment with alendronate in the osteoporosis of Cushing's disease. *Clin Endocrinol* **48**, 655–662.

Genco, R.J. (1999). Relationship of stress, distress and inadequate coping behaviors to periodontal disease. *J Periodontol* **70**, 711–723.

Granek, E., Baker, P.S., Abbey, H. *et al.* (1987). Medications and diagnoses in relation to falls in a long-term care facility. *J Am Geriatr Soc* **35**, 503–511.

Gyulai, L., Jaggi, J., Bauer, M.S. *et al.* (1997). Bone mineral density and L-thyroxine treatment in rapidly cycling bipolar disorder. *Biol Psychiatry* **41**, 503–506.

Halbreich, U., Rojansky, N., Palter, S. *et al.* (1995). Decreased bone mineral density in medicated psychiatric patients. *Psychosom Med* **57**, 485–491.

Hermus, A.D., Smals, A.G., Swinkdels, L.M. *et al.* (1995). Bone mineral density and bone turnover before and after surgical cure of Cushing's syndrome. *J Clin Endocrinol Metab* **80**, 2859–2865.

Hooper, M.B. (1998). Bone density measurements in major depression. *Neuropsychophar Biol Psychiatry* **22**, 267–277.

Horrobin, D.F. and Bennett, C.N. (1999). Depression and bipolar disorder: relationships to impaired fatty acid and phospolipids metabolism and to diabetes, cardiovascular disease, immunological abnormalities, cancer ageing, and osteoporosis. *Prostag Leukotr Ess* **60**, 217–234.

Leong, G.M., Leilani, M., Mercado-Asis, L.B. *et al.* (1996). The effect of Cushing's syndrome on bone mineral density, body composition, growth, and puberty: a report of an identical adolescent twin pair. *J Clin Endocrinol Metab* **81**, 1905–1911.

Licinio, J. and Wong, M.L. (1999). The role of inflammatory mediators in the biology of major depression: central nervous system cytokines modulate the biological substrate of depressive symptoms, regulate stress-responsive systems, and contribute to neurotoxicity and neuroprotection. *Mol Psychiatry* **4**, 317–327.

Liu, B., Anderson, G., Mittman, N. *et al.* (1998). Use of selective serotonin-reuptake inhibitors or tricyclic antidepressants and risk of hip fractures in elderly people. *Lancet* **351**, 1303–1307.

Michelson, D., Stratakis, C., Hill, L. *et al.* (1996). Bone mineral density in women with depression. *New Engl J Med* **335**, 1176–1181.

Pavlov, E.P., Harman, S.M., Chrousos, G.P., Loriaux, D.L. and Blackman, M.R. (1986). Responses of plasma ACTH, cortisol, and dehydroepiandrosterone to ovine CRH in healthy men. *J Clin Endocrinol Metab* **62**, 767–772.

Ravn, P., Bidstrup, M., Wasnich, M. *et al.* (1999a). Alendronate and estrogen-progestin in the long-term prevention of bone loss: four-year results from the early postmenopausal intervention cohort. *Ann Intern Med* **131**, 935–942.

Ravn, P., Cizza, G., Bjarnason, N.H. *et al.* (1999b). Low body mass index is an important risk factor for low bone mass and increased bone loss in early postmenopausal women. Early Postmenopausal Intervention Cohort (EPIC) study group. *J Bone Miner Res* **14**, 1622–1627.

Reginster, J.Y., Deroisy, R., Paul, I., Hansenne, M. and Ansseau, M. (1999). Depressive vulnerability is not an independent risk factor for osteoporosis in postmenopausal women. *Maturitas* **33**, 133–137.

Riggotti, N.A., Neer, R.M., Skates, S.J., Herzog, D.B. and Nussbaum, S.R. (1991). The clinical course of osteoporosis in anorexia nervosa. *JAMA* **265**, 1133–1138.

Robbins, L.N., Helzer, J.E., Weissman, M.M. *et al.* (1984) Lifetime prevalence of specific psychiatry disorders in three sites. *Arch Gen Psychiatry* **41**, 949–958.

Saag, K.G., Emkey, R., Schitzer, T.J. *et al.* (1998). Alendronate for the prevention and treatment of glucocorticoid-induced osteoporosis. *New Engl J Med* **339**, 292–299.

Sambrook, P., Birmingham, J., Kelly, P. *et al.* (1993). Prevention of corticosteroid osteoporosis, a comparison of calcium, calcitriol, and calcitonin. *New Engl J Med* **328**, 1747–1752.

Schweiger, U., Deuschle, M., Korner, A. *et al.* (1994). Low lumbar bone mineral density in patients with major depression. *Am J Psychiatry* **151**, 1691–1693.

Schweiger, U., Weber, B., Deuschle, M. and Heuser, I. (2000). Lumbar bone mineral density in patients with major depression: evidence of increased bone loss at follow-up. *Am J Psychiatry* **157**, 118–120.

Whooley, M.A., Kip, P.E., Cauley, J.A. *et al.* (1999). Depression, falls and risk of fracture in older women. *Arch Int Med* **159**, 484–490.

Yaffe, K., Browner, W., Cauley, J., Launer, L. and Harris, T. (1999). Association between bone mineral density and cognitive decline in older women. *J Am Geriatr Soc* **47**, 1176–1182.

Zheng, D., Macera, C.A., Croft, J.B. *et al.* (1997). Major depression and all-cause mortality among white adults in the United States. *Ann Epidemiol* **7**, 213–218.

7

Depression and Cardiovascular Disease

MICHAEL DEUSCHLE

Central Institute of Mental Health, Mannheim, Germany

INTRODUCTION

In most European languages a 'broken heart' is synonymous with bereavement and grief. This semantic association implies knowledge about a relationship between disordered mood and heart function. However, only recently has systematic research uncovered a bidirectional relationship between these conditions: not only does depression precede cardiovascular disease and serves as a negative predictor for the prognosis of manifest heart disease, but vascular disease also represents a risk factor for late-onset depression. Thus far, there is only very limited knowledge about the pathophysiological links between these conditions. This chapter will summarize existing knowledge regarding the comorbidity of depression and cardiovascular disease.

DOES DEPRESSION PRECEDE HEART DISEASE?

Early in the first half of the 20th century Malzberg described increased cardiac mortality in hospitalized patients with 'involutional' depression compared with the general population (Malzberg, 1937). However, due to the nature of this study, i.e. comparing the mortality rate among hospitalized patients with that of the general population, it remained unclear whether this association could be attributed to an effect of the psychiatric condition or rather, was due to hospitalization and treatment. Generally, studies based on clinical populations may give clues to causes of excess mortality in a specific group of, usually hospitalized, patients (for example see Black *et al.*, 1985; 1987; Rabins *et al.*, 1985). However, effects of hospitalization and, later on, of pharmacological treatment may confound comparisons between patients with affective disorder and psychiatrically healthy controls.

Clearly, community-based prospective studies were needed to test whether psychiatric illness puts people at an increased cardiac risk. The 1950s and 1960s, however, saw no work in this area of research. Instead, psychiatric research was dominated by psychoanalytical theories and, in this context, the 'type A personality' was related to cardiac death. In the meantime, heart disease became a major target of epidemiological studies and several identified risk behaviours and factors were the focus of health programmes. Today, ischaemic heart disease still represents the most important cause of death in adults and the three–year mortality of patients hospitalized for acute myocardial infarction (MI) remains at around 25% (McGovern et al., 1996). After Malzberg's pioneering study, it took another 50 years before adequate prospective trials were published which, again, supported the idea that affective disorders might play a significant role in the development of cardiovascular disease.

In the majority of these studies several symptoms of depression were independently associated with an increased risk for fatal and non-fatal heart disease, even after controlling for socioeconomic status and traditional cardiovascular risk factors. Usually, these studies did not include patients with pre-existing heart disease. The vast majority of depressed subjects in these studies did not receive antidepressive medication making any bias due to medication seem highly unlikely. Furthermore, studying community-based instead of institution-based populations in a prospective manner shifted the focus from severe to mild subtypes of affective disorders. Since most of these studies included rather large numbers of population-based subjects, selection biases could be excluded. Table 1 summarizes prospective studies employing the most rigorous methods, especially controlling for traditional risk factors for cardiovascular disease.

Major milestones in this series of large-scale community-based prospective studies were the National Health Examination Follow-up Study (Anda et al., 1993), the Kuopio Ischemic Heart Disease Study (Everson et al., 1996) as well as the Glostrup Study (Barefoot and Schroll, 1996). Altogether some 10 000 subjects were included in these observations with follow-up periods from 2 years to several decades. All of these studies controlled for the major risk factors of cardiovascular disease. Finally, all but one study with a remarkably low age (Vogt et al., 1994), found good evidence for depressive symptoms to be related to future cardiac disease.

In most of these studies, symptoms of depression were measured with instruments that ascertain the number of self-reported depressive symptoms present during the past week. Of course, these subjective measures may vary from week to week and are not comparable to an objective, categorical clinical diagnosis in terms of severity and duration. These facts, however, do not diminish the significance of the reported data. Clearly, a degree of depression less than that necessary for the diagnosis of major depression can also influence human health (Johnson et al., 1992). Moreover, these studies prove that even mild forms of depression will put people at increased risk of cardiac disease. It appears that even minor variations of mood may possibly make a subject vulnerable to coronary artery disease. In line with this observation, in a recent editorial, Appels remarked that DSM-defined depression obviously has a shorter predictive power than self-rated depression regarding subsequent heart disease (Appels, 1997). As Booth-Kewley and Friedman (1987) concluded from their meta-analysis, the coronary prone person, instead of being a 'type A personality' workaholic is more likely to be a person with negative emotions: depressed, aggressively competitive, easily frustrated, anxious and angry. Obviously, clinical depression is not necessary, although some studies found severity of depressive symptoms to be predictive for cardiac health (Wassertheil-Smoller et al., 1996).

But, what about clinical depression? The above-mentioned prospective aetiological studies were based on depressive symptoms rather than clinical depression. As shown in Table 1 quite different factors such as hopelessness, vital exhaustion, worrying and so on were related to and, possibly, contribute to the noted cardiovascular risk. The disadvantage of low specificity associated with these studies was to some degree outweighed by the large number of subjects included. However, the question of whether in addition to depressive symptoms, clinical depression is related to future heart disease remained unanswered. Some groups attempted to focus on clinical depression, which, of course, is not an easy endeavour regarding the necessary number of cases. Yet, several studies were based on clinical interviews carried out by trained nurses, general physicians or psychiatrists. Increased rates of fatal and non-fatal cardiac events clearly showed that, in addition to depressive symptoms, subjects with a clinical diagnosis of depression are at high risk for cardiac disease (Murphy et al., 1989; Aromaa et al., 1994; Ford et al., 1998; see also Table 1).

At this point, it should also briefly be mentioned that, unlike heart disease, there is only limited evidence that depression might also be a precipitating condition for the occurence of a stroke. However, there are some data in support of this hypothesis, such as the findings by Colantonio and colleagues (1992), who followed up 2812 elderly individuals and were able to show that frequently depressive symptoms, as measured by the CES-D scale, preceded future stroke.

There are several pitfalls that have to be considered with regard to the above-mentioned studies. First, depressed subjects may be more likely to complain about physical symptoms, i.e. chest pain, in the absence of coronary artery disease. Therefore, it is imperative to rely on 'hard' outcome measures such as documented myocardial infarction, which was the case in most of the studies summarized in Table 1. Secondly, both depression and heart disease may lead to similar symptoms, such as tiredness or feelings of weakness, so that subclinical heart disease may be mistaken for depressive symptomatology. It is possible to address this problem by excluding all coronary events occurring soon after baseline, as has been done by the groups led by Anda

Table 1. Large scale, community-based prospective studies to assess depression as a risk factor for cardiovascular disease.

Study	Sample size	Prognostic factors	Follow-up (years)	Endpoint	Relative risk
Prospective aetiological studies: based on symptoms of depression					
Hälström et al., 1986	795	Depression symptoms	12	AP	OR = 5.4
Hagman et al., 1987	5735	Anxiety ('stress')	2–7	AP	Strong predictor for angina
Haines et al., 1987	1457	Phobic anxiety	10	Cardiac death	OR = 3.77
Appels et al., 1993	3877	'Vital exhaustion'	4.2	Unstable AP	OR = 1.86
Anda et al., 1993	2832	Depression symptoms	12	Cardiac death	OR = 1.5
Vogt et al., 1994	2573	Depression symptoms	15	Stroke, CHD, hypertension	OR = 1.37 (hypertension)
Kawachi et al., 1994	33999	Phobic anxiety	2	Cardiac death	OR = 6.08
Everson et al., 1996	2428	Hopelessness	6	Non-fatal MI	OR = 2.05
Barefoot and Schroll, 1996	730	Depression symptoms	25	Non fatal MI	OR = 1.7 (2 SD increase in scale-D)
Wassertheil-Smoller et al., 1996	4367	Depression symptoms	4.5	Non-fatal MI	OR = 1.18 (per 5 units of CES-D)
Kubzansky et al., 1997	1759	Worrying	20	MI	OR = 2.41 (for 'high worries')
Jonas et al., 1997	2992	General well-being	7–19	Hypertension	OR = 1.82 (anxiety); OR = 1.80 (depression)

Prospective aetiological studies: based on clinical depression

Study	Sample	Follow-up	Measure	Outcome	OR
Murphy et al., 1989	1003	16	Depression	Circulatory death	OR = 2.1 (males); OR = 1.2 (females)
Aromaa et al., 1994	5355	6.6	Depression	Cardiac death	OR = 3.36
Pratt et al., 1996	1551	13	Depression	MI	OR = 4.54
Ford et al., 1998	1190	40	Depression	CHD, MI	OR = 2.12 (CHD); OR = 2.12 (MI)

Prognostic studies in patients with pre-existing heart disease

Study	Sample	Follow-up	Measure	Outcome	OR
Carney et al., 1988a, b	52 pts after angiography	1	Depression, DIS	Major cardiac events	OR = 2.2
Ahern et al., 1990	353	12	Depression	Cardiac death	OR = 1.3
Kop et al., 1994	127 pts after angioplasty	1.5	Vital exhaustion questionnaire	Major cardiac events	OR = 2.34
Ladwig et al., 1994	377 post-MI pts	0.5	Depression	AP	OR = 2.31
Frasure-Smith et al., 1995	222 post-MI pts	1.5	Depression	All-death mortality	OR = 6.64
Denollet et al., 1996	303 CHD pts	8	Type D personality	Cardiac death	OR = 4.1
Kaufmann et al., 1999	331 post-MI pts	1	Depression	All-death mortality	OR = 2.33

DIS, Diagnostic Interview Schedule; AP, angina pectoris; CHD, coronary heart disease; MI, myocardial infarction.

and Barefoot (Anda *et al.*, 1993; Barefoot and Schroll, 1996). Thirdly, 'vital exhaustion' is known to precede myocardial infarction, but its risk declines over time (Appels and Mulder 1989; Appels *et al.*, 1993; Kop *et al.*, 1994). Therefore, the depressive cluster should exclude symptoms of exhaustion, such as fatigue and irritability.

In a synopsis of the aforementioned studies, however, there is little doubt that depression may precede heart disease in a high proportion of depressed subjects. Of course, if depression in fact does present a risk factor for heart disease, it should also change the course of pre-existing heart disease.

DOES DEPRESSION CHANGE THE COURSE OF HEART DISEASE?

As summarized above, there is considerable evidence from epidemiological studies that depression precedes heart disease. However, since most of these population-based studies followed up physically healthy subjects, they do not allow us to draw any conclusions on whether depression changes the course of pre-existing heart disease. Only a few studies have been done in order to help clinicians anticipate coronary patients' outcome based on their psychiatric status. Interestingly, for a variety of chronic diseases it became increasingly clear that the additional diagnosis of depression further worsens the prognosis. Several authors found that among patients with a greater number of chronic medical conditions, outcomes were poorer for depressed patients (Moos, 1990; Swindle *et al.*, 1990).

Could depression impair the prognosis of patients with heart disease in a similar way? This question is especially important since a substantial proportion of post-infarction patients (Carney *et al.*, 1987; Schleifer *et al.*, 1989; Frasure-Smith *et al.*, 1993) and patients with coronary artery disease (Carney *et al.*, 1988b; Gonzalez *et al.*, 1996), as much as 15–23%, also suffer from major depression. Nearly every second post-MI patient and every third patient with coronary bypass grafting (McKhann *et al.*, 1997) suffers from depression, when minor forms of depressive disorders are included (Schleifer *et al.*, 1989). The mental state in post-MI depression has repeatedly been described to differ from depressed patients in psychiatric populations. Rather than negative images of the self and guilt, exhaustion and loss of energy are the predominant symptoms. In fact, a large proportion of patients were already depressed (8–16%; Lesperance *et al.*, 1996) or exhausted before the MI. Both of the aforementioned pre-MI conditions are significantly related to a subsequent high level of depression (Ladwig *et al.*, 1992). Furthermore, a prior history of depression is found in up to 44% of all patients with newly diagnosed coronary disease (Freedland *et al.*, 1992) and, similar to a post-MI depressive episode, is of prognostic value for the course of the heart disease (Frasure-Smith *et al.*, 1995). Is it possible that these affective syndromes change the prognosis of heart disease?

It is well documented that psychological distress in patients with a major cardiac event, as evidenced by high scores on symptom checklists, leads to a significantly increased rate of recurrence, especially of myocardial infarction within a six-month follow-up (Allison *et al.*, 1995). The same holds true for anxiety in the hours immediately following myocardial infarction. Those patients with high anxiety levels suffer more complications during follow-up than those with low anxiety (Moser and Dracup, 1996). Depression, conceptualized as a 'stress disorder' by many psychiatrists, may similarily lead to an increased risk in post-MI patients. In 1250 patients with established coronary artery disease self-rated severity of symptoms of depression were associated with increased risk of cardiac death within a follow-up ranging up to 20 years (Barefoot *et al.*, 1996). Similarly, Denollet and colleagues studied the cardiac prognosis for a distressed personality type, characterized by experiencing distress and by inhibited expression of emotions. This cluster of enduring personality traits significantly increased the mortality risk of patients during a two- to five–year follow-up after myocardial infarction (Denollet *et al.*, 1995) as well as in a six- to 10-year follow-up in patients with coronary heart disease (Denollet *et al.*, 1996). Thus, there is at the least evidence that acute stress and 'depressed personality' negatively affect the prognosis of heart disease.

However, not only 'stress' and 'traits of depression', but also clinical depression is known to be related to increased risk in cardiac patients. Frasure-Smith and colleagues performed milestone studies in patients with acute myocardial infarction. In 896 patients they found 50% of female patients and 25% of male patients to have significant depression scores in the first weeks after myocardial infarction. After a one-year follow-up, depressed patients had a significantly increased risk of cardiac death (odds ratio (OR) 3.23), arrhythmic events (OR: 3.11) and recurrent myocardial infarction (OR: 1.62), even after controlling for other post-MI risks (Frasure-Smith *et al.*, 1993; 1999). These findings were recently confirmed in an independent sample. Following up 331 patients with acute myocardial infarction, depression significantly predicted mortality within a 12-month follow-up period (Kaufmann *et al.*, 1999). Additionally, the Cardiac Arrhythmia Pilot Study showed self-rated depression to be related to death or cardiac arrest after acute myocardial infarction (Ahern *et al.*, 1990). Similarly, severe levels of post-MI depressive symptoms were found to be related to an increased risk of angina pectoris (OR: 2.31) in a six-month follow-up of 377 patients (Ladwig *et al.*, 1994). In a group of 52 patients with coronary artery disease as confirmed by angiography, the presence of a major depressive episode was related to an increased risk of a major cardiac event during a one-year follow-up, such as infarction, death, bypass surgery or angioplasty (Carney *et al.*, 1988a). What holds true in the months immediately following an infarction is also valid in the long run: the severity of depressive symptoms predicted incidence of angina in a 12-year follow-up of 795 females

(Hällström *et al.*, 1986). However, depression is related not only to impaired cardiac prognosis of patients with heart disease. It also leads to clinically significant functional disability and impaired self-maintenance in patients with coronary artery disease (Steffens *et al.*, 1999).

It seems that depression after myocardial infarction bears the same risk for cardiac death as heart failure, the strongest medical predictor of mortality after a heart attack. Thus, the relationship between affective disorders and heart disease has a second component. Not only does depression render patients prone to heart disease, but depression also is related to increased mortality in patients with manifest heart disease. Data for the second component are especially clear for post-MI patients. It should be mentioned that similar to what we have learned about coronary heart disease, depressive syndromes associated with stroke also modifies the health risks following the acute event. Accordingly, patients with post-stroke depression have a three-fold increased mortality rate within 10 years of follow-up compared with their non-depressed counterparts (Morris *et al.*, 1993).

Of course, the nature of the reviewed data does not fully explain the causal relationship between the associated disorders, depression and cardiovascular disease. Within this context, the following hypotheses seem possible: (a) depression may be a risk factor for cardiovascular disease by affecting behaviour related to cardiovascular health or by more directly influencing cardiovascular regulation; (b) cardiovascular disease may cause depressive symptoms and even clinical depression; (c) associations of depression and cardiovascular disease may be due either to common causes or to other reasons for the clustering of chronic diseases in the population.

These questions indicate that discovering an association between two conditions is not sufficient to provide clinicians with useful advice on how to improve treatment. Step by step we will have to work through possible factors mediating the relationship between the disorders. It is important to differentiate between 'classic' risk factors and 'non-classic' risk factors for heart disease, which may be differentially affected by psychiatric conditions. 'Classic' risk factors, such as hypertension, smoking, diabetes or dyslipidaemia, of course, may not fully explain the increased cardiovascular risk of depressed patients. It is safe to assume that in the end no single factor will be found to be responsible for the increased cardiac risk in depression.

CLASSIC RISK FACTORS

Blood pressure

Life circumstances and stress may affect blood pressure and cardiovascular morbidity. This has been illustrated elegantly by a 30-year follow-up study of 144 Italian nuns and a group of control subjects, matched for other risk factors (Timio *et al.*, 1997). During the observation period, the group of lay women, but not the group of nuns living in secluded order, showed the expected age-associated increase in diastolic blood pressure, which was associated with an elevated number of fatal and non-fatal cardiac events. The same may hold true for anxiety and depression, which in epidemiological studies have been shown to be independently predictive for the development of hypertension (Markovitz *et al.*, 1993; Jonas *et al.*, 1997). In several large-scale studies of psychiatric populations, depression and anxiety were found to be related to an increased risk of comorbid arterial hypertension (Friedman and Bennet, 1977; Rabkin *et al.*, 1983; Mezzich *et al.*, 1987).

Thus far, it has been difficult to show depressed patients, as a group, to suffer from increased blood pressure. However, independent of age, hypertension is more frequent among depressed dexamethasone nonsuppressors than among depressed suppressors (Pfohl *et al.*, 1991). Similar to Cushing's disease, it might be expected that patients with hypercortisolaemic depression, in particular, suffer from arterial hypertension.

These findings do not preclude that more subtle effects upon blood pressure reactivity and circadian rhythm may also contribute to the cardiovascular risk in subgroups of depressed patients. In patients with arterial hypertension a pattern of overshooting cardiovascular reactivity with retarded return to baseline activity has repeatedly been shown in response to standard triggers, such as the Cold-Pressure Test (Loyke, 1995) or mental stress (Matthews *et al.*, 1993). Similarily, in hypercortisolaemic depressed patients blood pressure and heart rate showed sustained increases after mental stress and needed longer to return to baseline values, when compared with healthy controls (Gotthardt *et al.*, 1995). In fact, one line of research follows the hypothesis that stress-induced impairment of autonomic cardiac control leads to increased blood pressure responses to challenges. In the long run, increased blood pressure throughout the day and, moreover, plaque formation and coronary events may follow (Sloan *et al.*, 1999).

Disturbance of the circadian function of blood pressure regulation may be an additional factor putting depressed patients at increased risk of cardiac events. An insufficient decrease of blood pressure during the night – 'nocturnal non-dipping' – is known to be associated with a significantly increased cardiovascular risk, both in subjects with normotension and hypertension (Ohkubo *et al.*, 1997). Depressed patients frequently exhibit a pattern of nocturnal non-dipping in blood pressure regulation (Deuschle *et al.*, unpublished). Nocturnal non-dipping in circadian blood pressure regulation is a feature which is commonly observed in patients suffering from secondary hypertension, such as, for example, in Cushing's disease (Imai *et al.*, 1988).

Taken together, it may be summarized that there is at least some evidence for the assumption that depression and anxiety render subjects more prone to the development of arterial hypertension. Although there is no generally increased rate of hypertension within depressed patients, dynamic measures, such as stress responses and ambulatory blood pressure monitoring, provide some hints to how disturbances of blood pressure regulation may affect the cardiovascular risk of depressed patients.

Nicotine abuse

Most of the epidemiological studies supporting the assumption that depression and heart disease are related disorders, are controlled for smoking. However, smoking itself may be considered a major additional factor contributing to and increasing depressed patients' coronary risk.

In general, psychiatric patients show significantly increased cigarette consumption. Several studies in particular have demonstrated a large proportion of heavy smokers among subjects even long after a period with depressive symptoms (Kandel and Davies, 1986). It has further been shown that lifetime cigarette consumption is strongly related to lifetime and prospectively assessed prevalence of major depression. In fact, the relationship with major depressive disorder is found across the entire spectrum of smoking behaviour with stronger use of nicotine being directly related to higher rates of depression (Kendler et al., 1993). Smokers with a mild level of nicotine dependence run an increased risk for lifetime prevalence of depression compared with non-dependent subjects (OR: 2.12) and this risk strongly increases with the degree of dependence. Moderately dependent smokers were shown to have an odds ratio of 5.69. Interestingly, the risk for major depression is not increased in non-dependent smokers (Breslau et al., 1991). Therefore, it may be concluded that it is rather nicotine dependence than abuse which is closely related to depression. However, similar to heart disease, not only clinically diagnosed depression, but also subsyndromal depressive symptomatology has been associated with cigarette smoking in adolescents (Patton et al., 1996) and adults (Pérez-Stable et al., 1990).

The causal relationship between smoking and depression has not been completely resolved. Nicotine use or withdrawal may (a) render subjects prone to depression, (b) depression may be causative for smoking or, (c) a non-causal relationship may exist due to common predisposing factors.

There is limited evidence for the aforementioned assumption that nicotine use or withdrawal renders subjects prone to depression (Glassman et al., 1988). For example, prospectively, there is a two-fold increase in the risk of depression in subjects with daily nicotine use (Breslau et al., 1998). However, at the same time nicotine has been reported to induce an elevation in mood and sense of well-being (Gilbert and Spielberger, 1987; Carmody, 1989). Thus, some authors have voiced the speculation that depressed patients tend to self-medicate with cigarettes and that the reinforcing effects of nicotine's mood altering properties are especially powerful in depressed smokers (Hughes, 1988).

Clearly, the initiation of smoking behaviour is primarily influenced by social–environmental factors, while a role for major depression in smoking initiation cannot be substantiated. The maintenance of the behaviour, however, is more dependent upon personality traits, among them neuroticism (Spielberger, 1986; Giovino et al., 1995). Dependent, but not non-dependent, smoking is strongly related to measures of vulnerability to depression, such as neuroticism, negative affect, hopelessness and emotional distress, which underscores the possibility of a common predisposition to nicotine dependence and depression (Breslau et al., 1993). In line with these findings, a study with a large number of female twins supports the view that depression and smoking are due to a common genetic predisposition (Kendler et al., 1993).

Some data, however may be interpreted in favour of the hypothesis that it is depression which actually increases the risk to become nicotine-dependent following initial abuse. The fact that during a five–year longitudinal study a three-fold risk of progression of smoking behaviour was found in subjects with depression at baseline is in accordance with this assumption (Breslau et al., 1993). The effort to quit smoking is obviously more difficult for depressed subjects than for non-depressed controls. This has to be concluded from a nine-year follow-up, in which successful smoking cessation was found to be 40% less likely in subjects with depressive symptoms present at baseline (Anda et al., 1990).

Taken together, smoking and depression are tightly intertwined and smoking behaviour may put a depressed subject at an even higher risk of developing heart disease. Within this context, especially, the risk of becoming nicotine addicted and to unsuccessfully attempt to quit smoking is increased in depressed subjects. As a consequence, most of the above-mentioned epidemiological studies controlled for smoking as an intervening variable. However, after adjustment for this risk factor, cardiac mortality of depressed patients was still elevated, which means that additional factors must be operating.

Diabetes mellitus

The prevalence of depressive disorders in patients with diabetes mellitus is markedly increased (Gavard et al., 1993). Furthermore, a particularly high lifetime prevalence of depression has been found in overweight diabetic patients (Lustman et al., 1992). Interestingly, the Epidemiologic Catchment Area Study found the prospective risk of developing type 2 diabetes mellitus within 13 years to be increased in depressed subjects (OR: 2.2) (Eaton et al., 1996). Therefore, it can be concluded that (1) there is a high co-occurence of both disorders and (2) that depression may be the preceding condition.

Physical impairment and the experience of threat may explain some variability in the prevalence of depression in diabetic patients (Connell et al.,

1994). However, depression itself may in turn also exacerbate or worsen the diabetic condition. In patients with affective disorders not only insulin resistance (Weber et al., 2000), but also a three-fold increase in the rate of diabetes has been found (Cassidy et al., 1999). Visceral obesity, which is discussed in a separate chapter, is the most probable pathophysiological link between disorders of glycaemic control and depression.

Finally, depression may impair the prognosis of diabetic patients by affecting compliance to treatment. Within this context, several studies in patients with non-insulin dependent (Marcus et al., 1992) and insulin dependent (Sachs et al., 1991) diabetes have shown compliance to treatment to be low in the case of comorbid depression. Furthermore, glycaemic control was found to be worse in depressed compared with non-depressed patients with diabetes (de Groot et al, 1999). There are some data supporting the hypothesis that the presence of depression is associated with increased risk of complications in patients with diabetes (Leedom et al., 1991).

Summarizing these findings, one can speculate that depression is associated with an increased risk for the onset of diabetes and its complications.

Dyslipidaemia

Hypercholesterolaemia represents one of the major risk factors for coronary artery disease among the general population. When primary prevention trials are being considered in the aggregate, cholesterol lowering had only moderate impact on total mortality as decreases in ischaemic heart disease had, at least partially, been negated by increases in cancer and violent deaths.

The association between low cholesterol and violent death including suicide, stimulated research about the association of depressive symptoms and plasma lipid levels. At present, there is general agreement that in subjects prone to depression cholesterol is not increased (Peet and Edwards, 1997). If changed at all, cholesterol levels in depressed patients are suspected to be decreased. The last epidemiological evaluation concerning this question is derived from the Alpha-Tocopherol, Beta-Carotene Cancer Prevention Study Group (Partonen et al., 1999). Within this study nearly 30 000 men were followed up for 5–8 years. Those probands with self-reported depression at baseline had lower total serum cholesterol compared with those with no self-reported depression. However, low baseline cholesterol was not related to subsequent depression, suggesting occurrence of depression to be the primary event. It may therefore be concluded that depression might either be related or lead to reduced serum cholesterol. The cause for this observed change in plasma cholesterol remains unclear, yet weight loss and malnutrition were both speculated to be involved. Due to this change of direction it cannot be assumed that plasma cholesterol contributes to the cardiovascular risk in depressed subjects.

More interestingly, polyunsaturated fatty acids (PUFAs) may be related to depression. A decrease in omega-3 PUFAs has been reported in serum cholesterol esters of depressed patients (Maes et al., 1996). An increased ratio of omega-6 to omega-3 PUFAs in plasma and erythrocyte membrane phospholipids seems to be related to the severity of depression in yet another population (Adams et al., 1996). In line with these findings, omega-3 PUFAs are depleted in depressed patients (Peet et al., 1998). As diets rich in omega-3 PUFAs, such as fish or fish oil, have been shown to be effective in prevention of heart disease (Kromhout et al., 1985), a reasonable and testable hypothesis is that both depression and heart disease are associated due to both being possible sequelae of abnormalities in fatty acids. However, there are insufficient data to draw any conclusions from these studies.

ATYPICAL RISK FACTORS

Cardiovascular response to stress

Experiences of bereavement or loss strongly correlate with the risk of developing a depressive condition as well as myocardial infarction. By far the most important event correlated with sudden cardiac death is bereavement. It has been shown that the mortality rate significantly increases in the year following the death of a loved one (Post, 1992). Thus, severe cardiovascular reactions may follow emotional stress – a fact, which is very descriptively captured in the term 'scared to death'.

Depression may also be associated with repeated situations of mental stress. In the presence of atherosclerotic damage, mental stress may lead to paradoxical constriction of the coronaries (Yeung et al., 1991). Similarly, in a laboratory mental stress setting, a high tendency for increased tension in patients with coronary artery disease (CAD) is associated with an increased likelihood of myocardial ischaemia compared with patients with low emotional responsivity (Carels et al., 1999). More importantly, in daily life patients with CAD have a high probability of myocardial ischaemia in the hour following negative emotions such as tension (OR: 3.0), sadness (OR: 2.9) or frustration (OR: 2.6) (Gullette et al., 1997). Additionally, in the long run, a high responsiveness to stress is of significant risk for the cardiovascular system. Accordingly, the prospective CARDIA study showed cardiovascular reactivity to predict subsequent blood pressure increases within the next 5 years (Markovitz et al., 1998). At the same time, the tendency, for example, to show an exaggerated blood pressure response to a mental stressor is known to be an independent risk factor for atherosclerosis (Kamarck et al., 1997) and to predict blood pressure increases (Markovitz et al., 1998) as well as left ventricular mass (Georgiades et al., 1997).

Taken together, 'emotional responsivity', i.e. a tendency for large variations of self-reported tension, is related to transient myocardial ischaemia
and increased cardiac risk. As emotional responsivity is thought to be related
to type A behaviour it has been studied extensively for quite some time.
However, several recent reports indicate that emotional responsivity and
transient myocardial ischaemia of coronary artery disease patients in stressful situations are also linked to depressive symptoms (Carels *et al.*, 1999).

Vagal control of the heart rate variability and baroflex sensitivity

Heart rate variability (HRV), the amount of heart rate fluctuation around
mean heart rate, can be used to probe the autonomic nervous system. In
patients with ischaemic heart disease, low HRV is associated with an
increased risk of sudden cardiac death (van Ravemswaaij-Arts *et al.*, 1993).
Fourier analysis of HRV into components allows differentiation of HRV in
bands that can be related to specific modulatory influences. While the high-
frequency band has been used to estimate cardiac vagal control (Saul *et al.*,
1991), HRV at lower frequencies is thought to reflect mixed sympathetic–
parasympathetic and thermoregulatory influcences upon heart rate.

Repeatedly it has been shown that depression is associated with significantly reduced HRV in patients with and without heart disease
(Krittayaphong *et al.*, 1997; Carney *et al.*, 1995b; 1988a). Additionally,
successful treatment of depression resulted in increased HRV (Balogh *et al.*,
1993), but treatment with anticholinergic antidepressants, such as tricyclics,
may further decrease HRV (Lederbogen *et al.*, 2001a).

Furthermore, reduced baroreceptor-mediated vagal reflex control of heart
rate is associated with threatening arrhythmias. Baroflex sensitivity was
found to be low in coronary artery disease patients with high depression
scores (Watkins and Grossman, 1999) and especially high anxiety scores
contributed to impairment of baroreflex cardiac control (Watkins *et al.*,
1999). Taken together, low HRV and low baroflex sensitivity in depressed
patients indicate a reduced influence of the stabilizing vagal control of the
heart, which may create an increased susceptibility to malignant arrhythmias
under conditions of myocardial ischaemia and, in doing so, predispose
patients to sudden cardiac death.

Ventricular arrhythmia

We know that emotional disturbances may predispose subjects to ventricular arrhythmic events. It has, for example, been shown for quite some time
that psychological stress and anger render subjects more prone to ventricular arrhythmia (Reich, 1985). Among others Follick *et al.* (1988) have demonstrated that distress during hospitalization for a myocardial infarction
predicted ventricular arrhythmias within the year following the infarction

(Follick *et al.*, 1988). In patients with implanted cardioverter-defibrillators stress within an arithmetic task may lead to clinically significant ventricular arrhythmia (Lampert *et al.*, 2000). Additionally, a depressed emotional state in healthy subjects has been associated with the risk of ventricular arrhythmias (Orth-Gomer *et al.*, 1980). This circumstance may be especially dangerous for patients with coronary artery disease. Within this group of patients, those with an additional diagnosis of depression exhibit a much higher rate of ventricular tachycardia than those with coronary artery disease alone (Carney *et al.*, 1993). Furthermore, there is some evidence that among patients suffering from ventricular arrhythmia, the additional diagnosis of depression leads to increased mortality (Kennedy *et al.*, 1987).

In summary, there is evidence that depression is frequently associated with proneness to arrhythmic events. In the least, this fact should seriously be taken into consideration when choosing the appropriate antidepressant. As a precautionary measure, TCA treatment should thus be avoided in patients with preexisting heart disease.

Platelet function

Thrombosis is recognized as the precipitant of acute coronary events. In arterial thrombosis, the platelet is a major factor and inhibiting platelet aggregation is a critical therapeutic intervention in order to prevent coronary events. Emotional stress is considered to increase platelet activity and to thereby predispose subjects to cardiovascular events (Markovitz and Matthews, 1991). Platelet factor 4 and β-thromboglobulin are proteins which are extruded when the platelet shifts into an activated state and a rise in the plasma concentrations of these proteins is associated with increased tendency of the platelet to aggregate. There is good evidence for acute stress to activate platelets and for β-thromboglobulin to be a marker for this activation (Malkoff *et al.*, 1993; Markovitz *et al.*, 1996). Interestingly, in depressed cardiac patients markedly elevated levels of these proteins were found compared with non-depressed cardiac patients, which may contribute to the increased risk for thrombotic events in these patients. Treatment with an SSRI, but not with a TCA, returned platelet factor 4 and β-thromboglobulin significantly toward control values (Laghrissi-Thode *et al.*, 1997), which is in line with the fact that SSRIs occasionally lead to bleeding due to impaired clotting. Using fluorescence-activated flow cytometric analysis, Musselman and colleagues (1996), discovered that, in comparison with healthy controls, depressed patients exhibited an enhanced platelet activation after a mild cardiovascular stressor. Our group found depression to be associated with a higher platelet aggregability after stimulation with thrombin and collagen. Thus, it could be demonstrated that not only biochemical surface markers of the platelet, but also its function due to physiological stimulation is different in depressed patients. Antidepressive treatment with either a tricyclic antidepressant or an SSRI did not significantly dampen this increase in platelet function (Lederbogen *et al.*, 2001b).

Although the mechanisms responsible for these changes in the activity of depressed patients' platelets remain unknown, it may be supposed that a heightened susceptibility to platelet activation and secretion underlies, at least in part, the increased vulnerability of depressed patients for developing cardiovascular disease.

Adherence to treatment after myocardial infarction

Post-myocardial infarction depressed patients not only have a poor cardiac prognosis, but their adjustment to life in a general sense is also impaired (Sykes *et al.*, 1999). This also includes, in a disproportionate number of patients, low adherence to medical treatment after myocardial infarction.

The failure of patients to comply with prescribed treatment is a major limiting factor in medical care and also holds true for post-MI treatment. Thus for example, exercise therapy is a central component of most cardiac rehabilitation programmes. However, the compliance to treatment is between 13 and 60% only. Patients scoring high in depression scales tend to drop prescribed treatment more often than non-depressed patients (Blumenthal *et al.*, 1982). Similarly, the adherence to prophylactic treatment with aspirin is thought to be low in depressed patients (Carney *et al.*, 1995a). To our knowledge, the compliance to other kinds of post-MI treatments has not been studied in depressed patients. However, it seems reasonable to assume that the situation is not much better with regard to beta-blockers, angiotensin converting enzymes (ACE) inhibitors and other prescribed medications. In compliant patients, the clinical response to anti-ischaemic medication is found to be smaller in patients with high baseline levels of stress.

There is not much knowledge about the role of depression in the use of revascularization interventions. Interestingly, it was reported recently that MI patients with an additional diagnosis of a mental disorder were less likely to undergo revascularization procedures such as angioplasty or bypass grafting (Druss *et al.*, 2000). So far, it is not understood to what degree patients and health care providers contribute to this difference.

Of course, we cannot judge the impact of use of adequate treatment and compliance upon the medical outcome in depressed post-MI patients. It may be assumed, however, that poor adherence to basic therapeutic interventions, such as aspirin, seriously impairs the prognosis of post-MI patients. Thus, this may be another factor contributing to the increased cardiovascular risk in depression.

Cardiovascular drug prescription and risk of depression

Interestingly, the control of cardiovascular risk factors itself may be at risk of causing depression. A number of antihypertensive drugs have been implicated as a cause of depression. Most of these data were not obtained in controlled clinical tirials, but are of casuistic nature or stem from the observation of sequential use of drugs. In particular, the prescription of β-blockers and calcium channel blockers has been found to be followed by a significantly increased use of antidepressants (Avorn et al., 1986; Hallas, 1996; Rathman et al., 1999). The fact that this phenomenon is related to the dosage of β-blockers and calcium channel blockers suggests that it is not due solely to an association of cardiovascular disease with depression. Although depression has been reported following the use of angiotensin converting enzyme blockers (Hallas, 1996), the risk seems to be lower than for β-blockers and calcium channel blockers. Therefore, diuretics and angiotensin converting enzyme blockers have to be considered drugs of choice for the treatment of hypertension in depressed patients. Finally, also the choice of antidepressant treatment is relevant to the cardiac patient with an affective disorder.

Therapeutic use of antidepressants

It is unlikely that the association between major depression and vascular disease is due to cardiotoxicity of antidepressants, since adequate treatment of depression appears either to lower (Avery and Winokur, 1976) or not to change (Pratt et al., 1996) the risk of heart disease. However, in two large-scale follow-up studies (Penttinen and Valonen, 1996; Thorogood et al., 1992) an increased risk of myocardial infarction (OR: 5.4/OR: 6.3) has been described for users of antidepressants. The nature of these data, however, precludes the possibility of testing whether this result was simply biased by an increased risk due to underlying depression. Generally, TCAs and SSRIs have clearly different effects upon cardiovascular function and bear a different cardiovascular risk, especially in patients with preexisting heart disease (Glassman, 1998).

TCAs were the most commonly used drug in suicide attempts during the 1960s. Over time it became increasingly evident that cardiovascular effects accounted for deaths due to TCA overdose. Also, the implications of cardiovascular effects at regular therapeutic levels have long been known to clinicians. In depressed patients without additional physical disease, the main cardiovascular side effect of TCAs is orthostatic hypotension causing falls in less than 5% of patients. In contrast, in patients with left ventricular impairment, a dramatic increase in orthostatic falls, affecting up to 50% of patients, has been reported (Glassman et al., 1983). Similarly, the TCA-induced prolongation of conduction is harmless in most patients, but can lead to severe complications in those who already suffer from conduction disease, such as bundle branch block (Roose et al., 1987). Next to orthostatic hypotension and conduction, antiarrhythmic properties of TCAs became a third field of concern. TCAs may be regarded as class 1 antiarrhythmic drugs which are suspected to increase mortality, especially of patients with low ejection fraction, in the long run, probably because they turn out to be proarrhyth-mogenic when cardiac tissue becomes anoxic. Based on these observations, it is generally agreed that TCAs might bear similar risks in patients with ischaemic heart disease (Glassman *et al.*, 1993).

In general, for SSRIs there is only limited evidence of cardiovascular toxic-ity, such as QRS widening in cases of overdose and sinus bradycardia in a small number of depressed patients without heart disease. More importantly, several studies in depressed patients with cardiovascular disease showed SSRIs to be almost devoid of negative effects upon heart rate, blood pressure or conduction. Possibly, antidepressant treatment with SSRIs instead leads to an increase in the ejection fraction (Roose *et al.*, 1998a, 1998b). The direct comparison of SSRIs with TCAs in depressed patients with heart disease provided clear evidence of fewer cardiovascular adverse events in the SSRI-treated subgroups (Nelson *et al.*, 1999). Recently, limited data have indicated that antidepressive treatment with SSRIs following myocardial infarction as early as 5–30 days after the event, is well tolerated by most patients (Shapiro *et al.*, 1999).

Keeping the aforementioned TCA-associated cardiac problems of ortho-static hypotension, prolongation of conduction and possible proarrhythmo-genic properties in anoxic cardiac tissue in mind, TCAs should be avoided in the initial treatment of a depressed patient with cardiac disease. Only recently, the first data about a direct comparison between a tricyclic antide-pressant (nortriptyline) and an SSRI (paroxetine) in depressed patients with documented ischaemic heart disease have been published (Roose *et al.*, 1998b). These data indicated both treatment modalities to be similarily effec-tive with regard to depressive symptoms, but that treatment with an SSRI seems to be preferable due to the observed lack of negative effects upon heart rate, heart rate variability and adverse cardiac events.

VASCULAR DISEASE: A RISK FACTOR FOR LATE-LIFE DEPRESSION?

The data summarized so far prove depression to be associated with heart disease. Moreover, depression clearly is a preceding factor for cardiovascu-lar disease and there is at least some evidence supporting the assumption that depression increases the proneness to heart disease. However, there is also evidence for an inverse relationship so that the question arises, whether it could be possible that vascular disease may be a preceding condition for affective disorders.

A major cause of cerebral white matter lesions is thought to be high blood pressure (de Leeuw *et al.*, 1999). In depressed patients with late onset, MRI studies found increased signal hyperintensities in T_2-weighted images of the brain, which were considered to be of vascular nature. These imaging findings are associated with a typical clinical picture in late-onset depressed patients mainly showing apathy, cognitive impairment, retardation and a few depressive cognitions (Alexopoulos *et al.*, 1997a). For this group of patients, the term 'vascular depression' has been coined. It is hypothesized that a disturbance at the level of prefrontal systems or their modulating pathways by vascular lesions represents the major pathophysiological mechanism (Alexopoulos *et al.*, 1997b).

Indeed, it may be of clinical relevance to better characterize this group of patients, since several outcome studies found sub-grouping patients into 'vascular depression' and 'non-vascular depression' to be of prognostic value. Most, but not all (Krishnan *et al.*, 1998), found 'vascular depression' to be related to poor clinical outcome (Yanai *et al.*, 1998; Simpson *et al.*, 1998). Similar to post-stroke depression, which goes beyond the scope of this overview, depression may follow silent infarctions, especially when localized in the left frontal grey matter areas (Greenwald *et al.*, 1998). We can conclude that controlling cardiovascular risk factors should also reduce the incidence of late-onset depression.

SUMMARY

The January 1994 Northridge Earthquake in Los Angeles made us aware that acute stress is dangerous for the heart. On the day of the earthquake the number of deaths from myocardial infarction increased from 73 to 125 per day in LA County (Kloner *et al.*, 1997). Depression, a condition of chronic stress, may similarly affect cardiac mortality. More than for any other psychosocial factor, such as type A personality, work characteristics and social support, there is epidemiological evidence for depression and anxiety to be associated with heart disease (Hemingway and Marmot, 1999). Clearly, (1) the high rate of co-occurence, (2) the often observed sequence: depression → heart disease, (3) the long-held observation of high mortality from cardiovascular disease in depressed subjects, and (4) the impact of affective disorder on the prognosis of heart disease, all provide good epidemiological evidence that depression predisposes subjects to be at high risk of developing heart disease and complications from heart disease.

At this time, the mechanisms of this association cannot be fully explained. Unfortunately, it seems too optimistic to assume that one single pathophysiological link between depression and heart disease will be identified. So far, at least, it rather appears as if an array of disturbances of the cardiovascular system render the depressed subject prone to heart disease. Mechanisms, as varied as platelet aggregation, heart rate variability, the cardiovascular stress response, subtle disturbances of blood pressure control, impaired glucose control and visceral obesity may all contribute to the association of affective and cardiovascular disorders. Of course, the diversity of these factors prevents any prophylactic intervention in depressed subjects. How should this spectrum of possible mediating factors be controlled? Thus, an integrative model of these disorders is clearly needed not only to promote awareness of depression as a possible risk factor for heart disease, but also to advance further studies and to overcome prophylactic and therapeutic fatalism.

Depression is considered, at least by one sector of the psychiatric community, as a condition of chronic stress. Clearly, within depressed populations a high rate of subjects will show activation of stress systems, e.g. the hypothalamic–pituitary–adrenal system and the sympathoadrenergic system. Interestingly, the same holds true for a large subgroup of patients with arterial hypertension. McEwen favours a concept of allostatic load, which may be considered the price the body pays for being forced to adapt to adverse situations (McEwen, 2000). Catecholamines and the adrenergic steroids cortisol, and dehydroepiandrosterone (DHEA), are seen as primary mediators of allostatic load. Activation of these stress-adaptive systems, however, may be considered a major cause of induction of increased platelet aggregation, low heart rate variability and increased cardiovascular stress response. Generally, stressed subjects show adaptations of cardiovascular autonomic control, which may be useful and considered stress-adaptive. In the long run, however, these changes in cardiovascular function may predispose the individual to cardiovascular disease. As has been reported earlier in this book, activation of the hypothalamic–pituitary–adrenal system in depressed subjects may be the pacemaker for an increment of visceral fat, which again may induce an array of metabolic changes, e.g. impairment of glucose control. Thus, at least so far, stress and its direct sequelae, activation of the hypothalamic–pituitary–adrenal system and the sympathoadrenergic system, seem to be the most important factors linking affective disorders and cardiovascular disease. This hypothesis provides a framework for further research. To relate heart disease and affective disorders as stress-associated conditions does not necessarily imply a causal relationship between both disorders. It also seems possible that, for example, in stress-prone subjects, depression is the first or only disease to manifest itself. Heart disease, if it appears at all, may follow, at least partly as a sequelae of an array of stress-related cardiovascular risk factors.

With regard to therapy, characterizing depression and heart disease as stress-related disorders also carries therapeutic implications. The activity of the stress-adaptive systems is dampened by TCAs and by SSRIs. Clinically, these drugs are termed 'antidepressants' but, of course, they also are 'antiobsessives', 'antipanics' and 'antianxious'. Ongoing studies will show, whether the dampening effect of these drugs upon the neuroendocrine and sympathetic stress systems also improves the cardiovascular prognosis of, first of all, subjects suffering from depression. The hypothesis outlined above is clearly in favour of such clinical trials.

The various forms of cardiovascular disease represent the main causes of mortality in western societies. If ongoing research confirms that depression is indeed associated with an increased risk for heart disease, this may not only open new approaches for preventing cardiac morbidity, but also change our concepts of 'mind' and 'body' diseases: heart disease and affective disorders might well be different, but overlapping sequelae of common vulnerabilities. Even the most recent diagnostic manuals (DSM-IV and ICD-10) hinder the acceptance of true psychobiological models. Patients with 'vascular depression', for example, thus far are considered to be suffering from major depressive disorder; a fact, which clearly neglects the proneness to an affective disorder due to a cardiovascular condition. Similarly, heart disease in depressed subjects may be considered to be just another aspect, a 'somatic' expression, of a stress-related condition. In my opinion, the conceptualization of 'stress-related' disorders should follow the advancement in clinical research. Without implementation of these models to clinical practice, it will be hard to improve the awareness of what happens on the other side of the 'blood–brain barrier'. More precise definitions of a subgroup of patients with 'stress-related disorder' with both affective and cardiovascular expression, may help these patients to receive adequate treatment by both cardiologists and psychiatrists open to a unitary understanding of mind and body.

REFERENCES

Adams, P.B., Lawson, S., Sanigorski, A. and Sinclair, A.J. (1996). Arachidonic acid to eicosapentanoic acid ratio in blood correlates positively with clinical symptoms of depression. *Lipids* **31**(Suppl), S157–S161.

Ahern, D.K., Gorkin, L., Anderson, J.L. *et al.* (1990). Biobehavioral variables and mortality or cardiac arrest in the Cardiac Arrhythmia Pilot Study (CAPS). *Am J Cardiol* **66**, 59–62.

Alexopoulos, G.S., Meyers, B.S., Young, R.C. *et al.* (1997a). Clinically defined vascular depression. *Am J Psychiatry* **154**, 562–565.

Alexopoulos, G.S., Meyers, B.S., Young, R.C. *et al.* (1997b). The 'vascular depression' hypothesis. *Arch Gen Psychiatry* **54**, 915–922.

Allison, T.G., Williams, D.E., Miller, T.D. *et al.* (1995). Medical and economic costs of psychologic distress in patients with coronary artery disease. *Mayo Clin Proc* **70**, 734–742.

Anda, R., Williamson, D., Escobedo, L.G. *et al.* (1990). Depression and the dynamics of smoking. A national perspective. *JAMA* **264**, 1541–1545.

Anda, R., Willliamson, D., Jones, D. *et al.* (1993). Depressed affect, hopelessness and the risk of ischemic heart disease in a cohort of U.S. adults. *Epidemiology* **4**, 285–294.

Appels, A. (1997). Depression and coronary heart disease: observations and questions. *J Psychosom Res* **43**, 443–452.

Appels, A. and Mulder, P. (1989). Fatigue and heart disease: the association between 'vital exhaustion' and past, present and future coronary heart disease. *J Psychosom Res* **33**, 727–738.

Appels, A., Falger, P.R. and Schouten, E.G. (1993). Vital exhaustion as risk indicator for myocardial infarction in women. *J Psychosom Res* **37**, 881–890.

Aromaa, A., Raitasalo, R., Reunanen, A. *et al.* (1994). Depression and cardiovascular diseases. *Acta Psychiatr Scand* **377**(Suppl), 77–82.

Avery, D. and Winokur, G. (1976). Mortality in depressed patients treated with electroconvulsive therapy and antidepressants. *Arch Gen Psychiatry* **33**, 1029–1037.

Avorn, J., Everitt, D.E. and Weiss, S. (1986). Increased antidepressant use in patients prescribed β-blockers. *JAMA* **255**, 357–360.

Balogh, S., Fitzpatrick, D.F., Hendricks, S.E. and Paige, S.R. (1993). Increases in heart rate variability with successful treatment in patients with major depressive disorder. *Psychopharmacol Bull* **29**, 201–206.

Barefoot, J.C. and Schroll, M. (1996). Symptoms of depression, acute myocardial infarction and total mortality in a community sample. *Circulation* **93**, 1976–1980.

Barefoot, J.C., Helms M.J., Mark D.B. *et al.* (1996). Depression and long-term mortality risk in patients with coronary artery disease. *Am J Cardiol* **78**, 613–617.

Black, D.W., Warrack, G. and Winokur, G. (1985). Excess mortality among psychiatric patients. The Iowa record-linkage study. *JAMA* **253**, 58–61.

Black, D.W., Winokur, G. and Masrallah, A. (1987). Is death from natural causes still excessive in psychiatric patients? *J Nerv Ment Dis* **175**, 674–680.

Blumenthal, J.A., Williams, R.S., Wallace, A.G., Williams, R.B. and Needles, T.L. (1982). Physiological and psychological variables predict compliance to prescribed therapy in patients recovering from myocardial infarction. *Psychosom Med* **44**, 519–527.

Booth-Kewley, S. and Friedman, H.S. (1987). Psychological predictors of heart disease: a quantitative review. *Psychol Bull* **101**, 342–362.

Breslau, N., Kilbey, M. and Andreski, P. (1991). Nicotine dependence, major depression and anxiety in young adults. *Arch Gen Psychiatry* **48**, 1069–1074.

Breslau, N., Kilbey, M.M. and Andreski, P. (1993). Vulnerability to psychopathology in nicotine-dependent smokers: an epidemiologic study of young adults. *Am J Psychiatry* **150**, 941–946.

Breslau, N., Peterson, E.L., Schultz, L.R., Chilcoat, H.K. and Andreski, P. (1998). Major depression and stages of smoking. A longitudinal investigation. *Arch Gen Psychiatry* **55**, 161–166.

Carels, R.A., Sherwood, A., Babyak, M. *et al.* (1999). Emotional responsivity and transient myocardial ischemia. *J Consult Clin Psychol* **67**, 605–610.

Carmody, T.P., Crossen, J.R. and Wiens, A.N. (1989). Hostility as a health risk factor: relationships with neuroticism, Type A behavior, attentional focus, and interpersonal style. *J Clin Physiol* **45**, 754–62.

Carney, R.M., Rich, M.W., Tevelde, A.J. *et al.* (1987). Major depressive disorders in coronary artery disease. *Am J Cardiol* **60**, 1273–1275.

Carney, R.M., Rich, M.W., te Velde, A. *et al.* (1988a). The relationship between heart rate, heart rate variability and depression in patients with coronary artery disease. *J Psychosom Res* **32**, 159–164.

Carney, R.M., Rich, M.W., Freedland, K.E. and Saini, J. (1988b). Major depressive disorder predicts cardiac events in patients with coronary artery disease. *Psychosom Med* **50**, 627–633.

Carney, R.M., Freedland, K.E., Rich, M.W. and Smith, L.J. (1993). Ventricular tachycardia and psychiatric depression in patients with coronary artery disease. *Am J Med* **95**, 23–28.

Carney, R.M., Freedland, K.E., Eisen, S.A., Rich, M.W. and Jaffe, A.S. (1995a). Major depression and medication adherence in elderly patients with coronary artery disease. *Health Psychol* **14**, 88–90.

Carney, R.M., Saunders, R.D., Freedland, K.E. *et al.* (1995b). Association of depression with reduced heart rate variability in coronary artery disease. *Am J Cardiol* **76**, 562–564.

Cassidy, F., Ahearn, E. and Carroll, B.J. (1999). Elevated frequency of diabetes mellitus in hospitalized manic-depressive patients. *Am J Psychiatry* **156**, 1417–1420.

Colantonio, A., Kasi, S.V. and Ostfeld, A.M. (1992). Depressive symptoms and other psychosocial factors as predictors of stroke in the elderly. *Am J Epidemiol* **136**, 884–894.

Connell, C.M., Davis, W.K., Galant, M.P. and Sharpe, P.A. (1994). Impact of social support, social cognitive variables, and perceived threat on depression among adults with diabetes. *Health Psychol* **13**, 263–273.

de Groot, M., Jacobson, A.M., Samson, J.A. and Welch, G. (1999). Glycemic control and major depression in patients with type 1 and type 2 diabetes mellitus. *J Psychosom Res* **46**, 425–435.

de Leeuw, F.E., de Groot, J.C., Oudkerk, M. *et al.* (1999). A follow-up study of blood pressure and cerebral white matter lesions. *Ann Neurol* **46**, 827–833.

Denollet, J., Sys, S.U. and Brutsaert, D.L. (1995). Personality and mortality after myocardial infarction. *Psychosom Med* **57**, 582–591.

Denollet, J., Sys, U.S. and Stroobant, N. *et al.* (1996). Personality as independent predictor of long-term mortality in patients with coronary heart disease. *Lancet* **347**, 417–421.

Druss, B.G., Bradford, D.W., Rosenheck, R.A., Radford, M.J. and Krumholz, H.M. (2000). Mental disorders and use of cardiovascular procedures after myocardial infarction. *JAMA* **283**, 506–11.

Eaton, W.W., Armenian, H., Gallo, J., Pratt, L. and Ford, D.E. (1996). Depression and the risk for onset of type II diabetes. *Diabet Care* **19**, 1097–1102.

Everson, S.A., Goldberg, D.E. and Kaplan, G.A. *et al.* (1996). Hopelessness and risk of mortality and incidence of myocardial infarction and cancer.*Psychosom Med* **58**, 113–121.

Follick, M.J., Gorkin, L. and Capone, R.J. *et al.* (1988). Psychological distress as a predictor of ventricular arrhythmias in a post-myocardial infarction population. *Am Heart J* **116**, 32–36.

Ford, D.E., Mead, L.A. and Chang, P.P. *et al.* (1998). Depression is a risk factor for coronary artery disease in men. *Arch Intern Med* **158**, 1422–1426.

Frasure-Smith, N., Lesperance, F. and Talajic, M. (1993): Depression following myocardial infarction. Impact on 6–month survival. *JAMA* **270**, 1819–1825.

Frasure-Smith, N., Lesperance, F. and Talajic, M. (1995). Depression and 18–month prognosis after myocardial infarction. *Circulation* **91**, 999–1005.

Frasure-Smith, N., Lesperance, F., Juneau, M., Talajic, M. and Bourassa, M.G. (1999). Gender, depression and one-year prognosis after myocardial infarction. *Psychosom Med* **61**, 26–37.

Freeland, K.E., Carney, R.M., Lustman, P.J., Rich, M.W. and Jaffe, A.S. (1992). Major depression in coronary artery disease patients with vs. without a prior history of depression. *Psychosom Med* **54**, 416–421.

Friedman, M.J. and Bennet, P.L. (1977). Depression and hypertension. *Psychosomatic Med* **39**, 134–142.

Gavard, J.A., Lustman, P.J. and Cluse, R.E. (1993). Prevalence of depression in adults with diabetes. *Diabet Care* **16**, 1167–1178.

Georgiades, A., Lemne, C., de Faire, U., Lindvall, K. and Fredrikson, M. (1997). Stress-induced blood pressure measurements predict left ventricular mass over three years among borderline hypertensive patients. *Eur J Clin Invest* **27**, 733–739.

Gilbert, D.G. and Spielberger, C.D. (1987). Effects of smoking on heart rate, anxiety, and feelings of success during social interaction. *J Behav Med* **10**, 629–638.

Giovino, G.A., Henningfield, J.E., Tomar, S.L., Escobedo, L.G. and Slade, J. (1995). Epidemiology of tobacco use and dependence. *Epidemiol Rev* **17**, 48–65.

Glassman, A.H. (1998). Cardiovascular effects of antidepressant drugs: updated. *J Clin Psychiatry* **59**(Suppl 15), 13–18.

Glassman, A.H., Johnson, L.L., Giardina, E.G. *et al.* (1983). The use of imipramine in depressed patients with congestive heart failure. *JAMA* **250**, 1997–2001.

Glassman, A.H., Roose S.P. and Bigger J.T. (1993). The safety of tricyclic antidepressants in cardiac patients: risk/benefit reconsidered. *JAMA* **269**, 2673–2675.

Glassman, A.H., Stener, F., Walsh, B.T. *et al.* (1998). Heavy smokers, smoking cessation, and clonidine. Results of a double-blind, randomized trial. *JAMA* **259**, 2863–2866.

Gonzalez, M.B., Snyderman, T.B., Colket, J.T. *et al.* (1996). Depression in patients with coronary artery disease. *Depression* **4**, 57–62.

Gotthardt, U., Schweiger, U., Farhenberg, J. *et al.* (1995). Cortisol, ACTH and cardiovascular response to a cognitive challenge paradigm in aging and depression. *Am J Physiol* **268**, R865–R873.

Greenwald, B.S., Kramer-Ginsburg, E., Krishnan, K.R.R. *et al.* (1998). Neuroanatomic localization of magnetic resonance imaging signal hyperintensities in geriatric depression. *Stroke* **29**, 613–617.

Gullette, E.C., Blumenthal, J.A., Babyak, M. *et al.* (1997). Effects of mental stress on myocardial ischemia during daily life. *JAMA* **277**, 1521–1526.

Hagman, M., Wilhelmsen, L., Wedel, H. and Pennert, K. (1987). Risk factors for angina pectoris in a population study of Swedish men. *J Chronic Dis* **40**, 265–275.

Haines, A.P., Ineson, J.D. and Meade, T.W. (1987). Phobic anxiety and ischemic heart disease. *Br Med J* **295**, 297–299.

Hallas, J. (1996): Evidence of depression provoked by cardiovascular medication: a prescription sequence symmetry analysis. *Epidemiology* **7**, 478–484.

Hällström, T., Lapidus, L., Bengtsson, C. and Edström, K. (1986). Psychosocial factors and risk of ichaemic heart disease and death in women: a twelve-year follow-up of participants in the population study of women in Gothenburg, Sweden. *J Psychosom Res* **30**, 451–459.

Hemingway, H. and Marmot, M. (1999). Evidence based cardiology: psychosocial factors in the aetiology and prognosis of coronary heart disease: systemic review of prospective cohort studies. *BMJ* **318**, 1460–1467.

Hughes, J.R. (1988). Clinodine, depression, and smoking cessation. *JAMA* **259**, 2901–2902.

Imai, Y., Abe, K., Sasaki, S. *et al.* (1988). altered circadian blood pressure rhythm in patients with Cushing's syndrome. *Hypertension* **12**, 11–19.

Johnson, J., Weissman, M.M. and Klerman, G.L. (1992). Service utilization and social morbidity associated with depressive symptoms in the community. *JAMA* **267**, 1478–1483.

Jonas, B.S., Franks, P. and Ingram, D.D. (1997). Are symptoms of anxiety and depression risk factors for hypertension? *Arch Fam Med* **6**, 43–49.

Kamarck, T.W., Everson, S.A., Kaplan, G.A. *et al.* (1997). Exaggerated blood pressure responses during mental stress are associated with enhanced carotid atherosclerosis in middle-aged Finnish men: findings from the Kuopio Ischemic Heart Disease Study. *Circulation* **96**, 3842–3848.

Kandel, D.B. and Davies, M. (1986). Adult sequelae of adolescent depressive symptoms. *Arch Gen Psychiatry* **43**, 255–262.

Kaufmann, M.W., Fitzgibbons, J.P., Sussman, E.J. *et al.* (1999). Relation between myocardial infarction, depression, hostility and death. *Am Heart J* **138**, 549–554.

Kawachi, I., Sparrow, D., Vokonas, P.S. and Weiss, S.T. (1994). Symptoms of anxiety and risk of coronary heart disease. The Normative Aging Study. *Circulation* **90**, 2225–2229.

Kendler, K.S., Neale, M.C., MacLean, C.J. *et al.* (1993). Smoking and major depression. A causal analysis. *Arch Gen Psychiatry* **50**, 36–43.

Kennedy, G.J., Hofer, M.A., Cohen, D., Shindledecker, R. and Fisher, J.D. (1987). Significance of depression and cognitive impairment in patients undergoing programed stimulation of cardiac arrhythmias. *Psychosom Med* **49**, 410–421.

Kop, W.J., Appels, A., de Leon, C.F., de Swart, H.B. and Bar, F.W. (1994). Vital exhaustion predicts new cardiac events after successful coronary angioplasty. *Psychosom Med* **56**, 281–287.

Kloner, R.A., Leor, J., Poole, W.K. and Perritt, R. (1997). Population-based analysis of the effect of the Northridge Earthquake on cardiac death in Los Angeles County, California. *J Am Coll Cardiol* **30**, 1174–1180.

Krishnan, K.R.R., Hays, J.C., George, L.K. and Blazer, D.G. (1998). Six-month outcomes for MRI-related vascular depression. *Depress Anxiety* **8**, 142–146.

Krittayaphong, R., Cascio, W.R., Light, K.C. *et al.* (1997). Heart rate variability in patients with coronary artery disease: differences in patients with higher and lower depression scores. *Psychosom Med* **59**, 231–235.

Kromhout, D., Bosschieter, E.B. and Coulander, C. (1985). The inverse relation between fish consumption and 20-year mortality from coronary heart disease. *New Engl J Med* **312**, 205–209.

Kubzansky, L.D., Kawachi, I., Spioro, A. *et al.* (1997). Is worrying bad for your brain? A prospective study of worry and coronary heart disease in the Normative Aging Study. *Circulation* **95**, 814–824.

Ladwig, K.H., Lewhmacher, W., Roth, R. *et al.* (1992). Factors which provoke post-infarction depression: results from the post-infacrtion late potential study. *J Psychosom Res* **36**, 723–729.

Ladwig, K.H., Breithardt, G., Budde, T. and Borggrefe, M. (1994). Post-infarction depression and incomplete recovery 6 months after acute myocardial infarction. *Lancet* **343**, 20–23.

Laghrissi-Thode, F., Wagner, W.R., Pollock, B.R., Johnson, P.C., Finkel, M.S. (1997). Elevated platelet factor 4 and β-thromboglobulin plasma levels in depressed patients with ischemic heart disease. *Biol Psychiatry* **42**, 290–295.

Lampert, R., Jain, D., Burg, M.M., Batsford, W.P. and McPherson, C.A. (2000). Destabilizing effects of mental stress on ventricular arrhythmias in patients with implantable cardioverter-defibrillators. *Circulation* **101**, 158–164.

Lederbogen, F., Gernoth, C., Weber, B. *et al.* (2001a). Antidepressive treatment with amitriptyline and paroxetine: similar effects upon heart rate variability. *J Clin Psychopharmacol* (in press).

Lederbogen, F., Maras, A., Weber, B. *et al.* (2001b). Increased platelet aggregability in major depression. *Submitted*.

Leedom, L., Meehan, W.P., Procci, W. and Zeidler, A. (1991). Symptoms of depression in patients with type II diabetes mellitus. *Psychosomatics* **32**, 280–286.

Lesperance, F., Frasure-Smith, N. and Talajic, M. (1996). Major depression before and after myocardial infarction: its nature and consequences. *Psychosom Med* **58**, 99–110.

Loyke, H.F. (1995). Cold pressure test as a predictor of the severity of hypertension. *South Med J* **88**, 300–304.

Lustman, P.J., Freedland, K.E., Carney, R.M., Hong, B.A. and Clouse, R.E. (1992). Similarity of depression in diabetic and psychiatric patients. *Psychosom Med* **54**, 602–611.

McEwen, B.S. (2000). Allostasis and allostatic load: implications for neuropsychopharmacology. *Neuropsychopharmacology* **22**, 108–124.

McGovern, P.G., Pankow, J.S., Shahar, E. *et al.* (1996). Recent trends in acute coronary heart disease. Mortality, morbidity, medical care and risk factors. *New Engl J Med* **334**, 884–890.

McKhann, G.M, Borowicz, L.M., Goldsborough, M.A., Enger, C. and Selnes, O.A. (1997). Depression and cognitive decline after coronary artery bypass grafting. *Lancet* **349**, 1282–1284.

Maes, M., Smith, R., Christophe, A. *et al.* (1996). Fatty acid composition in major depression: decreased w3 fractions in cholesteryl esters and increased C20:4omega6/C20:5omega3 ratio in cholesteryl esters and phospholipids. *J Affect Disord* **38**, 35–46.

Malkoff, S.B., Muldoon, M.F., Zeigler, Z.R. and Manuck, S.B. (1993). Blood platelet responsivity to acute mental stress. *Psychosom Med* **55**, 477–482.

Malzberg, B. (1937). Mortality among patients with involution melancholia. *Am J Psychiatry* **93**, 1231–1238.

Markovitz, J.H. and Matthews, K.A. (1991). Platelets and coronary heart disease: potential psychophysiological mechanisms. *Psychosom Med* **53**, 643–668.

Markovitz, J.H., Matthews, J.H., Kannel, W.B. and D'Agostino, R.B. (1993). Psychological predictors of hypertension in the Framingham Study: is there tension in hypertension? *JAMA* **270**, 2439–2443.

Markovitz, J.H., Matthews, K.A., Kiss, J. and Smitherman, T.C. (1996). Effects of hostility on platelet reactivity to psychological stress in coronary heart disease patients and in healthy controls. *Psychosom Med* **58**, 143–149.

Markovitz, J.H., Raczynski, J.M., Wallace, D., Chettur, V. and Chesney, M.A. (1998). Cardiovascular reactivity to video game predicts subsequent blood pressure increases in young men: the CARDIA study. *Psychosom Med* **60**, 186–191.

Marcus, M.D., Wing, R.R., Guare, J., Blair, E.H. and Jawad, A. (1992). Lifetime prevalence of major depression and its effect on treatment outcome in obese type II diabetic patients. *Diabet Care* **15**, 253–255.

Matthews, K.A., Woodall, K.L. and Allen, M.T. (1993). Cardiovascular reactivity to stress predicts future blood pressure status. *Hypertension* **22**, 479–485.

Mezzich, J.E., Fabegra, H. and Coffman, G.A. (1987). Multiaxial characterization of depressive patients. *J Nerv Ment Dis* **175**, 339–446.

Moos, R.H. (1990). Depressed outpatients' life contexts, amount of treatment and treatment outcome. *J Nerv Ment Dis* **178**, 105–112.

Morris, P.L.P., Robinson, R.G., Andrzejewski, Samuels, J. and Price, T.R. (1993). Association of depression with 10-year poststroke mortality. *Am J Psychiatry* **150** 124–129.

Moser, D.K. and Dracup, K. (1996). Is anxiety early after myocardial infarction associated with subsequent ischemic and arrhythmic events? *Psychosom Med* **58**, 395–401.

Murphy, J.M., Monson, R.R., Olivier, D.C. *et al.* (1989). Mortality risk and psychiatric disorders. *Soc Psychiatry Psychiatr Epidemiol* **24**, 134–142.

Musselman, D.L., Tomer, A., Manatunga, A.K. *et al.* (1996). Exaggerated platelet reactivity in major depression. *Am J Psychiatry* **153**, 1313–1317.

Nelson, J.C., Kennedy, J.S., Pollock, B.G. *et al.* (1999). Treatment of major depression with nortriptyline and paroxetine in patients with ischemic heart disease. *Am J Psychiatry* **156**, 1024–1028.

Ohkubo, T., Imai, Y., Tsuji, I. *et al.* (1997). Relation between nocturnal decline in blood pressure and mortality. The Ohasama Study. *Am J Hypertens* **10**, 1201–1207.

Orth-Gomer, K., Edwards, M., Erhardt, L., Sjorgren, A. and Theorell, T. (1980). Relation between ventricular arrhythmias and psychological profile. *Acta Med Scand* **207**, 31–36.

Partonen, T., Haukka, J., Virtamo, J., Taylor, P.R. and Lönnqvist, J. (1999). Association of low serum total cholesterol with major depression and suicide. *Br J Psychiatry* **175**, 259–262.

Patton, G.C., Hibbert, M., Rosier, M.J. *et al.* (1996). Is smoking associated with depression and anxiety in teenagers? *Am J Public Health* **86**, 225–230.

Peet, M. and Edwards, R.W. (1997). Lipids, depression and physical health. *Curr Opinion Psychiatry* **10**, 477–480.

Peet, M., Murphy, B., Shay, J. and Horrobin, D. (1998). Depleteion of omega-3 fatty acid levels in red blood cell membranes of depressive patients. *Biol Psychiatry* **43**, 315–319.

Penttinen, J. and Valonen, P. (1996). Use of psychotropic drugs and risk of myocardial infarction: a case-control study in Finnish farmers. *Int J Epidemiol* **25**, 760–762.

Pérez-Stable, E.J., Marín, G., Marín, B.V. and Katz, M.H. (1990). Depressive symptoms and cigarette smoking among latinos in San Francisco. *Am J Public Health* **80**, 1500–1502.

Pfohl, B., Rederer, M., Coryell, W. and Stangl, D. (1991). Association between post-dexamethasone cortisol level and blood pressure in depressed patients. *J Nerv Ment Dis* **178**, 44–47.

Post, R.M. (1992). Transduction of psychosocial stress into neurobiology of recurrent affective disorder. *Am J Psychiatry* **149**, 999–1010.

Pratt, L.A., Ford, D.E., Crum, R.M. *et al.* (1996). Depression, psychotropic medication and risk of myocardial infarction: prospective data from the Baltimore ECA follow-up. *Circulation* **94**, 3123–3129.

Rabins, P.V., Harvis, K. and Koven, S. (1985). High fatality rates of late-life depression associated with cardiovascular disease. *J Affective Disord* **9**, 165–167.

Rabkin, J.G., Charles, E. and Kass, F. (1983). Hypertension and DSM-III depression in psychiatric outpatients. *Am J Psychiatry* **140**, 1072–1074.

Rathman, W., Haastert, B., Roseman, J.M. and Giani, G. (1999). Cardiovascular drug prescriptions and risk of depression in diabetic patients. *J Clin Epidemiol* **52**, 1103–1109.

Reich, P. (1985). Psychological predisposition to life-threatening arrhythmias. *Annu Rev Med* **36**, 397–405.

Roose, S.P., Glassman, A.H., Giardina, E.G.V. *et al.* (1987). Tricyclic antidepressants in depressed patients with cardiac conduction disease. *Arch Gen Psychiatry* **44**, 273–275.

Roose, S.P., Glassman, A.H., Attia, E. *et al.* (1998a). Cardiovascular effects of fluoxetine in depressed patients with heart disease. *Am J Psychiatry* **155**, 660–665.

Roose, S.P., Laghrissi-Thode, F., Kennedy, J.S. *et al.* (1998b). Comparison of paroxetine and nortriptyline in depressed patients with ischemic heart disease. *JAMA* **279**, 287–291.

Roose, S.P., Dalack, G.W. and Woodring, S. (1991). Death, depression and heart disease. *J Clin Psychiatry* **52**(Suppl), 34–39.

Sachs, G., Spiess, K., Moser, G. *et al.* (1991). Glycosylated hemoglobin and diabetes self-monitoring (compliance) in depressed and non-depressed type I diabetic patients. *Psychother Psychosom Med Psychol* **41**, 306–312.

Saul, J.P., Berger, R.D., Albrecht, P. *et al.* (1991). Transfer function analysis of the circulation: unique insights into cardiovascular regulation. *Am J Physiol* **30**(4 Pt 2), H1231–1245.

Schleifer, S.J., Macari-Hinson, M.M., Coyle, D.A. *et al.* (1989). The nature and course of depression following myocardial infarction. *Arch Intern Med* **149**, 1785–1789.

Shapiro, P.A., Lesperance, F., Frasure-Smith, N. *et al.* (1999). An open-label preliminary trial of sertraline for treatment of major depression after acute myocardial infarction (the SADHAT Trial). *Am Heart J* **137**, 1100–1106.

Simpson, S., Baldwin, R.C., Jackson, A. and Burns, A.S. (1998). Is subcortical disease associated with poor response to antidepressants? Neurological, neuropsychological and neuroradiological findings in late-life depression. *Psychol Med* **28**, 1015–1026.

Sloan, R.P., Shapiro, P.A., Bagiella, E., Myers, M.M. and Gorman, J.M. (1999). Cardiac autonomic control buffers blood pressure variability responses to challenge: a psychophysiologic model of coronary artery disease. *Psychosomatic Med* **61**, 58–68.

Spielberger, C.D. (1986). Psychological determinants of smoking behavior. In: Tollison, R.D. (Ed.) *Smoking and Society: Toward a More Balanced Assessment.* Lexington Books, Lexington, Mass.

Steffens, D.C., O'Connor, C.M., Jiang, W.J. *et al.* (1999). The effect of major depression on functional status in patients with coronary artery disease. *J Am Geriatr Soc* **47**, 319–322.

Swindle, R.W., Cronkite, R.C. and Moos, R.H. (1990). Life stressors, social resources, coping and the 4–year course of unipolar depression. *J Abnorm Psychol* **98**, 468–477.

Sykes, D.H., Hanley, M., Boyle, D.M., Higginson, J.D.S. and Wilson, C. (1999). Socioeconomic status, social environment, depression and postdischarge adjustment of the cardiac patient. *J Psychosom Res* **46**, 83–99.

Timio, M., Lippi, G., Venanzi, S. *et al.* (1997). Blood pressure trend and cardiovascular events in nuns in a secluded order: a 30-year follow-up study. *Blood Press* **6**, 81–87.

Thorogood, M., Cowen, P., Mann, J., Murphy, M. and Vessey, M. (1992). Fatal myocardial infarction and use of psychotropic drugs in young women. *Lancet* **340**, 1067–1068.

van Ravemswaaij-Arts, C.M., Kollée, L.A., Hopman, J.C., Stoelinga, G.B. and van Geijn, H.P. (1993). Heart rate variability. *Ann Intern Med* **118**, 436–447.

Vogt, T., Pope, C., Mullooly, J. and Hollis, J. (1994). Mental health status as a predictor of morbidity and mortality: a 15–year follow-up of members of a health maintenance organization. *Am J Public Health* **84**, 227–231.

Wassertheil-Smoller, S., Applegate, W.B., Berge, K. *et al.* (1996). Change in depression as a precursor of cardiovascular events. SHEP Cooperative Research Group (Systolic Hypertension in the elderly). *Arch Intern Med* **156**, 553–561.

Watkins, L.L. and Grossman, P. (1999). Association of depressive symptoms with reduced baroreflex cardiac control in coronary artery disease. *Am Heart J* **137**, 453–457.

Watkins, L.L., Grossman, P., Krishnan, R. and Blumenthal, J.A. (1999b). Anxiety reduces baroreflex cardiac control in older adults with major depression. *Psychosom Med* **61**, 334–340.

Weber, B., Deuschle, M. and Schweiger, U. *et al.* (2000). Patients with depression have an impairment of glucose utilisation. *Exp Clin Endocrinol Diabet* **108**, 187–190.

Wells, K.B., Rogers, W., Burnam, M.A. and Camp, P. (1993). Course of depression in patients with hypertension, myocardial infarction or insulin-dependent diabetes. *Am J Psychiatry* **150**, 632–638.

Yanai, I., Fujikawa, T., Horiguchi, J., Yamawaki, S. and Touhouda, Y. (1998). The 3–year course and outcome of patients with major depression and silent cerebral infarction. *J Affect Disord* **47**, 25–30.

Yeung, A.C., Vekshtein, V.I., Krantz, D.S. *et al.* (1991). The effect of atherosclerosis on the vasomotor response of coronary arteries to mental stress. *New Engl J Med* **325**, 1551–1556.

8

The Impact of Depression on the Immune System and Immune-Related Disorders

JANE F. GUMNICK, BRADLEY D. PEARCE and ANDREW H. MILLER

Department of Psychiatry and Behavioral Sciences, Emory University School of Medicine, Atlanta, Georgia, USA

'This . . . is the great error of our day in the treatment of the human body, that the physicians separate the soul from the body.'

Plato

INTRODUCTION

A tremendous amount of data has been accumulated over the past several decades demonstrating the capacity of the immune system and the brain to have meaningful interactions that are relevant to the expression of both immunologic and neuropsychiatric disorders. Data have demonstrated that immune cells express receptors for transmitters, peptides and hormones derived from and/or regulated by the nervous system. In addition, direct innervation of lymphoid tissue by autonomic nervous system fibres has been described. Perturbations of nervous system function through exposure to a variety of stressors or direct brain lesions have also been reliably associated with alterations in immune system function. A host of studies have demonstrated that, like the nervous system, the immune system can be conditioned. More recently, data have documented that brain–immune system interactions are bidirectional. Immune system products (cytokines) and their receptors have been found throughout nervous and endocrine system tissues, and a multitude of studies have shown that cytokines can have powerful influences on nervous and endocrine system function including behaviour.

Given the prevalence of the depressive disorders in both healthy and medically ill individuals, the contribution of brain and immune system interactions in depressed patients has received a great deal of attention. Not only has research examined how depression may influence immune system function and the onset, course and outcome of immune-related disorders, but also the potential contribution of immune system activation to the development of depression has been explored. This chapter will summarize and discuss highlights of this research. It will also discuss possible mechanisms for a link between depression and the immune system. Finally, current knowledge of how antidepressant medications may affect immune functioning will be discussed.

IMPACT OF DEPRESSION ON IMMUNE SYSTEM PARAMETERS

Since the early 1980s, studies have examined immune parameters in an effort to elucidate what specific changes in the immune system may accompany major depression. Investigations can be divided into two major categories: enumerative studies and functional studies, both of which typically examine white cells (leukocytes) taken from the peripheral blood. The enumerative studies count immune cells of various types, and functional studies include those that measure immune cell activity such as natural killer cell activity, proliferation of lymphocytes in response to polyclonal mitogens, and the production of acute phase proteins and cytokines *in vivo* and/or *in vitro*.

Cell number

A multitude of investigators have examined the numbers of immune cells in the peripheral blood of depressed patients. These studies have counted cells in the major classes of leukocytes including neutrophils, lymphocytes, and monocytes. Subsets of lymphocytes also have been enumerated. Table 1 summarizes studies of patients diagnosed with acute major depression by DSM-III, -III-R, or -IV criteria (Sengar *et al.*, 1982; Schleifer *et al.*, 1984, 1985, 1989, 1996; Albrecht *et al.*, 1985; Syvalahti *et al.*, 1985; Calabrese *et al.*, 1986; Darko *et al.*, 1988; Evans *et al.*, 1988, 1992; Kronfol and House, 1989; Irwin *et al.*, 1990a; Caldwell *et al.*, 1991; Levy *et al.*, 1991; Maes *et al.*, 1992a, 1993; Andreoli *et al.*, 1993; Hickie *et al.*, 1993; McAdams and Leonard, 1993; Muller *et al.*, 1993; Landmann *et al.*, 1997; Kanba *et al.*, 1998; Ravindran *et al.*, 1998; Miller *et al.*, 1999). Only studies with a control group were included, and patients were not on medication at the time of study. The summary information includes only results for those patients with unipolar major depression. If patients with other diagnoses were studied, that portion of the data is not presented.

Table 1. Cell numbers.

Cell type	Increased	Decreased	No difference	Total
White blood cells	7	0	7	14
Neutrophils	5	0	7	12
Lymphocytes	2	3	13	18
Total T cells	2	2	12	16
Helper T cells	1	0	12	13
Suppressor T cells	1	0	12	13
Total B cells	0	1	9	10
NK cells	2	3	3	8
Monocytes	2	1	5	8

Although the design of these studies varies dramatically, making it difficult to compare across studies, general patterns of cell number alterations in depressed patients have emerged. White blood cell (WBC) counts were found to be increased in depressed subjects in seven out of 14 studies whereas neutrophil counts were increased in depressed subjects in five out of 12 studies. Lymphocytes and their subsets and monocytes have not exhibited consistent changes across studies. Eighteen studies examined lymphocyte count, and two found increases in depressed subjects while three found decreases. Natural killer (NK) cell number has been measured in eight studies and was found to be increased in depressed subjects in two studies and decreased in three studies. Worth noting is that gender-related differences in NK cell number were present in several studies (Evans *et al.*, 1992; Ravindran *et al.*, 1998), with more pronounced increases in NK number in male depressed patients compared with females. Monocyte count was increased in two and decreased in one out of eight studies.

Several studies warrant particular attention. The two largest studies (Schleifer *et al.*, 1989; Andreoli *et al.*, 1993) used paired, age- and gender-matched controls whose blood was drawn and assayed on the same day. Schleifer *et al.* found that when the variables of age, gender, inpatient versus outpatient hospitalization status, and severity of depression were taken into account, enumeration of the major classes of leukocytes did not differ significantly between depressed patients and controls. Andreoli *et al.* studied only outpatients and, in addition, obtained information about social history (including level of physical activity, ethanol use, tobacco use, and employment status). Their study also found no significant differences in immune cell numbers in patients with major depression after correcting for those lifestyle variables.

Given that the majority of cells in human peripheral blood are neutrophils, the increase in WBC that has been found in depressed patients is probably related to the increase in neutrophil count. Indeed, five out of the seven studies demonstrating an increased WBC also found increased neutrophils. Demargination of neutrophils by catecholamines and glucocorticoids, both hormones known to be increased in depression, may account for these changes. Decreased lymphocyte counts, a less reliable finding across studies, may be secondary to the relative increase in neutrophil number and percentage.

Although there is evidence that differences in WBC count and neutrophil count exist, the meaning of these changes remains obscure. Altered numbers of immune cells in the peripheral blood may represent immune activation or suppression depending on the relative distribution of leukocytes throughout bodily compartments and the functional capacity of these leukocytes. For example, a decreased number of peripheral blood lymphocytes may not necessarily indicate immune suppression but may, in fact, indicate increased lymphocyte migration or activity in immune compartments other than the blood, including the brain and/or peripheral immune tissues such as the skin.

Cell function

Lymphocyte proliferation

The ability of lymphocytes to proliferate in response to polyclonal mitogens has been examined in depressed patients. Mitogen responses involve crosslinking of lymphocyte surface receptors leading to the release of growth factors (cytokines) and cell proliferation and division. In these studies, peripheral blood lymphocytes are typically incubated with phytohaemagglutinin (PHA), concanavalin A (ConA), and/or pokeweed mitogen (PWM), and proliferation is assessed by incorporation of radioactive nucleosides. Table 2 presents a summary of results of studies examining patients with acute major depressive episode who were not taking medication at the time of study (Cappel et al., 1978; Sengar et al., 1982; Kronfol et al., 1983, 1986; Schleifer et al., 1984, 1985, 1989, 1996; Kronfol and House, 1985, 1989; Albrecht et al., 1985; Syvalahti et al., 1985; Calabrese et al., 1986; Altshuler et al., 1989; Darko et al. 1991; Levy et al., 1991; Maes et al., 1991a; Andreoli et al., 1993; Hickie et al., 1993; McAdams and Leonard, 1993; Bauer et al., 1995; Miller et al., 1999). Only studies of patients with unipolar major depression including a control group are listed.

Table 2. Lymphocyte proliferation.

Mitogen	Increased	Decreased	No difference	Total
Phytohaemagglutinin (PHA)	3	9	9	21
Concanavalin A (ConA)	0	9	10	19
Pokeweed mitogen (PWM)	0	6	10	16

Of the 21 studies using PHA, nine showed a decrease, three found an increase, and nine showed no significant difference between depressed patients and controls. Nine of the 19 studies using ConA found a decrease in depressed subjects compared with controls while the rest detected no change. Of the PWM studies, six of 16 showed a decrease in depressed subjects while the 10 other studies found no significant difference. These data demonstrate an association between depression and decreased lymphocyte proliferation in response to mitogens in approximately half of the studies; however, it should be noted that the most well-controlled studies have not detected significant differences.

Schleifer et al. (1989) and Andreoli et al. (1993), as described previously, found no significant differences in lymphocyte proliferation following mitogen stimulation in depressed patients compared with healthy controls. The study by Schleifer et al. did show significant age-related changes in lymphocyte proliferation. While the control subjects exhibited increased mitogen responses with increasing age, the depressed subjects did not. A well-controlled study by Miller et al. (1999) found that much of the variability in proliferative responses could be accounted for by subjects' level of physical activity. Moreover, this study found that depression was associated with increased use of tobacco and that smoking was associated with decreased PHA but unchanged ConA responses. Numerous interacting variables thus appear to contribute to altered lymphocyte proliferation and confound the ability to detect differences due solely to the physiological state of depression.

Natural killer cell activity

Natural killer cells are peripheral blood lymphocytes that play an important role in the recognition and destruction of virally-infected and certain malignant cells. Many studies have examined the functioning of NK cells in depressed patients. Typically, NK cells are isolated from the peripheral blood and their activity is measured in vitro against a radiolabelled tumour cell line.

Table 3 summarizes the studies measuring NK cell activity in patients with major depression compared with controls. Reduction in NK activity was found in 11 out of 15 studies, while one study (Miller et al., 1999) found NK activity to be increased in younger depressed patients and decreased in older depressed patients. The age at which this difference occurred was approximately 40 years old. The study by Evans et al. (1992) found a significant decrease in NK activity in male patients only. These results indicate that alterations in NK cell activity of depressed patients are more consistent than those of other measures and appear more likely to be found in older depressed patients who are male. Caldwell et al. (1991) examined hospitalized depressed and schizophrenic patients and found decreased NK activity

Table 3. NK cell activity.

Study	N (patients/controls)	Interassay control	Dose	Result
Mohl et al., 1987	10/10	Yes	DR	NS
Irwin et al., 1987	19/19	Yes	DR	dec
Urch et al., 1988	29/27	Yes	DR	dec
Kronfol et al., 1989	12/12	Yes	DR	dec
Nerozzi et al., 1989	22/22	Yes	DR	dec
Schleifer et al., 1989	91/91	Yes	DR	NS
Irwin et al., 1990b	36/36	Yes	DR	dec
Irwin et al., 1991	19/19	Yes	DR	dec
Caldwell et al., 1991	10/10	Yes	DR	dec
Miller et al., 1991	34/21	No	DR	NS
Levy et al., 1991	18/18	Yes	DR	NS
Evans et al., 1992	30/19	No	DR	dec[a]
Maes et al., 1992b	37/37	No	O	dec
Bauer et al., 1995	27/27	Yes	DR	dec
Schleifer et al., 1996	21/21	Yes	DR	dec
Miller et al., 1999	32/32	No	DR	inc/dec[b]

[a] Male patients only.
[b] Increased in younger patients, decreased in older patients.
NS, not significant; DR, dose response assay; o, optimal dose assay.

only in the depressed patients, suggesting that these findings are not simply related to hospitalization status and may be more specific to depression.

Cytokines and acute phase proteins

Cytokines are soluble peptides produced by immune cells that help regulate inflammatory and immune responses (Muller and Ackenheil, 1998). During the early stages of an inflammatory response, proinflammatory cytokines including tumour necrosis factor (TNF), interleukin (IL)-1 and IL-6 mediate protection against invading pathogens, recruit immune cells, activate the release of chemical mediators of inflammation, and stimulate the liver to produce acute phase proteins (Baumann and Gauldie, 1994). The induction of acute phase proteins from the liver is mediated in large part by IL-6 and is designed to limit tissue damage, isolate and destroy invading pathogens and stimulate repair pathways.

Of great interest to neurobiologists is that experimental administration of proinflammatory cytokines to laboratory animals has been observed to cause a set of neurobehavioural sequelae that has been termed 'sickness behaviour' (Anisman and Merali, 1999). As cytokine therapies have been developed for clinical use, including the treatment of cancer and viruses such as hepatitis C, physicians have noted similar neuropsychiatric effects in humans. These effects resemble the signs and symptoms of major depression (Dantzer et al.,

Table 4. Immune messengers – acute phase proteins and cytokines.

	Increased	Decreased	No difference	Total
Acute phase protein				
C-reactive protein	3	0	1	4
Haptoglobin	5	0	0	5
C4	3	0	0	3
α-1-acid glycoprotein	3	0	1	4
α-1-antitrypsin	2	0	1	3
Ceruloplasmin	2	0	0	2
Transferrin receptor	2	0	0	2
Transferrin	1	0	0	1
α-1-antichymotrypsin	1	0	0	1
Fibrinogen	1	0	0	1
Haemopexin	1	0	0	1
Cytokine				
IL-2	0	2	1	3
Soluble IL-2-receptor	4	0	2	6
IL-6	3	0	3	6
IL-1-β	1	1	4	6
TNF-α	0	1	2	3
Soluble IL-6-receptor	2	0	0	2
Soluble CD8 molecule	1	0	0	1

1999, Meyers, 1999), and therefore, researchers have looked for increased levels of cytokines and related acute phase proteins in humans with depression to determine whether these immune mediators may be involved in the pathophysiology of the depressive disorders. It should also be noted that proinflammatory cytokines are potent stimulators of the hypothalamic–pituitary–adrenal (HPA) axis, in large part through the induction of corticotrophin releasing hormone (CRH). HPA axis abnormalities including CRH hypersecretion are a hallmark of the neurobiological changes of major depression. Table 4 summarizes significant findings of relevant studies (Healy *et al.*, 1991; Maes *et al.*, 1991a, b, 1992c, 1995, 1996, 1997; Joyce *et al.*, 1992; Song *et al.*, 1994; Weizman *et al.*, 1994; Seidel *et al.*, 1995; Sluzewska *et al.*, 1996; Berk *et al.*, 1997; Landmann *et al.*, 1997; Brambilla and Maggioni, 1998; Anisman *et al.*, 1999; Haack *et al.*, 1999; Miller *et al.*, 1999).

Two general classes of studies – *in vitro* and *in vivo* – were included. *In vivo* studies measured plasma or serum levels of acute phase proteins or cytokines. *In vitro* studies measured production of cytokines by mitogen-stimulated peripheral blood leukocytes grown in culture.

More studies are available measuring acute phase proteins than cytokines. Of acute phase proteins that have been examined in at least three studies, C-reactive protein was found to be increased in three out of four studies, serum haptoglobin was increased in five out of five, C4 was increased in three out of three studies, α-1-acid-glycoprotein was increased in three out of four, and α-1-antitrypsin was increased in two out of three studies. No study reported a decrease in these acute phase reactants.

As for cytokines and their receptors, IL-2 has been found to be decreased in depressed patients in two out of three studies, while soluble IL-2 receptor (sIL-2R) was increased in depressed subjects in four out of six studies; two studies found no difference. IL-6 has been found to be increased in depressed patients in three out of six studies and unchanged in the remainder. Related to the IL-6 changes, sIL-6R has been increased in two out of two studies. Results with IL-1-beta (interleukin-1-β) and TNF-α (tumor necrosis factor-α) have been more mixed with increases in IL-1β in depressives in one of six studies, decreases in one of six, and no differences in four out of six studies. TNFα (tumor necrosis factor-alpha) was decreased in one out of three studies, while two out of three studies found it to be unchanged. In summary, the overall pattern in depressed patients appears to be an increase in acute phase proteins, IL-6, sIL-6R and sIL-2R with an associated decrease in IL-2.

Discussion of studies on immune measures

Drawing conclusions from the now large body of information regarding depression and measurements of immune parameters is a difficult task. Differences in the design of these studies limit comparison across studies. A large meta-analysis (Herbert and Cohen, 1993) has been conducted on this literature and the following conclusions are drawn: patients with depression were found to have increased total white blood cell count, increased neutrophil number, and decreased lymphocyte number. Depression was associated with decreased B, T and helper/suppressor T cells. The analysis concluded that depression was related to decreased lymphocyte proliferative responses to mitogens and decreased NK cell activity. We would argue, however, that the studies included in this analysis were too heterogeneous to enable one to combine studies in this way and draw such conclusions.

One must take into account many factors in evaluating the data from these studies. Interassay variability has been large, especially in mitogen-induced lymphocyte proliferation assays, accounting for approximately 50% of the variance in one study (Schleifer et al., 1989). Studies which use appropriately matched controls studied on the same day and in the same assay seem to find fewer significant differences in immune responses, suggesting that immune differences, when found, may not be due solely to the presence of depression but to other factors. Consistency of diagnosis and absence of comorbid diagnoses are also important issues in these studies. Some studies included patients with diagnoses as varied as unipolar, bipolar and psychotic depression, and combined results under the label 'depression'. Severity and course of a patient's illness have been associated with alterations in immune parameters, and therefore, recurrent, longstanding, or severe depressive illness may alter immune parameters more than a single or brief episode of less severe depression. A few studies such as those by Schleifer et al. (1989), Irwin et al. (1990a), Evans et al. (1992) and Andreoli et al. (1993) report information on characteristics such as chronicity of the depressive illness. Some studies do not exclude comorbid diagnoses such as anxiety disorders, although at least one study (Andreoli et al., 1992) has found that the presence or absence of comorbid panic disorder in depressed patients seems to have specific and significant effects on immune parameters.

Lack of adequate controls calls into question the usefulness of the data of some investigations. Appropriate controls are necessary because individual characteristics have been shown to affect measurements of immune function dramatically. Variables such as age, gender, use of tobacco, presence of recent infectious disease, body mass index, and use of medication have all been shown to affect these parameters (Haack et al., 1999; Miller et al., 1999.) Nutritional status has been suggested to play a role, at least in natural killer cell activity (Ravindran et al., 1998.) Sex hormones have been shown to affect immune parameters (Bauer et al., 1995), and it is important in studying female patients to control for variables such as ingestion of oral contraceptives and premenopausal or postmenopausal status. Both sleep and immune function have been shown to vary with hormonal changes of the menstrual cycle and ingestion of oral contraceptives (Moldofsky et al., 1995.) Some authors have looked at how sleep changes may mediate alterations in immune functioning (Irwin et al., 1994; Hall et al., 1998; Savard et al., 1999) and how diurnal body rhythm can change in depression (Irwin 1999; Petitto et al., 1993). Cover and Irwin (1994) demonstrated that NK cell activity was decreased in depressed patients as a function of sleep disturbance and increased as a function of retardation symptoms. Socioeconomic status is increasingly being studied because of its association with altered immune function (Morag et al., 1998). Physical activity has also been shown to alter immune functioning (Miller et al., 1999). Rarely have subjects been matched for level of exercise or sleep quality in studies of immune function in depression.

One of the largest studies to date (Haack et al.,1999) studied 351 psychiatric inpatients, 113 of whom were diagnosed with unipolar major depression by DSM-III-R criteria, and 64 controls. This very large sample did not use typical exclusion criteria such as presence of infection, use of tobacco, use of psychotropic medications, or severe medical illness. Because of the large sample size and the inclusion of patients who would otherwise be excluded, the researchers were able to examine effects of multiple variables on immune parameters. They found few significant differences in cytokine levels when these variables were taken into account.

Aside from the variability of results found here, the question presents itself: if some differences exist and are reliably associated with depression, what is their significance? It is unclear what relationship these immune parameters have with the functioning of the immune system in depressed patients who are otherwise healthy. The immune system is a network of specialized cells that have specific functions in immune compartments throughout the body. The number or function of cells in one compartment does not necessarily reflect the functioning of the immune cells in other compartments. The studies that were included here all measured peripheral blood or cells from peripheral blood. The local environment of the brain and immune tissues including the spleen, thymus and lymph nodes is undoubtedly another matter. Two recent studies examined cerebrospinal fluid (CSF) of patients with depression versus controls (Stubner et al., 1999; Levine et al., 1999). Stubner et al. studied 20 elderly patients and 20 matched controls, and all except one patient were taking psychotropic medication. They found decreased IL-6 and soluble IL-6-receptor in the depressed patients compared with controls. Levine studied 13 hospitalized depressed patients compared with 10 controls and found higher CSF IL-1β, lower IL-6, and no change in TNF-α levels. For obvious reasons it is more difficult to obtain CSF than peripheral blood, and such studies are rare. They can also be as difficult to interpret as studies of peripheral blood

Another important point pertaining to the clinical relevance of the depression–immune studies is that even though immune parameters have been shown to be changed in depressives compared with controls in some studies, in most cases, the immune measures in depressives are within the normal range. Other measures that assess in vivo functioning of the immune system might be of help in identifying clinical differences in these patients. A study in 1993 by Hickie et al. looked at in vivo delayed-type hypersensitivity (DTH) in depressed patients with and without melancholia compared with normal healthy controls. This study found decreased DTH only in the subgroup of patients with melancholic depression.

In conclusion, studies have found a variety of alterations in immune function in depressed patients (see Figure 1). Because of the heterogeneity of presentations of depression, it is possible that different subtypes of depression exist which have distinctive immune profiles. There also may exist a type of 'immune-based' depression initiated or perpetuated by immune dysfunction. This hypothetical immune-based depression would probably be accompanied by both hyperactivity and suppression of various parts of the immune system, in which disturbed homeostasis tries to right itself via multiple feedback pathways.

IMPACT OF DEPRESSION ON IMMUNE-RELATED DISORDERS

Based on the changes in immune parameters found in some studies of depressed patients, attention has been paid to the potential impact of

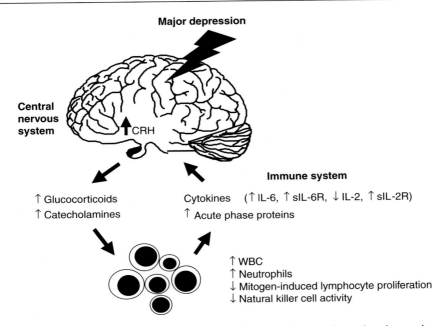

Figure 1. Overview of neuroendocrine and immune changes in major depression.

depression on the onset, course and outcome of diseases related to the immune system including cancer and infectious diseases such as HIV/AIDS. Conventional wisdom for physicians is that certain personality traits or psychological characteristics put one at risk for these diseases. This notion has been championed by physicians as far back as the Greeks.

Depression and cancer

Several clinical questions arise in looking at the relationship between depression and cancer. Does the presence of depression put one at increased risk for developing cancer? Does the development of depression in a patient with cancer affect the course or outcome of the cancer? Does the treatment of depression affect the outcome in a patient with cancer?

Depression and the development of cancer

The connection between the presence of specific personality traits or psychiatric symptoms and later development of cancer has been examined throughout the middle and late part of the 20th century. As shown in Table 5, few studies have documented robust increases in the likelihood of developing

Table 5. Depression and cancer incidence.

Study	Sample characteristics	Depression measures	Length of follow-up (years)	Findings for patients with depressive symptoms or diagnosis
Shekelle et al., 1981[a]	40–55 year old working men	MMPI-D	17	Increased incidence cancer mortality during entire follow up (OR 2.3)
Persky et al., 1987[a]	40–55 year old working men	MMPI-D	20	High D profile associated with increased incidence cancer over first 10 years (OR 1.9–2.0), increased mortality during entire follow-up (OR 1.9)
Hahn and Petitti, 1988	Women – general population	MMPI-D	14	No increased incidence breast cancer
Kaplan and Reynolds, 1988	Community sample	HPL questionnaire	17	No increased cancer mortality
Zonderman et al., 1989	Community sample	GWB-D, CES-D	10	No increased cancer morbidity or mortality
Linkins and Comstock, 1990	General population	CES-D	12	Increased morbidity and mortality in depressed smokers only (4.5-fold risk at highest level of smoking)
Friedman, 1994	Depressed patients and general pharmacy patients	Physician clinical diagnosis	19	Slight increased cancer incidence (OR 1.38)
Everson et al., 1996	Men, ages 42–60	Hopelessness questions	6	Increased cancer morbidity (OR 1.80) and mortality (OR 2.61)
Knekt et al., 1996	General population – Finland	General Health Questionnaire, Present State Exam	14	No increased overall cancer incidence, but increased risk of lung cancer in depressed men (OR 3.32)
Penninx et al., 1998	General population age 71 and older	CES-D	Mean follow-up 3.8	Increased incidence cancer in chronically depressed elderly (OR 1.88)
Whooley and Browner, 1998	Women, age 67 and older	Geriatric Depression Scale	6	No increased cancer mortality

[a] Western Electric Health Study.
HPL, California Human Population Laboratory-California Department of Health Services; GWB-D, General Well Being Schedule-Depressed Subscale; CES-D, Center for Epidemiologic Studies Depression Scale; MMPI-D, Minnesota Multiphasic Personality Inventory-Depression Subscale; OR, odds ratio.

cancer in patients with depression. The majority of studies have found small or statistically insignificant increases in cancer risk in depressed cohorts compared with non-depressed controls. Interestingly, depressed patients do exhibit increased morbidity and mortality, but this increase is best accounted for by cardiovascular disease, accidents, and suicides.

There are many challenges that must be faced in determining the impact of depression on the onset of cancer. Sample sizes must be large and follow-up periods must be long due to the relatively lower incidence and slower development of cancer compared with other illnesses such as cardiovascular disease. In addition, depressive symptoms must be identified prospectively, i.e. depression must be diagnosed prior to the diagnosis of cancer. Prior identification is essential because the diagnosis of cancer may confound the recall of previous emotional states. Other difficulties include the quantification of depressive symptoms as well as assessment over time. The majority of studies have used large cohorts and measured depression by standardized rating scales. Most did not diagnose clinical depression and only examined depressive symptoms at one point in time. Furthermore, although other risk factors such as cigarette smoking were controlled, it is worth noting that Linkins and Comstock (1990) found that depression and smoking together had a significant and additive effect on one's risk for cancer morbidity or mortality. It is well known that depressed patients are more likely to smoke and have a hard time quitting smoking. Future studies in carefully diagnosed depressed patients followed over time may yield a more significant relationship between depression and cancer; however, it does not appear likely that the strength of this association will reach the already apparent strong association between depression and the development of cardiovascular disease.

Effects of depression on cancer outcome

Of equal importance to the development of cancer is the question: Once a patient has been diagnosed with cancer, what effect does mood state or other psychosocial variables have on their survival? While many studies have examined how coping style, presence of depressive symptoms, and other psychological factors influence disease outcome in cancer patients, the majority of studies have methodological weaknesses which limit our interpretation of their conclusions. Many studies have not controlled for basic prognostic variables such as cancer staging, steroid receptor status (in breast cancer), and other variables known to affect outcomes. Some of the more well-controlled studies are reviewed in Table 6. These studies have measured a variety of patient characteristics related to depression such as mood symptoms, helplessness, and ways of coping. Some also measured stressors such as relationship difficulties and severe life events such as divorce or death of a child. Outcome variables included time to relapse or time to death. The data demonstrate that severe stressors and depressive symptoms have been

Table 6. Depression and cancer-survival.

Study	Sample	Depression measure	Findings
Cassileth et al., 1985	N=204 unresectable cancer, N=155 stage I or II melanoma, stage II breast cancer	Hopelessness/helplessness	Hopelessness/helplessness not associated with decreased survival or time to recurrence
Jamison et al., 1987	N=49 metastatic breast cancer	Zung, other psychosocial measures	Zung score and other measures not related to survival time
Ramirez et al., 1989	N=50 breast cancer in relapse, N=50 breast cancer in remission	Bedford College Life Events and Difficulties Schedule	Severe life events/difficulties associated with increased risk of breast cancer relapse
Tross et al., 1996	N=280 breast cancer stage II	Symptom Checklist-90-Revised	Psychological factors including level of distress not associated with disease-free or overall survival
Schulz et al., 1996	N=238 patients receiving palliative radiation therapy	Pessimism, optimism	Pessimism was a risk factor for mortality in ages 30–39 years old only, depression not associated with mortality
Buccheri et al., 1998	N=133 lung cancer patients	Zung scale	Survival in lung cancer patients with depression significantly decreased
Watson et al., 1999	N=578 early stage breast cancer	Mental Adjustment to Cancer scale, Courtauld Emotional Control Scale, Hospital Anxiety and Depression Scale	Increased risk of death association with increased hopelessness, helplessness
Faller et al., 1999	N=103 lung cancer patients	Freidberg Questionnaire	Depressive coping associated with decreased survival

related to increased recurrence and reduced survival in patients with cancer; however, the results have not been consistent across all studies, and more well-controlled investigations are warranted.

Effects of treatment of depression or psychosocial intervention on cancer outcome

Complementing the data on the impact of depression and stress on cancer outcome are the studies that have examined whether treatment of depression or other psychosocial interventions in cancer patients affect their survival. A group psychotherapy intervention by Spiegel *et al.* (1989) resulted in improved quality of life and increased survival for subjects participating in group psychotherapy compared with control subjects who received standard treatment. Spiegel *et al.* studied patients with metastatic breast cancer who received an intervention of weekly group psychotherapy in addition to their standard treatment. Patients in the intervention group exhibited significant decreases in depressive symptoms over time and surprisingly exhibited a mean survival time 18 months greater than non-treated control subjects. Fawzy *et al.* (1990, 1993) studied patients with stage I or II malignant melanoma who attended nine-hours of group psychotherapy and standard treatment compared with control group patients who received standard treatment only. Interestingly, the intervention group was found to have significantly increased populations of the CD57 subtype of NK cells and increased NK cell responses to interferon-α 6 months after the intervention compared with the control group. Moreover, similar to the Spiegel study, there was a significantly lower rate of cancer recurrence in patients who underwent psychotherapy in combination with standard treatment compared with those given standard treatment alone. It should be emphasized however, that these studies were conducted with a general population of cancer patients who were not diagnosed with major depression. The mechanism of the improved outcome in the Spiegel and Fawzy studies remains unclear and the impact of psychotherapy on both immune variables and treatment compliance are currently underway. Studies examining the impact of antidepressant therapy on cancer outcome in depressed subjects are also in progress.

Depression and infection: focus on HIV/AIDS

Knowledge about HIV and AIDS has progressed immeasurably since the beginning of the epidemic. This disease is of special interest to the field of brain–immune interactions because of the multitude of associated immunologic derangements and psychiatric sequelae. One question is whether depression affects disease progression and survival in patients with HIV or AIDS. The hypothesis is that if depression is accompanied by immune dysfunction (suppression or activation), patients who are already immuno-suppressed may be at special risk for further immune alterations.

Studies of depressed patients with HIV/AIDS have varied in their results and in how they measure depressive symptoms and health outcomes. Some studies of patients with HIV but not clinical AIDS have failed to find a significant association between depressive symptoms and disease progression as measured by decline in CD-4 or WHO disease stage rating (Rabkin *et al.*, 1991; Perry *et al.*, 1992; Lyketsos *et al.*, 1996). Other studies have found an association between depressive symptoms and more rapid disease progression as measured by CD-4 count, but have not found a difference in mortality (Burack *et al.*, 1993; Lyketsos *et al.*, 1993). Still others have found increased mortality associated with depression (Mayne *et al.*, 1996.) Severe life stress and bereavement have also been associated with more rapid disease progression or increased AIDS mortality (Evans *et al.*, 1997; Leserman, 1997; Leserman *et al.*, 1999.) Bereavement may present a special immune mediator for HIV patients because of the high death rate within HIV-infected samples. Taken together, the data indicate that depression and severe life stress are capable of altering immune function and exacerbating disease progression in HIV-infected individuals. Thus, treatment strategies targeting depressed mood may have beneficial effects on disease outcome in this population.

ANTIDEPRESSANTS AND IMMUNITY

In the context of data suggesting that depression may be associated with worse outcome of medical illnesses such as cancer and HIV/AIDS, there has been considerable interest in the role of antidepressants in treating mood symptoms in patients with immune-related disorders. Moreover, given that receptors for neurotransmitters are present on the surface of immune cells, investigators have examined whether antidepressants might have direct effects on immune responses.

A number of studies have demonstrated altered immune function following *in vitro* treatment with a range of antidepressants including tricyclic antidepressants (TCAs) and selective serotonin reuptake inhibitors (SSRIs). For reviews on this topic, see Miller and Lackner (1989) and Neveu and Castanon (1999). TCAs have been shown to inhibit mitogen-induced lymphocyte proliferation and NK cell activity (Miller *et al.*, 1986), while at least one report has suggested that SSRIs may increase NK activity *in vitro* (Frank *et al.*, 1999). Both TCAs and SSRIs have been associated with decreased monocyte or lymphocyte production of cytokines including TNF-α, IL-1-α, IL-2, and interferon-γ. The TCA, clomipramine, and the SSRI, sertraline, were found to increase IL-10 secretion.

In vivo studies examining the immune changes that accompany treatment with antidepressant medications are summarized in Table 7. Control groups are not possible in such studies because of the ethical issue of leaving patients with depression untreated. Therefore, patients to a degree act as their own controls. Results from these studies have been mixed, ranging from no immunologic effect of antidepressant treatment (Maes *et al.*, 1995; Landmann *et al.*, 1997; Brambilla and Maggioni, 1998; Schleifer *et al.*, 1999) to normalization of altered immune parameters (Pariante and Miller, 1995; Sluzewska *et al.*, 1995; Ravindran *et al.*, 1998; Frank *et al.*, 1999), to decreases in immune function after treatment (Albrecht *et al.*, 1985). Pariante and Miller (1995) found that initially increased NK activity in depressed patients decreased over time only in those patients who remained depressed, i.e. medication non-responders. Weizman *et al.* (1994) noted increases in IL-1-β and IL-3-like activity with antidepressant treatment, while Seidel *et al.* (1995) reported that initially increased acute phase proteins C-reactive protein, haemopexin, and α-2-macroglobulin remained high after treatment, and initially increased IL-2, IL-10, and IFN-γ decreased to normal after treatment. These *in vivo* studies present more questions than they answer. Some immune parameters normalize with treatment while others remain abnormal. Also, when normalization of values occurs, this change has not necessarily coincided with recovery from depression, i.e. response to antidepressant. Therefore, it remains unclear whether antidepressant medications directly cause changes in immune variables over time, accompany the physiological changes of remission from depression, or accompany physiological changes independent of depression status.

DEPRESSION AND THE IMMUNE SYSTEM: POTENTIAL MECHANISMS OF OBSERVED IMMUNE CHANGES

In considering the potential pathways by which immune changes might occur in the depressive disorders much of the focus has been on the HPA axis. Hyperactivity of the HPA axis in patients with major depression is one of the most consistent findings in biological psychiatry. Patients with major depression exhibit elevated cortisol concentrations in plasma, urine and CSF, an enlargement of the pituitary and adrenal glands, and an exaggerated cortisol response to ACTH (Owens and Nemeroff, 1993; Holsboer and Barden, 1996). The aetiology of these HPA axis alterations is believed to be a function of hypersecretion of CRH. CRH is a key regulatory peptide in HPA axis regulation and has a multitude of behavioural effects in animals which are similar to those seen in patients suffering from depression including alterations in activity, appetite, and sleep (Owens and Nemeroff, 1993). Moreover, patients with depression have been found to exhibit increased concentrations of CRH in the CSF, increased mRNA in the paraventricular nucleus of the hypothalamus, and a blunted adrenocorticotrophic hormone (ACTH) response to CRH challenge (probably reflecting downregulation of

Table 7. Antidepressants and immunity.

Study	Study description	Antidepressant	Outcome
Albrecht et al., 1985	In vivo, 3–6 weeks of treatment	Tricyclic antidepressants or ECT	Reduction in lymphocyte response to mitogens after treatment/clinical remission
Irwin et al., 1992	In vivo, 6 months follow-up	Various antidepressants	Initially decreased NK activity increased to normal after treatment
Rabkin et al., 1994	In vivo, HIV/AIDS patients, 6 weeks of treatment	Imipramine v. placebo	No effect of imipramine on CD4 count
Weizman et al., 1994	In vivo, 4 weeks of treatment	Clomipramine	Decreased IL-1-β, IL-2, IL-3-like activity initially Post-treatment- significant increase in IL-1-β, IL-3-like activity
Maes et al., 1995	In vivo, mean treatment duration 85.4 days	Fluoxetine or tricyclic antidepressants	No treatment effect on IL-6, sIL-6-R, sIL-2R, or transferrin receptor
Pariante and Miller, 1995	In vivo, average 12 weeks of treatment	Desmethylimipramine	NK activity initially higher in depressed patients, non-responders only had decrease in NK activity over treatment
Seidel et al., 1995	In vivo, 6 weeks of treatment	Tricyclic antidepressants	Increased initial serum CRP and Hp, α-2-macroglobulin: all remained high post-treatment. Increased initial IL-2, IL-10, IFN-γ, all normalized post-treatment.

Reference	Conditions	Treatment	Results
Sluzewska et al., 1995	In vivo, 8 weeks of treatment	Fluoxetine	Initial increase in IL-6, normalized after treatment
Landmann et al., 1997	In vivo, 12 weeks of treatment	Moclobemide	No treatment effect on cell numbers, plasma TNF, IFN-γ
Brambilla and Maggioni, 1998	In vivo, 30 days treatment	Phosphatidylserine	No initial changes IL-1-β, IL-6, TNF-α
Ravindran et al., 1998	In vivo, 12 weeks of treatment	Various antidepressants	No treatment effect on parameters. Initial increase NK, post-treatment decrease to normal in subset of patients with positive drug response
Frank et al., 1999	In vivo, over 4 weeks of treatment. Human lymphocytes	Fluoxetine (in vivo)	In vivo, fluoxetine treatment augmented NK cell activity only in patients with low levels at baseline
Schleifer et al., 1999	In vivo, 6 weeks medication treatment	Nortriptyline	Initial increased leukocytes, decreased NK number and activity. T cell count, CD4+, CD29+, CD45RA+ subsets and mitogen responses decreased significantly with treatment. No change NK activity or number compared with pre-treatment

pituitary CRH receptors) (Owens and Nemeroff, 1993; Holsboer and Barden, 1996). Finally, downregulation of receptors for CRH in the frontal cortex of victims of suicide (presumably secondary to hypersecretion of CRH) has been described (Owens and Nemeroff, 1993).

The immunologic effects of CRH on a wide range of immune functions have been well characterized (Irwin et al., 1988, 1990b; Irwin, 1993). In laboratory animals, intracerebroventricular (ICV) administration of CRH has been shown to lead to suppression of splenic NK activity (Irwin et al., 1988). Follow-up studies have shown that CRH is also capable of inhibiting in vivo and in vitro antibody formation, including the generation of an IgG response to immunization with keyhole limpet haemocyanin (KLH) (Irwin, 1993; Leu and Singh, 1993). The influence of CRH on antibody responses is also apparent in CRH overproducing mice whose immune deficits are characterized by a profound decrease in the number of B cells and severely diminished primary and memory antibody responses (Stenzel-Poore et al., 1996). Chronic ICV administration of CRH and acute infusion of CRH into the locus coeruleus have been shown to suppress lymphocyte proliferative responses to nonspecific mitogens and antibody to the T cell receptor (Labeur et al., 1995; Rassnick et al., 1994; Caroleo et al., 1993).

Interestingly, CRH also has been found to stimulate the release of proinflammatory cytokines in both laboratory animals and humans. For example, chronic ICV administration of CRH to rats led to induction of IL-1 mRNA in splenocytes, and acute intravenous infusion of CRH in humans led to an almost four-fold induction of IL-1 (Labeur et al., 1995; Schulte et al., 1994). Both treatments also led to significant increases in the immunoregulatory cytokine, IL-2 (Labeur et al., 1995; Schulte et al., 1994). In addition, CRH has also been found to induce the release of IL-1 and IL-6 from human mononuclear cells in vitro (Leu and Singh, 1993; Paez Pereda et al., 1995).

CRH is also capable of directly modulating immune and inflammatory responses (Karalis et al., 1991, 1997). Local production of CRH has been demonstrated in inflammatory diseases such as ulcerative colitis (Kawahito et al., 1995) and arthritis, where it is proposed to act as a local proinflammatory agent. Recent evidence also suggests that CRH may act as a protective factor against inflammation-induced pain (Schafer et al., 1994) and plasma extravasation (Yoshihara et al., 1995). Taken together, these results demonstrate that CRH has well-documented immunosuppressive effects on in vivo cellular and humoral responses while having a stimulatory effect on cytokine production and local inflammation.

As for the neuroendocrine mechanisms by which CRH influences immune responses, activation of the sympathetic nervous system (SNS) by ICV CRH has been found to be a major regulator of the effects of CRH on splenic NK activity (Irwin et al., 1988). In particular, the sympathetic ganglionic blocker, chlorisandamine, has been shown to reverse the inhibitory effect of ICV CRH on NK activity in the spleen (Irwin *et al.*, 1988). The HPA axis is also involved in CRH immune effects as shown by Labeur and coworkers (1995) who demonstrated that the effects of chronic ICV CRH on splenocyte proliferative responses are eliminated by adrenalectomy. In addition, the B cell decreases found in CRH overproducing mice are very consistent with the marked reduction of rodent B cells found following chronic exposure to glucocorticoids (Miller *et al.*, 1994).

CONCLUSIONS

The literature on brain–immune interactions is large and growing. How depression affects the immune system is of great interest because of the prevalence of this disorder in the population of healthy and medically ill individuals. A large number of studies on generally physically healthy patients with depression have been summarized here, and some general trends have emerged. Numbers of white blood cells in the peripheral blood are increased, associated with an increase in neutrophil count. Lymphoproliferative responses to PHA, ConA, and PWM have been decreased in a number of studies as has NK cell activity. Acute phase proteins such as C-reactive protein, haptoglobin, and α-1-acid-glycoprotein have been found to be consistently increased while cytokines present a more mixed picture with increases in IL-6 and IL-2R and decreases in IL-2 being reproducible across reports.

Depression in healthy patients is physiologically heterogeneous and accompanied by evidence of both increased and decreased immune activity. Whether these changes represent overall immune activation or suppression has been a question of interest. While the existing evidence does not suggest that depression significantly predisposes an individual to cancer, the patient with cancer and depressive symptoms or severe life stress appears to have higher risk of cancer morbidity and mortality. The data for HIV/AIDS are mixed but suggest a similar increased risk of medical deterioration associated with depressive symptoms or life stress. Data on the role of antidepressant treatment in these medical illnesses have not been resolved. Nevertheless, it should be emphasized that whether or not the presence of depression or treatment affects morbidity and mortality from these diseases, the importance of treating depression for the patient's quality of life cannot be overemphasized. Further research is needed based on testable hypotheses regarding depression and the immune system. Much may be gained in studying both medically well and ill patients, taking into account individual variables such as course and severity of depression, depression symptom patterns, lifestyle factors, hormonal status, and comorbid psychiatric illnesses.

REFERENCES

Albrecht, J., Helderman, J.H., Schlesser, M.A. and Rush, A.J. (1985). A controlled study of cellular immune function in affective disorders before and during somatic therapy. *Psychiatry Res* **15**, 185–193.

Altshuler, L.L., Plaeger-Marshall, S., Richeimer, S., Daniels, M, Jr and Baxter, L.R. (1989). Lymphocyte function in major depression. *Acta Psychiatr Scand* **80**, 132–136.

Andreoli, A., Keller, S.E., Rabaeus, M. *et al.* (1992). Immunity, major depression, and panic disorder comorbidity. *Biol Psychiatry* **31**, 896–908.

Andreoli, A.V., Keller, S.E., Rabaeus, M. *et al.* (1993). Depression and immunity: age, severity, and clinical course. *Brain Behav Immun* **7**, 279–292.

Anisman, H. and Merali, Z. (1999). Anhedonic and anxiogenic effects of cytokine exposure. *Adv Exp Med Biol* **461**, 199–233.

Anisman, H., Ravindran, A.V., Griffiths, J. and Merali, Z. (1999). Endocrine and cytokine correlates of major depression and dysthymia with typical or atypical features. *Mol Psychiatry* **4**, 182–188.

Bauer, M.E., Gauer, G.J., Luz, C., *et al.* (1995). Evaluation of immune parameters in depressed patients. *Life Sci* **57**, 665–674.

Baumann, H. and Gauldie, J. (1994). The acute phase response. *Immunol Today* **15**, 74–80.

Berk, M., Wadee, A.A., Kuschke, R.H. and O'Neill-Kerr, A. (1997). Acute phase proteins in major depression. *J Psychosom Res* **43**, 529–534.

Brambilla, F. and Maggioni, M. (1998). Blood levels of cytokines in elderly patients with major depressive disorder. *Acta Psychiatr Scand* **97**, 309–313.

Buccheri, G. (1998). Depressive reactions to lung cancer are common and often followed by a poor outcome. *Eur Respir J* **11**, 173–178.

Burack, J.H., Barrett, D.C., Stall, R.D. *et al.* (1993). Depressive symptoms and CD4 lymphocyte decline among HIV-infected men. *JAMA* **270**, 2568–2573.

Calabrese, J.R., Skwerer, R.G., Barna, B. *et al.* (1986). Depression, immunocompetence, and prostaglandins of the E series. *Psychiatry Res* **17**, 41–47.

Caldwell, C.L., Irwin, M. and Lohr, J. (1991). Reduced natural killer cell cytotoxicity in depression but not in schizophrenia. *Biol Psychiatry* **30**, 1131–1138.

Cappel, R., Gregoire, F., Thiry, L. and Sprecher, S. (1978). Antibody and cell-mediated immunity to herpes simplex virus in psychotic depression. *J Clin Psychiatry* **39**, 266–268.

Caroleo, M.C., Pulvirenti, L., Arbitrio, M. *et al.* (1993). Evidance that CRH microinfused into the locus coeruleus decreases cell-mediated immune response in rats. *Funct Neurol* **8**, 271–277.

Cassileth, B.R., Lusk, E.J., Miller, D.S., Brown, L.L. and Miller, C. (1985). Psychosocial correlates of survival in advanced malignant disease? *New Engl J Med* **312**, 1551–1555.

Cover, H. and Irwin, M. (1994). Immunity and depression: insomnia, retardation, and reduction of natural killer cell activity. *J Behav Med* **17**, 217–223.

Dantzer, R., Aubert, A., Bluthe, R.-M. *et al.* (1999). Mechanisms of the behavioural effects of cytokines. *Adv Exp Med Biol* **461**, 83–105.

Darko, D.F., Gillin, J.C., Risch, S.C. *et al.* (1988). Immune cells and the hypothalamic-pituitary axis in major depression. *Psychiatry Res* **25**, 173–179.

Darko, D.F., Wilson, N.W., Gillin, J.C. and Golshan, S. (1991). A critical appraisal of mitogen-induced lymphocyte proliferation in depressed patients. *Am J Psychiatry* **148**, 337–344.

Evans, D.L., Pedersen, C.A. and Folds, J.D. (1988). Major depression and immunity: preliminary evidence of decreased natural killer cell populations. *Prog Neuropsychopharmacol Biol Psychiatry* **12**, 739–748.

Evans, D.L., Folds, J.D., Pettito, J.M. *et al.* (1992). Circulating natural killer cell phenotypes in men and women with major depression: relation to cytotoxic activity and severity of depression. *Arch Gen Psychiatry* **49**, 388–395.

Evans, D.L., Leserman, J., Perkins, D.O. *et al.* (1997). Severe life stress as a predictor of early disease progression in HIV infection. *Am J Psychiatry* **154**, 630–634.

Everson, S.A., Goldberg, D.E., Kaplan, G.A. *et al.* (1996). Hopelessness and risk of mortality and incidence of myocardial infarction and cancer. *Psychosom Med* **58**, 113–121.

Faller, H., Bulzebruck, H., Drings, P. and Lang, H. (1999). Coping, distress, and survival among patients with lung cancer. *Arch Gen Psychiatry* **56**, 756–762.

Fawzy, F.I., Kemeny, M.E., Fawzy, N.W. *et al.* (1990). A structured psychiatric intervention for cancer patients. II. Changes over time in immunological measures. *Arch Gen Psychiatry* **47**, 729–735.

Fawzy, F.I., Fawzy, N.W., Hyun, C.S. *et al.* (1993). Malignant melanoma: effects of an early structured psychiatric intervention, coping, and affective state on recurrence and survival 6 years later. *Arch Gen Psychiatry* **50**, 681–689.

Frank, M.G., Hendricks, S.E., Johnson, D.R., Wieseler, J.L. and Burke, W.J. (1999). Antidepressants augment natural killer cell activity: in vivo and in vitro. *Neuropsychobiology* **39**, 18–24.

Friedman, G.D. (1994). Psychiatrically-diagnosed depression and subsequent cancer. *Cancer Epidemiol Biomarkers Prev* **3**, 11–13.

Haack, M., Hinze-Selch, D., Fenzel, T. *et al.* (1999). Plasma levels of cytokines and soluble cytokine receptors in psychiatric patients upon hospital admission: effects of confounding factors and diagnosis. *J Psychiatr Res* **33**, 407–418.

Hahn, R.C. and Petitti, D.B. (1988). Minnesota multiphasic personality inventory-rated depression and the incidence of breast cancer. *Cancer* **61**, 845–848.

Hall, M., Baum, A., Buysse, D.J. *et al.* (1998). Sleep as a mediator of the stress-immune relationship. *Psychosom Med* **60**, 48–51.

Healy, D., Calvin, J., Whitehouse, A.M. *et al.* (1991). Alpha-1–acid glycoprotein in major depressive and eating disorders. *J Affect Disord* **22**, 13–20.

Herbert, T.B. and Cohen, S. (1993). Depression and immunity: a meta-analytic review. *Psychol Bull* **113**, 472–486.

Hickie, I., Hickie, C., Lloyd, A., Silove, D. and Wakefield, D. (1993). Impaired *in vivo* immune responses in patients with melancholia. *Br J Psychiatry* **162**, 651–657.

Holsboer, F. and Barden, N. (1996). Antidepressants and hypothalamic-pituitary-adrenocortical regulation. *Endocr Rev* **17**, 187–205.

Irwin, M. (1993). Brain corticotropin-releasing-hormone and interleukin-1-beta-induced suppression of specific antibody production. *Endocrinology* **133**, 1352–1360.

Irwin, M. (1999). Immune correlates of depression. *Adv Exp Med Biol* **461**, 1–24.

Irwin, M., Smith, T.L. and Gillin, J.C. (1987). Low natural killer cytotoxicity in major depression. *Life Sci* **41**, 2127–2133.

Irwin, M., Hauger, R.L., Brown, M. *et al.* (1988).CRF activates autonomic nervous system and reduces natural killer cell cytotoxicity. *Am J Physiol* **255**, R744–747.

Irwin, M., Patterson, T., Smith, T.L. *et al.* (1990a). Reduction of immune function in life stress and depression. *Biol Psychiatry* **27**, 22–30.

Irwin, M., Vale, W. and Rivier, C. (1990b). Central corticotropin-releasing factor mediates the suppressive effects of stress on natural killer cytotoxicity. *Endocrinology* **126**, 2837–2844.

Irwin, M., Brown, M., Patterson, T. *et al.* (1991). Neuropeptide Y and natural killer cell activity: findings in depression and Alzheimer caregiver stress. *FASEB J* **5**, 3100–3107.

Irwin, M., Lacher, U. and Caldwell, C. (1992). Depression and reduced natural killer cytotoxicity: a longitudinal study of depressed patients and control subjects. *Psychol Med* **22**, 1045–1050.

Irwin, M, Mascovich, A, Gillin, J.C., *et al.* (1994). Partial sleep deprivation reduces natural killer cell activity in humans. *Psychosom Med* **56**, 493–498.

Jamison, R.N., Burish, T.G. and Wallston, K.A. (1987). Psychogenic factors in predicting survival of breast cancer patients. *J Clin Oncol* **5**, 768–772.

Joyce, P.R., Hawes, C.R., Mulder, R.T. *et al.* (1992). Elevated levels of acute phase plasma proteins in major depression. *Biol Psychiatry* **32**, 1035–1041.

Kanba, S., Manki, H., Shintani, F. *et al.* (1998). Aberrant interleukin-2 receptor-mediated blastoformation of peripheral blood lymphocytes in a severe major depressive episode. *Psycholog Med* **28**, 481–484.

Kaplan, G.A. and Reynolds, P. (1988). Depression and cancer mortality and morbidity: prospective evidence from the Alameda County study. *J Behav Med* **11**, 1–13.

Karalis, K., Sano, H., Redwine, J. *et al.* (1991). Autocrine or paracrine inflammatory actions of corticotropin-releasing hormone *in vivo*. *Science* **254**, 421–423.

Karalis, K., Muglia, L.J., Bae, D. *et al.* (1997). CRH and the immune system. *J Neuroimmunol* **72**, 131–136.

Kawahito, Y., Sano, H. and Mukai, S. (1995). Corticotropin releasing hormone in colonic mucosa in patients with ulcerative colitis. *Gut* **37**, 544–551.

Knekt, P., Raitasalo, R., Heliovaara, M. *et al.* (1996). Elevated lung cancer risk among persons with depressed mood. *Am J Epid* **144**, 1096–1103.

Kronfol, Z. and House, J.D. (1985). Depression, hypothalamic-pituitary-adrenocortical activity, and lymphocyte function. *Psychopharm Bull* **21**, 476–478.

Kronfol, Z. and House, J.D. (1989). Lymphocyte mitogenesis, immunoglobulin and complement levels in depressed patients and normal controls. *Acta Psychiatr Scand* **80**, 142–147.

Kronfol, Z., Silva, J., Greden, J. *et al.* (1983). Impaired lymphocyte function in depressive illness. *Life Sci* **33**, 241–247.

Kronfol, Z., House, J.D., Silva, J., Greden, J. and Carroll, B.J. (1986). Depression, urinary free cortisol excretion and lymphocyte function. *Br J Psychiatry* **148**, 70–73.

Kronfol, Z., Nair, M., Goodson, J. *et al.* (1989). Natural killer cell activity in depressive illness: preliminary report. *Biol Psychiatry* **26**, 753–756.

Labeur, M.S., Arzt, E. and Wiegers, G.J. (1995). Long-term intracerebroventricular corticotropin-releasing hormone administration induces distinct changes in rat splenocyte activation and cytokine expression. *Endocrinology* **136**, 2678–2688.

Landmann, R., Schaub, B., Link, S. and Wacker, H.R. (1997). Unaltered monocyte function in patients with major depression before and after three months of antidepressive therapy. *Biol Psychiatry* **41**, 675–681.

Leserman, J., Petitto, J.M., Perkins, D.O. *et al.* (1997). Severe stress, depressive symptoms, and changes in lymphocyte subsets in human immunodeficiency virus-infected men. A 2-year follow-up study. *Arch Gen Psychiatry* **54**, 279–285.

Leserman, J., Jackson, E.D., Petitto, J.M. *et al.* (1999). Progression to AIDS: the effects of stress, depressive symptoms, and social support. *Psychosom Med* **61**, 397–406.

Leu, S.-J.C. and Singh, V.K. (1993). Suppression of in vitro antibody production by corticotropin-releasing factor neurohormone. *J Neuroimmunol* **45**, 23–29.

Levine, J., Barak, Y., Chengappa, K.N. *et al.* (1999). Cerebrospinal cytokine levels in patients with acute depression. *Neuropsychobiology* **40**, 171–176.

Levy, E.M., Borrelli, D.J., Mirin, S.M. *et al.* (1991). Biological measures and cellular immunological function in depressed psychiatric inpatients. *Psychiatry Res* **36**, 157–167.

Linkins, R.W. and Comstock, G.W. (1990). Depressed mood and development of cancer. *Am J Epidemiol* **132**, 962–972.

Lyketsos, C.G., Hoover, D.R., Guccione, M. *et al.* (1993). Depressive symptoms as predictors of medical outcomes in HIV infection. Multicenter AIDS Cohort Study. *JAMA* **270**, 2563–2567.

Lyketsos, C.G., Hoover, D.R. and Guccione, M. (1996). Depression and survival among HIV-infected persons. *JAMA* **275**, 35–36.

Maes, M., Bosmans, E., Suy, E. *et al.* (1991a). Depression-related disturbances in mitogen-induced lymphocyte responses and interleukin-1beta and soluble inter-leukin-2 receptor production. *Acta Psychiatr Scand* **84**, 379–386.

Maes, M., Bosmans, E., Suy, E. *et al.* (1991b). Antiphospholipid, antinuclear, Epstein-Barr and cytomegalovirus antibodies, and soluble interleukin-2 receptors in depressive patients. *J Affect Disord* **21**, 133–140.

Maes, M., Lambrechts, J., Bosmans, E. *et al.* (1992a). Evidence for a systemic immune activation during depression: results of leukocyte enumeration by flow cytometry in conjunction with monoclonal antibody staining. *Psychol Med* **22**, 45–53.

Maes, M., Stevens, W., Peeters, D. *et al.* (1992b). A study on the blunted natural killer cell activity in severely depressed patients. *Life Sci* **50**, 505–513.

Maes, M., Scharpe, S. and Van Grootel, L. (1992c). Higher alpha-1-antitrypsin, haptoglobin, ceruloplasmin and lower retinol binding protein plasma levels during depression: Further evidence for the existence of an inflammatory response during that illness. *J Affect Disord* **24**, 183–192.

Maes, M., Stevens, W.J., Declerck, L.S. *et al.* (1993). Significantly increased expression of T-cell activation markers (interleukin-2 and HLA-DR) in depression: further evidence for an inflammatory process during that illness. *Prog Neuropsychopharmacol Biol Psychiatry* **17**, 241–255.

Maes, M., Meltzer, H.Y. and Bosmans, E. (1995). Increased plasma concentrations of interleukin-6, soluble interleukin-6, soluble interleukin-2, and transferrin receptor in major depression. *J Affect Disord* **34**, 301–309.

Maes, M., Vandoolaeghe, E., Ranjan, R. *et al.* (1996). Increased serum soluble CD8 or suppressor/cytotoxic antigen concentrations in depression: suppressive effects of glucocorticoids. *Biol Psychiatry* **40**, 1273–1281.

Maes, M., Delange, J., Ranjan, R. *et al.* (1997). Acute phase proteins in schizophrenia, mania and major depression: modulation by psychotropic drugs. *Psychiatry Res* **66**, 1–11.

Maes, M., Song, C., Lin, A.H. *et al.* (1999). Negative immunoregulatory effects of antidepressants: inhibition of interferon-gamma and stimulation of interleukin-10 secretion. *Neuropsychopharmacology* **20**, 370–379.

Mayne, T.J., Vittinghoff, E., Chesney., M.A., Barrett, D.C. and Coates, T.J. (1996). Depressive affect and survival among gay and bisexual men infected with HIV. *Arch Intern Med* **156**, 2233–2238.

McAdams, C. and Leonard, B.E. (1993). Neutrophil and monocyte phagocytosis in depressed patients. *Prog Neuropsychopharmacol Biol Psychiatry* **17**, 971–984.

Meyers, C.A. (1999). Mood and cognitive disorders in cancer patients receiving cytokine therapy. *Adv Exp Med Biol* **461**, 75–81.

Miller, A.H. and Lackner, C. (1989). Tricyclic antidepressants and immunity. In: Miller, A.H. (Ed.) *Depressive Disorders and Immunity,* American Psychiatric Press, Washington DC, pp. 85–104.

Miller, A.H., Asnis, G.M., van Pragg, H.M. *et al.* (1986). The influence of desmethylimipramine on natural killer cell activity. *Psychiatry Res* **19**, 9–15.

Miller, A.H., Asnis, G.M., Lackner, C., Halbreich, U. and Norin, A.J. (1991)

Depression, natural killer cell activity, and cortisol secretion. *Biol Psychiatry* **29**, 878–886.

Miller, A.H., Spencer, R.L., Hassett, J. *et al.* (1994). Effects of selective type I and II adrenal steroid receptor agonists on immune cell distribution. *Endocrinology* **135**, 1934–1944.

Miller, G.E., Cohen, S. and Herbert, T.B. (1999). Pathways linking major depression and immunity in ambulatory female patients. *Psychosom Med* **61**, 850–860.

Mohl, P.C., Huang, L., Bowden, C. *et al.* (1987). Natural killer cell activity in major depression. *Am J Psychiatry* **144**, 1619.

Moldofsky, H., Lue., F.A., Shahal, B., Jiang, C.G. and Gorczynski, R.M. (1995). Diurnal sleep/wake-related immune functions during the menstrual cycle of healthy young women. *J Sleep Res* **4**, 150–159.

Morag, M., Yirmiya, R., Lerer, B. and Morag, A. (1998). Influence of socioeconomic status on behavioral, emotional, and cognitive effects of rubella vaccination: a prospective, double blind study. *Psychoneuroendocrinology* **23**, 337–351.

Muller, N. and Ackenheil, M. (1998). Psychoneuroimmunology and the cytokine action in the CNS: implications for psychiatric disorders. *Prog Neuropsychopharmacol Biol Psychiatry* **22**, 1–33.

Muller, N., Hofschuster, E., Ackenheil, M., Mempel, W. and Eckstein, R. (1993). Investigations of the cellular immunity during depression and the free interval: evidence for an immune activation in affective psychosis. *Prog Neuropsychopharm Biol Psychiatry* **17**, 713–730.

Nerozzi, D., Santoni, A., Bersani, G. *et al.* (1989). Reduced natural killer cell activity in major depression: neuroendocrine implications. *Psychoneuroendocrinology* **14**, 295–301.

Neveu, P.J. and Castanon, N. (1999). Is there evidence for an effect of antidepressant drugs on immune function? *Adv Exp Med Biol* **461**, 267–282.

Owens, M.J. and Nemeroff, C.B. (1993). The role of corticotropin-releasing factor in the pathophysiology of affective and anxiety disorder: laboratory and clinical studies. *Ciba Found Symp* **172**, 296–308.

Pariante, C.M. and Miller, A.H. (1995). Natural killer cell activity in major depression: a prospective study of the *in vivo* effects of desmethylimipramine treatment. *Eur Neuropsychopharm* **5**(Suppl), 83–88.

Penninx, B.W., Guralnik, J.M., Pahor, M. *et al.* (1998). Chronically depressed mood and cancer risk in older persons. *J Natl Cancer Inst* **90**, 1888–1893.

Paez Pereda, M.P., Sauer, J., Perez Castro, C.P. *et al.* (1995). Corticotropin-releasing hormone differentially modulates the interleukin-1 system according to the level of monocyte activation by endotoxin. *Endocrinology* **136**, 5504–5510.

Perry, S., Fishman, B., Jacobsberg, L. and Frances, A. (1992). Relationships over 1 year between lymphocyte subsets and psychosocial variables among adults with infection by human immunodeficiency virus. *Arch Gen Psychiatry* **49**, 396–401.

Persky, V.W., Kempthorne-Rawson, J. and Shekelle, R.B. (1987). Personality and risk of cancer: 20-year follow-up of the Western Electric Study. *Psychosom Med* **49**, 435–449.

Petitto, J.M., Folds, J.D. and Evans, D.L. (1993). Abnormal diurnal variation of B lymphocyte circulation patterns in major depression. *Biol Psychiatry* **34**, 268–270.

Rabkin, J.G., Williams, J.B.W., Remien, R.H. *et al.* (1991). Depression, distress, lymphocyte subsets, and human immunodeficiency virus symptoms on two occasions in HIV-positive homosexual men. *Arch Gen Psychiatry* **48**, 111–119.

Rabkin, J.G., Wagner, G. and Rabkin, R. (1994). Effects of sertraline on mood and immune status in patients with major depression and HIV illness: an open trial. *J Clin Psychiatry* **55**, 433–439.

Ramirez, A.J., Craig, T.K.J., Watson, J.P. *et al.* (1989). Stress and relapse of breast cancer. *Br Med J* **298**, 291–293.

Rassnick, S., Sved, A.F. and Rabin, B.S. (1994). Locus coeruleus stimulation by corticotropin-releasing hormone suppresses in vitro cellular immune responses. *J Neurosci* **14**, 6033–6040.

Ravindran, A.V., Griffiths, J., Merali, Z. and Anisman, H. (1998). Circulating lymphocyte subsets in major depression and dysthymia with typical or atypical features. *Psychosomatic Med* **60**, 283–289.

Savard, J., Miller, S.M., Mills, M. *et al.* (1999). Association between subjective sleep quality and depression on immunocompetence in low-income women at risk for cervical cancer. *Psychosom Med* **61**, 496–507.

Schafer, M., Carter, L. and Stein, C. (1994). Interleukin 1 beta and corticotropin-releasing factor inhibit pain by releasing opioids from immune cells in inflamed tissue. *Proc Natl Acad Sci USA* **91**, 4219–4223.

Schleifer, S.J., Keller, S.E., Meyerson, A.T. *et al.* (1984). Lymphocyte function in major depressive disorder. *Arch Gen Psychiatry* **41**, 484–486.

Schleifer, S.J., Keller, S.E., Siris, S.G., Davis, K.L. and Stein, M. (1985). Depression and immunity: lymphocyte function in ambulatory depressed patients, hospitalized schizophrenic patients, and patients hospitalized for herniorrhaphy. *Arch Gen Psychiatry* **42**, 129–133.

Schleifer, S.J., Keller, S.E., Bond, R.N., Cohen, J. and Stein, M. (1989). Major depressive disorder and immunity: role of age, sex, severity and hospitalization. *Arch Gen Psychiatry* **46**, 81–87.

Schleifer, S.J., Keller, S.E., Bartlett, J.A., Eckholdt, H.M. and Delaney, B.R. (1996). Immunity in young adults with major depressive disorder. *Am J Psychiatry* **153**, 477–482.

Schleifer, S.J., Keller, S.E. and Bartlett, J.A. (1999). Depression and immunity: clinical factors and therapeutic course. *Psychiatry Res* **85**, 63–69.

Schulte, H.M., Bamberger, C.M., Elsen, H. *et al.* (1994). Systemic interleukin-1 alpha and interleukin-2 secretion in response to acute stress and to corticotropin-releasing hormone in humans. *Eur J Clin Invest* **24**, 773–777.

Schulz, R., Bookwala, J., Knapp, J.E., Scheier, M. and Williamson, G.M. (1996). Pessimism, age, and cancer mortality. *Psychol Aging* **11**, 304–309.

Seidel, A., Arolt, V., Hunstiger, M. *et al.* (1995). Cytokine production and serum proteins in depression. *Scand J Immunol* **41**, 534–538.

Sengar, D.P.S., Waters, B.G.H., Dunne, J.V. and Bouer, I.M. (1982). Lymphocyte subpopulations and mitogenic responses of lymphocytes in manic-depressive disorders. *Biol Psychiatry* **17**, 1017–1022.

Shekelle, R.B., Raynor, W.J. Jr, Ostfeld, A.M. *et al.* (1981). Psychological depression and 17-year risk of death from cancer. *Psychosom Med* **43**, 117–125.

Sluzewska, A., Rybakowski, J.K., Laciak, M. *et al.* (1995). Interleukin-6 serum levels in depressed patients before and after treatment with fluoxetine. *Ann NY Acad Sci* **762**, 474–476.

Sluzewska, A., Rybakowski, J., Bosmans, E. *et al.* (1996). Indicators of immune activation in major depression. *Psychiatry Res* **64**, 161–167.

Song, C., Dinan, T. and Leonard, B.E. (1994). Changes in immunoglobulin, complement and acute phase protein levels in the depressed patients and normal controls. *J Affect Disord* **30**, 283–288.

Spiegel, D., Bloom, J.R., Kraemer, H.C. and Gottheil, E. (1989). Effect of psychosocial treatment on survival of patients with metastatic breast cancer. *Lancet* **2**, 888–891.

Stenzel-Poore, M.P., Duncan, J.E., Rittenberg, M.B. *et al.* (1996). CRH overproduction in transgenic mice: behavioral and immune system modulation. *Ann NY Acad Sci* **780**, 36–48.

Stubner, S., Schon, T. and Padberg, F. (1999). Interleukin-6 and the soluble IL-6 receptor are decreased in cerebrospinal fluid of geriatric patients with major depression: no alteration of soluble gp130. *Neurosci Lett* **259**, 145–148.

Syvalahti, E., Eskola, J., Ruuskanen, O. and Laine, T. (1985). Nonsuppression of cortisol in depression and immune function. *Prog Neuropsychopharmacol Biol Psychiatry* **9**, 413–422.

Tross, S., Herndon, J 2nd., Korzun, A. *et al.* (1996). Psychological symptoms and disease-free and overall survival in women with stage II breast cancer. Cancer and Leukemia Group B. *J Natl Cancer Inst* **88**, 661–667.

Urch, A., Muller, C., Aschauer, H., Resch, F. and Zielinski, C.C. (1988). Lytic effector cell function in schizophrenia and depression. *J Neuroimmunol* **18**, 291–301.

Watson, M., Haviland, J.S., Greer, S., Davidson, J. and Bliss, J.M. (1999). Influence of psychological response on survival in breast cancer: a population-based cohort study. *Lancet* **354**, 1331–1336.

Weizman, R., Laor, N., Podliszewski, E. *et al.* (1994). Cytokine production in major depressed patients before and after clomipramine treatment. *Biol Psychiatry* **35**, 42–47.

Whooley, M.A. and Browner, W.S. (1998). Association between depressive symptoms and mortality in older women. *Arch Intern Med* **158**, 2129–2135.

Xia, Z., DePierre, J.W. and Nassberger, L. (1996). Tricyclic antidepressants inhibit IL-6, IL-1beta and TNF-alpha release in human blood monocytes and IL-2 and interferon-gamma in T cells. *Immunopharmacology* **34**, 27–37.

Yoshihara, S., Ricciardolo, F.L.M., Geppetti, P. *et al.* (1995). Corticotropin-releasing factor inhibits antigen-induced plasma extravasation in airways. *Eur J Pharmacol* **280**, 113–118.

Zonderman, A.B., Costa, P.T. and McCrae, R.R. (1989). Depression as a risk for cancer morbidity and mortality in a nationally representative sample. *JAMA* **262**, 1191–1195.

9

Antiglucocorticoid Strategies in Treating Major Depression and 'Allostatic Load'

OWEN M. WOLKOWITZ, ELISSA S. EPEL and VICTOR I. REUS

*Department of Psychiatry, School of Medicine,
University of California, San Francisco, USA*

We are on our guard against external intoxicants, but hormones are parts of our bodies; it takes more wisdom to recognize and overcome the foe who fights from within ... (But) what can we do about this? ... We do not yet know enough about their workings to justify any attempt at regulating our emotional key by taking hormones.

The Stress of Life (Selye, 1956)

INTRODUCTION

Forty-five years after Hans Selye, the 'Father of Stress Physiology', wrote these words, we are seemingly in a much stronger position to 'regulate our emotional key' by recognizing and correcting hormonal imbalances that are associated with behavioural disturbances. The purpose of this chapter is to summarize our current understanding of the role of stress hormone dysregulation in precipitating depressive symptoms and poor health outcomes, as well as to speculate on the role of novel hormonal interventions in treating such disorders.

Adrenocortical responses to acutely stressful situations are critical for successful adaptation, and, indeed, for life itself. Nonetheless, when such responses are excessive or remain elevated for extended periods of time, detrimental effects on both emotional well-being and physical health may ensue (McEwen *et al.*, 1992; Raber, 1998). The successful adaptation to acute stress has been termed 'allostasis', and the toll exerted on the organism by excessive allostatic demands has been termed 'allostatic load' (McEwen, 2000). The major premises of this chapter are that: (1) to the extent that inappropriate adrenocortical output has direct adverse health effects, interventions that normalize adrenocortical hormone levels should have salutary ones (Wolkowitz and Reus, 1999), and (2) understanding the biological mechanisms by which chronically activated limbic–hypothalamic–pituitary–adrenal (LHPA) axis activity leads to depression and poor health will likely prompt the development of new and specific therapeutic interventions (Raber, 1998).

In this chapter we review in greater detail the concepts of allostasis and allostatic load and how they might bear upon depressive and certain physical symptoms. We then review the evidence that hypercortisolaemia and other hormonal aberrations are associated with depressive illness and with risk factors for poor health. Finally, we review empirical data suggesting that clinical interventions that restore adrenocortical hormones to healthy levels have antidepressant and health promoting effects. The major focus of this chapter is the relationship of stress hormone activity to depression. Where pertinent, we also briefly review the peripheral health consequences of allostatic load and their potential sensitivity to antiglucocorticoid treatments. Also, while pharmacological treatment strategies are the primary focus of this review, we additionally review evidence suggesting that behavioural interventions have comparable effects, perhaps via similar endocrinologic mechanisms.

ALLOSTASIS AND ALLOSTATIC LOAD

Given the pervasive and varied effects of the stress response on regulatory systems, it has been difficult to show common mechanisms leading to disease. Allostasis or 'stability through change', describes the body's facile and efficient adaptation to demands of the moment (Sterling and Eyer, 1988). When no challenge is present, healthy allostasis is reflected by low levels of physiological arousal. When a threat is present, maintaining allostasis necessitates mounting a rapid stress response (including increased secretion of cortisol), and a rapid recovery back to resting state when the threat has resolved (Eriksen et al., 1999). However, cortisol can have harmful effects when its actions are prolonged and unopposed by counter-regulating or anabolic hormones. During stress and recovery from stress, counter-regulatory hormones, such as dehydroepiandrosterone (DHEA) and growth hormone (GH), can be elevated or suppressed and can play important roles in restoring equilibrium and repairing stress-related damage. Indeed, with ongoing stress, DHEA levels, which are initially elevated, decrease to levels below baseline (Stahl et al., 1992). As we demonstrate, this finely tuned response may go awry in depression and other states of chronic stress, during which catabolic stress hormones such as cortisol become damaging rather than protective (McEwen and Stellar, 1993).

The overall balance of anabolic to catabolic activity could be an informative index of health status. We refer to relative levels of DHEA or other anabolic hormones (e.g. testosterone, growth hormone, or insulin-like growth factor (IGF-1) to cortisol as 'anabolic balance' (Epel *et al.*, 1998). This ratio describes the net catabolic or anabolic effect on physiology. A catabolic profile (e.g. high cortisol and low DHEA) is often associated with depression, chronic stress and certain conditions of maladaptive response to ongoing stress (Goodyer *et al.*, 1996; Hechter *et al.*, 1997; Herbert 1997, 1998; McEwen and Seeman, 1999; Wolkowitz, 1999). High cortisol or a low anabolic balance is thought to be a primary response to stress that underlies pathogenic processes and leads to a cascade of dysregulation across systems and allostatic load (McEwen, 1998).

Allostatic load markers are thought to precede the expression of diagnosable chronic diseases (McEwen and Seeman, 1999; Eriksen *et al.*, 1999). The concept of allostatic load has only been tested in preliminary ways so far. To date, allostatic load markers have included indices of high cortisol, catecholamines and blood pressure, poor blood sugar control, visceral fat and low dehydroepiandrosterone-sulphate (DHEA-S). In the MacArthur Aging Study, this index predicted development of cardiovascular disease and cognitive decline in 1189 elderly people, 2.5 years (Seeman *et al.*, 1997) and 7 years later (Seeman *et al.*, 2001). Most strikingly, what appear to be subtle and subclinical signs of dysregulation may be pathophysiological. For example, *relatively* higher levels of stress mediators, such as cortisol and catecholamines, rather than clinically abnormal levels, confer risk of disease (Seeman *et al.*, 1997; McEwen, 2000). In this study, a measure of anabolic balance or stress mediators (high levels of cortisol and catecholamines, and low levels of DHEA-S) was compared with traditional risk factors (visceral fat, blood pressure and blood lipids). Stress mediators were equally predictive of allostatic load, supporting the importance of stress arousal in contributing to disease processes.

Similarly, in a population-based study of Swedish men, Rosmond and Björntorp discerned an overriding function of pathological LHPA axis activity on other, established risk factors for cardiovascular disease, type 2 diabetes and stroke (Rosmond and Björntorp, 2000). Further, they identified a polymorphism of the glucocorticoid receptor gene, with 13.7% homozygotes in the Swedish population, that might be responsible for the observed relationship between endocrine dysregulation and the observed anthropometric and metabolic abnormalities, such as central obesity, insulin resistance and hypertension; they termed this construct the 'hypothalamic arousal syndrome' (Björntorp *et al.*, 1999). This may be a similar construct as allostatic load, in that primary stress mediators are dysregulated. A full allostatic load battery – reflecting functioning across multiple regulatory systems – has not been tested on a depressed sample. However, when taking a wide lens view across studies relating physical symptoms and diseases to depression, they are conditions linked to overexposure to cortisol and other stress mediators. Thus, allostatic load may serve as a unifying theme to explain certain syndrome-like effects of altered cortisol levels.

Several of the basic mechanisms of steroid action, such as acute effects on neurotransmission, chronic effects on genomic transcription and on glucose disposition and possible trophic or atrophic effects on hippocampal neurons, may directly bear upon the sequelae of allostatic load. While a discussion of these mechanisms is beyond the scope of the present chapter, the interested reader is referred to several other articles (McEwen et al., 1979, 1992; Sapolsky et al., 1986, 1990; Majewska, 1987; Biegon, 1990; Wolkowitz et al., 1990; McEwen, 1991, 1997, 2000; Sapolsky, 1992; Wolkowitz, 1994; De Kloet et al., 1998).

EXOGENOUS CORTICOSTEROID EFFECTS

Several lines of evidence suggest that corticosteroids significantly regulate human behaviour as well as physical health. Among the earliest indications was the observation of behavioural changes, occasionally profound (e.g. delirium, confusion, insomnia, emotional lability, depression, hypomania, memory and attentional impairments, sensory flooding, psychosis and even suicidality) in some medically ill patients prescribed cortisone, dexamethasone, prednisone and other synthetic corticosteroids (Boston Collaborative Drug Surveillance Program, 1972); (Hall et al., 1979; Ling et al., 1981; Reus and Wolkowitz, 1993; Pies, 1995; Naber et al., 1996; Keenan et al., 1996; Wolkowitz et al., 1990, 1997a). Also of potential concern are isolated reports of individual patients suffering long-lasting cognitive impairment suggestive of hippocampal dysfunction after corticosteroid treatment (Wolkowitz et al., 1997a). While these studies demonstrate the potential of corticosteroids to induce psychiatric symptoms, it is problematic to directly extrapolate from the effects of exogenous corticosteroids to those of endogenous hypercortisolaemia (Wolkowitz, 1994; Plihal et al., 1996; Wolkowitz et al., 1997a).

Prolonged pharmacologic steroid treatment is also often accompanied by multiple somatic side-effects, including hypertension, hypernatraemia, hypokalaemia, central adiposity, nuchal fat pad deposition, 'moon facies', muscle wasting, cataracts, immune suppression, haematologic and bleeding disorders, gastric ulceration, skin thinning, stunted growth (in children) and osteoporosis (Nesbitt, 1995). Some of these side-effects are similar to those seen with severe, naturally occurring allostatic load. Interestingly, some of the catabolic effects of prednisone can be reversed by administration of the anabolic hormones GH or IGF-1 (Moxley, 1994).

ENDOGENOUS HYPERCORTISOLAEMIA: CUSHING'S SYNDROME

Excessively high levels of endogenously produced cortisol (or dysregulation of LHPA axis negative feedback), as seen in Cushing's syndrome, are also associated with altered psychological status, generally in the direction of depression and cognitive impairment, and with impaired health.

Depression in Cushing's syndrome

Cushing's syndrome is associated with a high incidence of fatigue, decreased energy, irritability, decreased memory and concentration, depressed or labile mood, decreased libido, insomnia and crying (Trethowen and Cobb, 1952; Whelan et al., 1980; Starkman et al., 1981). These symptoms are reminiscent of those commonly seen in major depression (Haskett, 1985), although certain differences, such as a preponderance of 'atypical' depressive features in Cushing's syndrome patients, may exist (Kling et al., 1991; Loosen, 1992). These symptoms in Cushing's syndrome patients are directly correlated with circulating cortisol levels (Cohen, 1980; Starkman et al., 1981). Cushing's syndrome patients also seemingly have hippocampal formation volume loss (assessed radiographically) (Starkman et al., 1992) or atrophy of the hypothalamic paraventricular nucleus (assessed at autopsy) (Spillane, 1951). The hippocampal formation volume in these patients is directly related to cognitive performance and is inversely related to urinary free cortisol levels (Starkman et al., 1992). The incidence of depression (approximately 62–67%) is not significantly different in patients with Cushing's syndrome (which is non-ACTH dependent) v. Cushing's disease (which is ACTH dependent) (Kathol, 1985; Murphy, 1991a; Sonino et al., 1993), suggesting a stronger relationship with circulating cortisol levels than with circulating ACTH levels. This suggestion is supported by the relatively low incidence of depression in patients with Nelson's syndrome, a post-adrenalectomy condition characterized by high CRH and ACTH levels but low cortisol levels (Kelly et al., 1980, 1983). Some studies, however, have found higher neuropsychiatric impairment in patients with elevated cortisol and ACTH levels than in patients with elevations in cortisol levels alone (Starkman et al., 1981).

Antiglucocorticoid treatment of Cushing's syndrome

Depressive and cognitive symptoms in Cushing's disease and Cushing's syndrome typically resolve with treatment of the hypercortisolaemia (Trethowen and Cobb, 1952; Hamm, 1955; Gifford and Gunderson, 1970; Taft et al., 1970; Welbourn et al., 1971; Regestein et al., 1972; Kelly et al., 1980, 1983, 1996; Jeffcoate et al., 1979; Cohen, 1980; Angeli and Frairia, 1985; Kramlinger et al., 1985; Nieman et al., 1985; Voigt et al., 1985; Loli et al., 1986; Sonino et al., 1986; Starkman et al., 1986; Ravaris et al., 1988, 1994; Arteaga *et al.*, 1989; Sonino *et al.*, 1991, 1993; van der Lely *et al.*, 1991; Verhelst *et al.*, 1991; Mauri *et al.*, 1993; Zeiger *et al.*, 1993; Li *et al.*, 1996) in direct relationship to the reductions in circulating cortisol levels. At least 28 separate reports have documented decreased depression, anxiety, suicidality, irritability, psychosis and cognitive impairment, and even complete psychiatric remission, in Cushing's patients who received either surgical or medical (e.g. ketoconazole, metyrapone, aminoglutethimide, RU-486) treatment aimed at lowering cortisol levels or cortisol activity. The largest two case series documented a response rate of 70–73% of treated patients (Verhelst *et al.*, 1991; Sonino *et al.*, 1993), although in several cases, psychiatric improvement was erratic, delayed or incomplete. Hippocampal volume loss may also eventually recover subsequent to normalization of cortisol levels (Starkman *et al.*, 1999). However, in some cases, brain damage may be irreversible or only partially reversible (Trethowen and Cobb, 1952). These treatment trials have been reviewed in greater detail elsewhere (Wolkowitz and Reus, 1999). These observations are quite suggestive of an aetiological role of cortisol elevations in psychiatric symptomatology, although it remains difficult to factor out non-specific illness-related contributions to the clinical presentation in patients with Cushing's disease and Cushing's syndrome. Additionally, levels of steroid hormones other than cortisol, which are also abnormal in Cushing's syndrome patients and which also have neuroactive properties, such as DHEA, have received virtually no attention to date (Levine and Mitty, 1988; Dubrovsky, 1991; Murphy, 1991a). The anabolic balance may be more important than cortisol alone in determining severity of depression. Another difficulty in interpreting the literature in Cushing's syndrome patients is that patients with Addison's disease (adrenocortical insufficiency) may also present with depression (Cleghorn, 1951; Leigh and Kramer, 1984); in such patients, psychiatric disturbances are negatively correlated with serum cortisol levels (Lobo *et al.*, 1988), and glucocorticoid administration as well as administration of the androgenic precursor hormone, DHEA (Arlt *et al.*, 1998; 1999), typically relieves the psychiatric symptoms. The relationship between cortisol and mood is undoubtedly complex and may even resemble an inverted U-shaped dose–response curve, with optimal functioning at mid-range levels (McEwen, 1987).

ENDOGENOUS HYPERCORTISOLAEMIA: MAJOR DEPRESSION

Hypercortisolaemia (either basally or following dexamethasone suppression) has been repeatedly demonstrated in many patients with major depression (Carroll *et al.*, 1981; Reus, 1985; Murphy, 1991a; Nelson and Davis, 1997) and has been directly correlated with symptoms such as sleep disturbance, decreased energy, impaired cognitive performance, psychosis, suicidality, decreased libido, psychomotor disturbance and anxiety (Reus, 1982; Winokur *et al.*, 1987; Meador-Woodruff *et al.*, 1990; Wolkowitz *et al.*, 1994). Further, continued hypercortisolaemia (in the face of seemingly adequate treatment) in depressed patients is a sign of incomplete recovery (Greden *et al.*, 1983; Ribeiro *et al.*, 1993). High cortisol-to-DHEA ratios may also predict persistence of depressive states (Goodyer *et al.*, 1998); this may be relevant to the notion of 'anabolic balance' described earlier. Consistent with a direct pathophysiologic role of hypecortisolaemia in depression are suggestions that common mechanisms of action of effective antidepressant treatments are increases in brain corticosteroid receptor levels, rendering individuals more sensitive to corticosteroid negative feedback (Barden *et al.*, 1995) or else the direct inhibition of glucocorticoid receptor-mediated gene transcription (Budziszewska *et al.*, 2000).

Antiglucocorticoid treatment of major depression

As reviewed above, excessive exposure to cortisol is often associated with depression and cognitive impairment, as well as with health risk factors such as low bone mineral density, cardiovascular alterations, insulin resistance and central body fat deposition. If these are causal relationships, as they appear to be, then hormones and other drugs considered antiglucocorticoids should have opposite effects on many of these health outcomes. We now review the effects of antiglucocorticoids and exogenous DHEA as well as effects of behavioural interventions on depression, stress hormones and certain health outcomes.

It is surprising that, until 1991, few studies had assessed the behavioural effects of direct pharmacological lowering of cortisol levels in patients with major depression. At present, there are 12 studies of antiglucocorticoids (used alone) in treating depression; only four of these were single or double-blinded. In interpreting the studies presented below, it is important to consider that, although cortisol was the major endocrinologic 'target' of the endocrinological interventions, the synthesis of other steroid hormones was invariably also affected by these drugs (Figure 1). Figure 1 displays the metabolic pathway of a number of adrenally-derived corticosteroids, along with the sites of enzymatic blockade of steroid biosynthesis inhibitors. As is evident, enzymatic blockade with these agents affects the synthesis of multiple steroid hormones, rendering the actual mechanism of any observed health effects indeterminate.

In each of the studies utilizing the antiglucocorticoid approach (Murphy, 1991a, b, 1997; Murphy *et al.*, 1991, 1993, 1998; Murphy and Wolkowitz, 1993; Wolkowitz *et al.*, 1993, 1999a; Amsterdam *et al.*, 1994; Anand *et al.*, 1995; Ghadirian *et al.*, 1995; O'Dwyer *et al.*, 1995; Thakore and Dinan, 1995; Iizuka *et al.*, 1996; Raven *et al.*, 1996; Sovner and Fogelman, 1996; Reus *et al.*, 1997; Malison *et al.*, 1999) antidepressant effects were reported in at least some patients. Across the 12 studies reviewed, an average of 67.5% of the treated

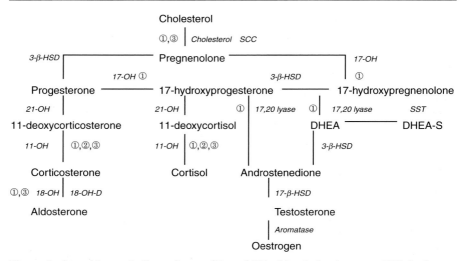

Figure 1. Steroid metabolic pathway. (Key: SCC, side chain cleavage; OH, hydroxylase; HSD, hydroxysteroid dehydrogenase; SST, steroid sulphotransferase; ①, site of blockade by ketoconazole; ②, site of blockade by metyrapone; ③, site of blockade by aminoglutethimide

patients showed at least a partial antidepressant response, and 55% showed a 'full' or clinically meaningful response. Of the studies that were single or double-blinded, 50% of the treated patients showed at least a partial antidepressant response, and 46.2% showed a 'full' or clinically meaningful response. These studies are described in greater detail elsewhere (Wolkowitz and Reus, 1999). These results must be interpreted very cautiously due to the small sample sizes in all of the studies.

Endocrinological predictors and correlates of antiglucocorticoid response remain uncertain. While it is appealing to postulate that patients who are hypercortisolaemic (or DST non-suppressing) at baseline are most likely to respond to this approach, few studies have meaningfully assessed this. In an early study by Murphy (1991b), five of six treatment responders who were DST non-suppressors before starting therapy had reverted to normal suppression when tested after completion of therapy; the one patient who did not revert to normal suppression suffered an early relapse (Murphy and Wolkowitz, 1993). Baseline 8.00 a.m. serum cortisol levels, however, did not predict treatment response, and treatment-associated decreases in 8.00 a.m. serum cortisol levels were inconsistent and not statistically significant. Other studies, however, have noted significant correlations between antidepressant effects and changes in cortisol levels. Anand *et al.* (1995), for example, in a double-blind case report utilizing ketoconazole, noted clinically significant improvements in depression and memory in one treatment-resistant patient. There was a close correlation between treatment-associated decreases in cortisol levels and decreases in Hamilton Depression Rating Scale (HDRS) ratings. Wolkowitz *et al.* (1993) also reported that ketoconazole, administered to medication-free depressed patients in an open-label manner for 3–6 weeks, significantly improved depression ratings and significantly decreased 4.00 p.m. serum cortisol levels. Changes in Beck Depression Inventory ratings were directly correlated with changes in serum cortisol levels. This research group subsequently reported on a sample of depressed patients treated with ketoconazole in a double-blind, placebo-controlled trial (Wolkowitz *et al.*, 1999a). Of 20 patients studied, eight were hypercortisolaemic at baseline (4.00 p.m. serum cortisol > 10 µg/dl) and 12 were eucortisolaemic. Whereas no significant main effect of ketoconazole v. placebo on depression ratings was observed, there was a significant interaction of drug (ketoconazole v. placebo) and baseline cortisol status (eucortisolaemic v. hypercortisolaemic). Specifically, ketoconazole was superior to placebo in alleviating depressive symptoms in the hypercortisolaemic but not in the eucortisolaemic patients. These findings are consistent with the hypothesized specificity of antiglucocorticoid benefits in hypercortisolaemic states and raise the possibility of biologically distinct sub-groups of patients with major depression. Such conclusions must remain tentative, however, due to the very small sample size of this and other studies.

Two other studies have attempted to clarify the mechanisms by which antiglucocorticoids might alleviate depression. Thakore and Dinan (1995) treated eight depressed patients with ketoconazole for four weeks and noted significant antidepressant effects (average decrease in HDRS ratings = 60%) and significant decreases in serum cortisol levels. They had postulated that elevated cortisol activity might provoke or maintain depressive symptoms via the induction of serotonin system sub-sensitivity. They based their hypothesis partially on observations that, in depressed patients, baseline cortisol levels are inversely related to the magnitude of serum prolactin (PRL) responses to 5HT agonists such as D-fenfluramine (a putative marker of serotonin system sensitivity). To test this hypothesis, they administered the D-fenfluramine challenge to their subjects at baseline and after four weeks of ketoconazole treatment. Ketoconazole normalized the PRL response to D-fenfluramine (i.e. increased the response relative to baseline), and the increases in PRL responses were significantly correlated with reductions in HDRS ratings. These findings are consistent with the notion that hypercortisolaemia down-regulates 5HT system sensitivity, and that antiglucocorticoid treatments may have antidepressant effects via a normalization (increase) of 5HT sensitivity. Lastly, O'Dwyer *et al.* (1995) treated eight depressed patients with metyrapone (plus replacement doses of hydrocortisone) v. placebo in a single-blind manner in a two week per-arm crossover design and noted significant decreases in depression ratings as well as in serum cortisol levels during metyrapone treatment. After discontinuation of metyrapone, depression ratings remained low despite return of cortisol to baseline levels. Checkley *et al.* (1994), commenting on the same group of subjects as O'Dwyer *et al.* (1995), noted that, in addition to normalizing cortisol levels, metyrapone led to an increased urinary excretion of the neuroactive steroids, tetrahydro-11-deoxycortisol and tetrahydrodeoxycortisone. They suggested that either the decreases in cortisol levels or the increases in levels of these 'neurosteroids' may have been related to the antidepressant effects (Checkley *et al.*, 1994; Raven *et al.*, 1996).

In addition to studies of antiglucocorticoids used alone in depression, other small-scale studies have examined their utility as augmentation agents in patients with treatment-resistant depression and other psychiatric illnesses. Beneficial effects of such treatment have been noted in patients with refractory bipolar II depression (Ravaris *et al.*, 1994) and severe refractory obsessive compulsive disorder (Chouinard *et al.*, 1996), in depressed schizophrenic and schizoaffective disorder patients, and in a patient with treatment-resistant depression and a coexisting 'metabolic syndrome' comprised of hypercortisolaemia, hypertension and insulin resistance (Bech *et al.*, 1999).

ALTERNATIVE ANTIGLUCOCORTICOID AND GLUCOCORTICOID TREATMENT APPROACHES TO DEPRESSION

Steroid receptor blockers (RU-486)

RU-486 (Mifepristone) does not inhibit steroid biosynthesis but blocks progesterone and, at higher doses, cortisol receptors in the brain. Indeed, circulating cortisol levels may significantly increase secondarily to RU-486's receptor blockade. Studies in animals have shown that RU-486 blocks stress- and corticosterone-induced impairments in synaptic plasticity and memory (Xu *et al.*, 1998) but not the development of learned helplessness (Papolos *et al.*, 1993). Early trials treating depressed patients with RU-486 in Canada showed promising results, but studies were curtailed due to unavailability of the drug at that time (Murphy *et al.*, 1993). Ongoing studies at Stanford University, using 4 days of RU-486 treatment v. placebo in the treatment of psychotic depression, have reportedly found some signs of efficacy in the small number of patients treated to-date, although psychotic and cognitive symptoms seemed to respond better than depressive ones (Belanoff and Schatzberg., 2000). The use of RU-486 for other than acute administration has been poorly studied and has been associated with rashes in some subjects (Murphy *et al.*, 1993). Other corticosteroid receptor blocking compounds, such as ORG-34116, are currently in development (Karst *et al.*, 1997).

CRH receptor blockers

Elevated CSF CRH levels have been frequently described in depressed patients compared with controls (Nemeroff, 1988, 2000), although in some studies (Kling *et al.*, 1991; Wong *et al.*, 2000), including an especially comprehensive one (Geracioti *et al.*, 1992), this finding was not replicated. It is possible that different subtypes of major depression differ in patterns of hyper-, normal or hyposecretion of CRH (Gold and Chrousos, 1985, 1999; Kling *et al.*, 1989, 1991). A compelling role can be posited for the aetiologic involvement of CRH hypersecretion in symptoms such as anxiety, fear, over-arousal, decreased slow wave sleep, decreased eating and decreased libido (Gold and Chrousos, 1985, 1999; Holsboer, 1988, 1999, 2000; Kling *et al.*, 1991; Schulkin *et al.*, 1994). Additionally, chronic CRH hypersecretion may lead to certain long-term medical consequences of depression such as premature coronary artery disease, osteoporosis and altered immune and inflammatory responses (Linthorst *et al.*, 1997; Gold and Chrousos, 1999). Such findings support the notion that chronic CRH hypersecretion is an important factor in the aetiology of anxiety, depression and stress-related disorders.

To the extent CRH hypersecretion does play a pathophysiological role in the development or maintenance of major depression, CRH receptor antagonists should also be therapeutic (Holsboer, 1999). Rats and non-human primates administered the CRH-1 antagonist, R121919/ NBI 30775 show diminished anxiety and lowered ACTH and corticosterone responses to novelty (Gutman *et al.*, 2000; Habib *et al* 2000). Early open-label human trials with the same CRH-1 receptor antagonist have suggested a significant antidepressant and anti-anxiety effect in depressed patients (Holsboer, 2000; Nemeroff, 2000; Zobel *et al.*, 2000).

Dexamethasone and hydrocortisone

In what seems a diametrically opposite approach to altering steroidal activity in depressed patients, Arana and colleagues (Arana, 1991; Arana *et al.*, 1995; Beale and Arana, 1995) reported antidepressant effects of acute high dose dexamethasone administration. In this paradigm, dexamethasone was administered intravenously as a one-time bolus of 4–8 mg or orally as 4 mg per day for 4 days. Results of the open-label intravenous dexamethasone trial indicated on average 56% improvement within 10 days in 75% of depressed subjects, including five of seven treatment-refractory ones who had failed at least two prior antidepressant trials. In the blinded oral dexamethasone trial, dexamethasone was associated with only a 27.5% improvement in depression ratings compared with a 13.6% improvement with placebo. A significantly greater number of dexamethasone-treated subjects responded to treatment (defined as a ≥50% decrease in depression ratings or a final Hamilton depression score of ≤14) compared with placebo-treated subjects.

The authors suggested that the beneficial effect of dexamethasone was secondary to regulation of CRH receptors, increased serotonergic activity or other genomically mediated changes in neurotransmission.

Similar results were obtained by another group using an open-label design. Dinan et al. (1997) studied 10 depressed patients who had not responded to sertraline or fluoxetine, and added dexamethasone, 3 mg p.o. daily for 4 days, to the ongoing antidepressant regimen. By the following day (day 5), three of the six sertraline patients and three of the four fluoxetine patients demonstrated significant antidepressant responses (50% reduction in depression ratings). Remarkably, this initial improvement was maintained through day 21, the last assessed day. Cortisol changes in response to dexamethasone treatment were not reported, but baseline morning serum cortisol levels were directly correlated with antidepressant responses (viz., higher baseline cortisol was associated with better responses to dexamethasone). The dexamethasone was relatively well tolerated, but several patients reported sleep disruption, nausea and/or anxiety during dexamethasone treatment.

More recently, Bodani et al. (1999) described two elderly patients with resistant depression who appeared to benefit from dexamethasone treatment. Finally, Wolkowitz et al. (1996) reported negative results in a very small, double-blind replication study. Five depressed patients received one-time intravenous infusions of either 6 mg dexamethasone or placebo and were evaluated 10 days later. The three subjects who received dexamethasone all fared more poorly than the two who received placebo; two of the three dexamethasone-treated subjects actually worsened following treatment, and the trial was discontinued. The one dexamethasone-treated subject who showed any antidepressant effect had the lowest baseline serum cortisol concentration of the group.

In a related strategy, several investigators have assessed the mood-altering effects of cortisol (hydrocortisone) (Cameron et al., 1985). In one small-scale study, Goodwin et al. (1992) noted that an acute cortisol infusion transiently improved self-rated mood in 12 depressed patients. These patients were not hypercortisolaemic at baseline, and long-term antidepressant effects were not assessed. DeBattista et al. (2000) acutely treated, in a double-blind manner, six depressed patients with hydrocortisone (15 mg i.v. over 2 hours), six patients with ovine CRH (1 μg/kg i.v.) and 10 patients with placebo at 7.00 p.m. and assessed depression ratings the following day at 4.00 p.m. Hydrocortisone-treated patients, compared with both placebo and CRH-treated ones, showed a significant acute antidepressant response. It was not reported whether the antidepressant responses were related to baseline cortisol levels, whether they were correlated with increases in circulating cortisol levels, or whether the antidepressant responses persisted beyond one day.

If acute dexamethasone treatment proves to have antidepressant effects, how might this be reconciled with antiglucocorticoids having similar effects?

Antiglucocorticoids and dexamethasone administration could both have antidepressant effects via: (1) their common effect of curtailing endogenous cortisol synthesis; (2) inducing up-regulation of brain corticosteroid receptors (with the effect of re-establishing effective negative feedback); (3) altering levels of other adrenal or neurosteroid hormones (e.g. shifting cholesterol metabolism in the direction of increased synthesis of certain GABAergic neurosteroids) (Raven et al., 1996; Romeo et al., 1998); or (4) increasing ACTH levels (with acute high dose dexamethasone treatment, this might occur after dexamethasone's acute inhibitory effects are terminated and the suppressed LHPA axis signals increased ACTH output). Additionally, recent evidence suggests that dexamethasone is actively excluded from brain and does not replace endogenous corticosteroids at hippocampal mineralocorticoid (MR) and glucocorticoid receptor (GR) sites (De Kloet et al., 1998). Its behavioural effects, therefore, may result from indirect effects of dexamethasone-induced ACTH suppression on the balance of occupation of the two corticosteroid receptor types in the hippocampus (De Kloet et al., 1998). Further, chronic dexamethasone has been shown to result in variable increases in GR mRNA levels in cortical neurons, an effect that parallels changes observed over the course of antidepressant treatment (Pepin et al., 1990).

The beneficial effects of hydrocortisone, if confirmed, are more difficult to explain, unless the effects are transient and are secondary, perhaps, to increased dopamine levels (Wolkowitz et al., 1986; DeBattista et al., 2000). Alternatively, even in the face of static hypercortisolaemia, phasic ('burst') increases in cortisol levels may induce a rapid 're-setting' of LHPA axis negative feedback control (Murphy, 1991a; DeBattista et al., 2000). Lastly, it is possible that different subgroups of depressed patients respond differentially to corticosteroid augmentation v. suppression, perhaps related to their baseline adrenocortical output (Wolkowitz et al., 1996; DeBattista et al., 2000). Considerably more work needs to be done to determine the predictors and mediators of glucocorticoid-based treatments of depression.

Dehydroepiandrosterone (DHEA)

We have discussed previously that DHEA may serve as one of the body's endogenous 'anti-cortisol' hormones and that the ratio of DHEA-to-cortisol (the 'anabolic balance') may be more informative regarding depression and health status than levels of either hormone alone (Leblhuber et al., 1992; Wolkowitz et al., 1992; Hechter et al., 1997). Indeed, multiple studies have verified DHEA's ability, both in vitro and in vivo, to antagonize certain of cortisol's physiological effects (Browne et al., 1992; Kalimi et al., 1994; Hechter et al., 1997; Patchev and Almeida, 1997; Svec and Porter, 1998). Several animal studies show that DHEA administration can reverse certain important effects of cortisol in the CNS (Dubrovsky, 1997; Kimonides et al.,

1999), and can have neuroprotective and cognition-enhancing effects and counteract the development of 'depression'-like behaviours (reviewed by Svec and Porter (1998), Kroboth et al. (1999), Wolkowitz et al. (2000a)). In the periphery, DHEA can also prevent the development of stress-induced changes in total body and adrenal gland weight, glucocorticoid receptor levels and free-radical generation (Hu et al., 2000). DHEA, in rodent studies, also has anti-obesity and insulin sensitizing effects (Dong-Ho et al., 1998) and leads to decreases in atherosclerosis (Gordon et al., 1988), improved immune function (Spencer et al., 1995; Loria, 1997), prevention or amelioration of diabetes (Coleman et al., 1982) and reduction of fat mass (Dong-Ho et al., 1998), as reviewed elsewhere (Nippoldt and Sreekumaran Nair, 1998; Svec and Porter, 1998). However, an often overlooked caveat to these results is that rats and mice produce little adrenal DHEA naturally, so these findings may be of limited generalizability to humans. Further, in humans, some of these effects may be gender-specific (Kroboth et al., 1999). Nonetheless, several studies reviewed in detail elsewhere raise the possibility that decreased DHEA(S) levels (or decreased DHEA(S)-to-cortisol ratios) contribute to the development or progression of cognitive decline, affective disturbance and impaired physical and emotional well-being in humans (Svec and Porter, 1998; Kroboth et al., 1999; Wolkowitz et al., 2000a).

Regardless of whether low endogenous levels of DHEA are associated with depression, cognitive impairment or physical disease risk factors, exogenous supplementation with DHEA may have therapeutic effects and may counteract certain deleterious effects of allostatic load. DHEA treatment (aimed at restoring levels to those seen physiologically in healthy young individuals) reportedly has antidepressant effects in patients with major depression (Wolkowitz et al., 1995, 1997b, 1999b) and dysthymia (Bloch et al., 1999), mildly and transiently improves cognitive performance in patients with Alzheimer's disease (Wolkowitz et al., 2000b) and enhances well-being, energy and libido in hypo-adrenal women with Addison's disease (Arlt et al., 1998, 1999).

Beneficial mood and memory effects of DHEA treatment in non-diseased or only mildly symptomatic populations have been demonstrated less consistently (Morales et al., 1994; Diamond et al., 1996; Wolf et al., 1997; Barnhart et al., 1999), but improvements in anthropometric indices of allostatic load, such as muscle-to-fat ratio, fasting glucose and insulin levels and bone mineral density, have been noted in some studies (Nestler et al., 1988; Diamond et al., 1996; Labrie et al., 1997). In one study, administration of topical DHEA for one year increased bone density in 14 post-menopausal women (Labrie et al., 1997). Although there was no control group, it is the natural course for bone density to decrease over time. In a six-month trial of 100 mg DHEA per day, there were increases in strength and decreases in fat mass for men only, but no changes in bone density, glucose, insulin, lipids, or cortisol for either gender (Morales et al., 1998). However, many subjects did not have low levels of DHEA to begin with. In another double-blind placebo-controlled study, elderly men and women received 50 mg/day of DHEA for a year. The greatest improvements were found in women over 70 years, who showed increases in bone mineral density, skin tone and libido compared with a placebo control group (Baulieu et al., 2000). In a six-month trial, DHEA increased IGF-1 levels but decreased high density lipoproteins (Casson et al., 1998). Finally, in a recent study of perimenopausal women, 50 mg/day of DHEA for 3 months produced no effects over placebo in terms of mood or blood lipids (Barnhart et al., 1999). Despite the widespread use of DHEA, more studies are needed before any conclusions are made about beneficial effects for a particular age, gender and target symptom (van Vollenhoven, 1997; Katz and Morales, 1998; Kroboth et al., 1999; Wolkowitz and Reus, 2000; Wolkowitz et al., 2000a;).

BEHAVIOURAL TREATMENT APPROACHES TO DEPRESSION, HORMONAL DYSREGULATION AND ALLOSTATIC LOAD

To the extent that altered stress hormone secretion underlies or perpetuates depressive symptoms and physical illness, behavioural as well as pharmacological interventions that normalize the hormonal milieu should prove therapeutic (Sapolsky, 1993; Drugan et al., 1994). In this section, we explore evidence for the psychoneuroendocrine mediation of some of the health benefits of 'stress-reduction' and other behavioural treatment modalities.

Decreasing cortisol

Numerous studies have examined the effects of relaxation techniques on cortisol and other stress-responsive hormones. Controlled studies of short-term interventions such as listening to music (Escher et al., 1993; Miluk-Kolasa et al., 1994; Mockel et al., 1994; McKinney et al., 1997), biofeedback (McGrady et al., 1987), yoga (Platania-Solazzo et al., 1992) and massage therapy (Field et al., 1992; Platania-Solazzo et al., 1992) have shown decreases in cortisol levels. Acupuncture, however, has not been shown to significantly decrease cortisol levels (Chiu et al., 1997; Kho et al., 1999). In one study, massage was given for a five-day period to 52 youths with depression or adjustment disorder. Compared with a control group, they showed significant reductions in depressive mood and salivary cortisol both immediately after the massage and after 5 days (Field et al., 1992). Experimental groups who learned to meditate regularly suppressed cortisol compared with controls (Jevning et al., 1978; Gallois et al., 1984; Sudsuang et al., 1991); however, see Michaels et al. (1979). Long-term meditators (average of 8.5 years), had 50% lower urinary free cortisol levels than a control group (Walton and Pugh, 1995; Walton et al., 1995), although these results are affected by selection bias. In a prospective random-assignment study, meditators showed lower basal cortisol over four months as well as slightly increased acute cortisol and growth hormone responses to stress (Maclean *et al.*, 1997). The biological significance of these increases is unknown, but a rapid stress response may indicate a more 'healthy' allostasis. Behaviourally-induced decreases in circulating cortisol levels have been associated with decreased anxiety and depression ratings (Platania-Solazzo *et al.*, 1992; Field *et al.*, 1996, 1998a, c), decreased acute stress responses (Miluk-Kolasa *et al.*, 1994; McKinney *et al.*, 1997), decreased pain (Field *et al.*, 1997, 1998b), enhanced immune (Ironson *et al.*, 1996) and pulmonary (Field *et al.*, 1998a) function, enhanced alertness and mathematical performance (Field *et al.*, 1996), increased brain alpha wave activity (Kamei *et al.*, 2000) and improved sleep (Field *et al.*, 1992).

Increasing DHEA

Behavioural treatment programmes have also been demonstrated to significantly alter DHEA(S) levels. Cognitive-behavioural treatment of depressed patients increased urinary DHEA-S levels, in comparison with imipramine, which lowered levels (Tollefson *et al.*, 1990). In a prospective study, Army officers participating in a stress-reduction programme showed significant increases in DHEA-S levels compared with non-participants (Littman *et al.*, 1993). Similarly, Cruess *et al.* (1999) reported that 10 weeks of 'cognitive-behavioural stress management' (comprised of treatments such as identification of cognitive distortions, assertiveness training, anger management, social support, group discussions, experiential exercises, progressive muscle relaxation, autogenic training, meditation and guided imagery), compared with a 10 week control 'wait list' condition, significantly increased plasma DHEA-S levels and decreased cortisol-to-DHEA-S ratios in HIV-seropositive men. Treated subjects, compared with control subjects, also showed significant improvements in mood disturbance and perceived stress that were directly correlated with the decreases in plasma cortisol-to-DHEA-S ratios. Since DHEA-S may functionally antagonize cortisol-induced immunosuppression in HIV-seropositive individuals (Hechter *et al.*, 1997), the authors postulated that the biochemical effects they observed may also underlie the purported efficacy of cognitive-behavioural stress management therapy in slowing the rate of progression of HIV disease.

Consistent with these studies, Arnetz *et al.* (1983) assigned elderly individuals from a senior citizen apartment building to either a 'social enrichment' programme (e.g. study groups in botany, history, music and geography, as well as outings, picnics and visits to the opera and theatre) or to a programme of normal pre-existing activities for 6 months. The experimental group, compared with the control group, showed significant increases in DHEA, testosterone, oestradiol and GH levels, as well as significantly attenuated decreases in height (suggestive of slowing of osteoporosis progression). The authors speculated that social isolation in the elderly decreases anabolic-to-catabolic hormone ratios, leading to increased susceptibility to illness (such as osteoporosis), and that social enrichment counteracts this process. Lökk (1998) presented confirmatory data in an uncontrolled study of 17 non-demented geriatric day-care attendees who participated in a new rehabilitation programme designed to decrease the 'stress of uncertainty and passivity' by giving patients greater control and responsibility over their own rehabilitation programmes. Patients were assessed at entry into the programme, after 3 months of treatment and again 3 months after discharge. Prolactin and cortisol levels significantly decreased over the 3 months of treatment, while DHEA and oestradiol levels significantly increased. These changes coincided with improvements in Activities of Daily Living ratings and with increases in 'optimism' ratings. By 3 months after discharge from the programme, prolactin, cortisol and oestradiol levels had returned to pre-treatment levels, but DHEA levels remained elevated. In another prospective study, but one lacking a control group for the hormonal determinations, healthy adult participants in an 'emotional self-management programme' experienced a 100% increase in salivary DHEA(S) levels; these levels were significantly correlated with the psychological variable 'warmheartedness' (McCraty et al., 1998). Experienced practitioners of transcendental meditation (TM) were also found to have elevated DHEA-S levels (Glaser et al., 1992; Walton et al., 1995), generally comparable to the levels seen in non-practitioners 5–10 years younger, increased urinary 5-HIAA (the major 5HT metabolite) levels and decreased urinary free cortisol levels compared with 'average stress' non-TM practitioners. The authors of the former report noted that extraneous factors, such as diet, body mass index and exercise, did not account for the difference in hormone levels (Glaser et al., 1992), and the authors of the latter report noted that DHEA-S levels in women varied directly with the months of TM practice (Walton et al., 1995). In contrast with chronic behavioural interventions, one session of Qigong training (a 'stress coping' method) did not alter DHEA(S) or cortisol levels (Ryu et al., 1996).

Clinical implications of behavioural treatment approaches

Stress reduction interventions usually reduce physiological arousal levels and lead to cognitive changes, such as increased perceptions of controllability and predictability. In this way, they may have direct antidepressant effects as well as indirect ones by restoring balance to the endocrine milieu (e.g. decreasing cortisol and increasing DHEA levels). In a complementary way, restoring cortisol and DHEA levels to normal may alter cognitive function and social behaviour in a direction less conducive to depression and to future disappointing life events (Goodyer et al., 1998).

It remains unclear whether patients with disturbed LHPA activity are more or less likely to respond to such behavioural interventions. However, behavioural treatments alone may be less appropriate for patients with clinically significant LHPA axis dysregulation. Thase and colleagues, for example, found that depressed inpatients with elevated urinary free cortisol levels showed poorer responses to cognitive-behavioural therapy (CBT) compared to those with normal urinary free cortisol levels (Thase *et al.*, 1993; Thase, 1994).

There is some evidence that stress reduction interventions like those described above also have direct impact on reducing physical disease or risk for disease (Fahrion *et al* 1987). Stress reduction programmes, including relaxation or meditation, can enhance immune response (Whitehouse *et al.*, 1996) and diabetic glycaemic control (Lustman *et al.*, 1998; McGrady and Horner, 1999) and reduce atherosclerosis (Castillo-Richmond *et al.*, 2000). In preliminary data, reducing depressive symptoms and stress in type 2 diabetics can significantly reduce visceral fat up to 6 months later, compared with a control group (Epel *et al.*, 2000).

CHOICE OF ANTIGLUCOCORTICOID DRUGS AND RISK OF SIDE EFFECTS

Whereas the stress reduction and CBT techniques outlined here are already in routine clinical use, the pharmacological antiglucocorticoid approaches reviewed in this chapter remain largely experimental, and their full risk/benefit ratios remain to be determined. They are not yet recommended for routine clinical use (other than in the treatment of Cushing's syndrome). A more detailed discussion of the clinical differences between existing antiglucocorticoid drugs and the risk of side effects with each one is presented elsewhere (Wolkowitz and Reus, 1999).

CONCLUSIONS

The data reviewed here raise the possibility that antiglucocorticoid drug treatments ameliorate depressive symptoms in some patients with major depression or other psychiatric disorders, and additionally, can reduce certain signs of allostatic load in the periphery. Such effects would be consistent with those observed in Cushing's syndrome patients treated with the same drugs. The majority of the reviewed trials, however, were non-blinded or small-scale. Therefore, any conclusions at this point must be considered tentative. Behavioural techniques, which also normalize elevated cortisol levels and/or increase DHEA levels, have proven clinical efficacy, but whether their efficacy is related to their hormonal effects is unknown.

If this endocrinological model of depression and allostatic load is correct, it provides several novel sites for therapeutic intervention. 'Biopsychosocial' interventions could be understood as having in common actions leading to normalization of stress hormone secretion, with attendant downstream normalization of neurotransmitter and neuropeptide levels and restoration of the balance between catabolic and anabolic processes.

The studies reviewed here cumulatively suggest the dual importance of further studying antiglucocorticoid strategies in major depression:

1. On a practical clinical level, it may lead to novel pharmacotherapeutic approaches for certain psychiatric patients. In many of the reviewed studies, good responses to antiglucocorticoid agents were seen in patients refractory to traditional antidepressants. Improvements often occurred rapidly (as early as 1–3 weeks), and remission occasionally persisted for long periods of time (in some cases even after antiglucocorticoid treatment was stopped). Since a substantial proportion of depressed patients is resistant to, or intolerant of, traditional antidepressants, the availability of a new class of antidepressant medication would be significant.

2. On a theoretical level, it may lead to a better understanding of the role of hyperactivity of the LHPA axis in major depression and other psychiatric disorders. This issue has been discussed and considered for over 45 years (Quarton et al., 1955), but until the availability and use of relatively safe antiglucocorticoid drugs, no suitable paradigm has existed to test it. It may also help clarify whether neurotransmitter and neuropeptide dysregulation and insensitivity to corticosteroid negative feedback are primary or secondary pathological events in the development of depression. The well-replicated finding that persistent DST non-suppression after antidepressant treatment portends poorly for long-term outcome (Ribeiro et al., 1993), suggests that re-establishment of LHPA axis negative feedback may itself be an important therapeutic goal.

Further studies will be needed to determine the appropriate clinical role of antiglucocorticoids in psychiatric treatment and of their role (as well as the role of certain behavioural interventions) in reducing the 'allostatic load' sequelae of depression and other stressful conditions. Confirmation of antidepressant and health-promoting effects of the antiglucocorticoid drugs reviewed here would undoubtedly spur the development of safer compounds and would refine our notions of appropriate targets of pharmacotherapy. Finally, elucidation of the relationship of hormonal normalization to clinical improvement might lead to a laboratory 'yardstick' by which to measure (and perhaps predict) incipient clinical response to drug or psychotherapeutic interventions.

ACKNOWLEDGEMENTS

The authors gratefully acknowledge support from the National Institute on Aging (Grant R41-AG13334-01), the National Alliance for Research in Schizophrenia and Affective Disorders (NARSAD), the Stanley Foundation of the National Alliance for the Mentally Ill (NAMI), the Scottish Rite Foundation and the UCSF Research Evaluation and Allocation Committee (REAC) as well as helpful discussions about allostasis and antiglucocorticoid treatments with Bruce S. McEwen, PhD and Eugene Roberts, PhD.

REFERENCES

Amsterdam, J., Mosley, P.D. and Rosenzweig, M. (1994). Assessment of adrenocortical activity in refractory depression: steroid suppression with ketoconazole. In: Nolan, W., Zohar, J., Roose, S. and Amsterdam, J. (Eds), *Refractory Depression*. John Wiley, Chichester, pp. 199–210.

Anand, A., Malison, R., McDougle, C.J. and Price, L.H. (1995). Antiglucocorticoid treatment of refractory depression with ketoconazole: a case report. *Biol Psychiatry* **37**, 338–340.

Angeli, A. and Frairia, R. (1985). Ketoconazole therapy in Cushing's disease [letter]. *Lancet* **1**, 821.

Arana, G.W. (1991). Intravenous dexamethasone for symptoms of major depressive disorder [letter]. *Am J Psychiatry* **148**, 1401–1402.

Arana, G.W., Santos, A.B., Laraia, M.T. *et al.* (1995). Dexamethasone for the treatment of depression: a randomized, placebo-controlled, double-blind trial. *Am J Psychiatry* **152**, 265–267.

Arlt, W., Justl, H.G., Callies, F. *et al.* (1998). Oral dehydroepiandrosterone for adrenal androgen replacement: pharmacokinetics and peripheral conversion to androgens and estrogens in young healthy females after dexamethasone suppression. *J Clin Endocrinol Metab* **83**, 1928–1934.

Arlt, W., Callies, F., van Vlijmen J.C. *et al.* (1999). Dehydroepiandrosterone replacement in women with adrenal insufficiency [see comments]. *New Engl J Med* **341**, 1013–1020.

Arnetz, B.B., Theorell, T., Levi, L., Kallner, A. and Eneroth, P. (1983). An experimental study of social isolation of elderly people: psychoendocrine and metabolic effects. *Psychosom Med* **45**, 395–406.

Arteaga, E., Mahana, D., Gonzalez, R. and Martinez, P. (1989). Cushing syndrome caused by macronodular adrenal hyperplasia, independent of ACTH: report of a case. *Rev Med Chil* **117**, 1398–1402.

Barden, N., Reul, J.M. and Holsboer, F. (1995). Do antidepressants stabilize mood through actions on the hypothalamic–pituitary–adrenocortical system? *Trends Neurosci* **18**, 6–11.

Barnhart, K.T., Freeman, E., Grisso, J.A. *et al.* (1999). The effect of dehydroepiandrosterone supplementation to symptomatic perimenopausal women on serum endocrine profiles, lipid parameters, and health-related quality of life. *J Clin Endocrinol Metab* **84**, 3896–3902.

Baulieu, E., Thomas, G., Legrain, S. *et al.* (2000). Dehydroepiandrosterone (DHEA), DHEA sulfate, and aging: Contribution of the DHEAge Study to a sociobiomedical issue. *Proc Natl Acad Sci USA* **97**, 4279–4284.

Beale, M.D. and Arana G.W. (1995). Dexamethasone for treatment of major depression in patients with bipolar disorder [letter]. *Am J Psychiatry* **152**, 959–960.

Bech, P., Raabaek Olsen, L. *et al.* (1999). A case of sequential anti-stress medication in a patient with major depression resistant to amine-reuptake inhibitors. *Acta Psychiatr Scand* **100**, 76–78.

Belanoff, J. and Schatzberg, A.F. (2000). Glucocorticoid antagonists. *Neuropsychopharmacology* **23**, S56.

Biegon, A. (1990). Effects of steroid hormones on the serotonergic system. *Ann NY Acad Sci* **600**, 427–432.

Björntorp, P., Holm, G. and Rosmond, R. (1999). Hypothalamic arousal, insulin resistance and type 2 diabetes mellitus. *Diabet Med* **16**, 373–383.

Bloch, M., Schmidt, P.J., Danaceau, M.A., Adams, L.F. and Rubinow, D.R. (1999). Dehydroepiandrosterone treatment of mid-life dysthymia. *Biol Psychiatry* **45**, 1533–1541.

Bodani, M., Sheehan, B. and Philpot, M. (1999). The use of dexamethasone in elderly patients with antidepressant-resistant depressive illness. *J Psychopharmacol* **13**, 196–197.

Boston Collaborative Drug Surveillance Program (1972). Acute adverse reactions to prednisone in relation to dosage. *Clin Pharmacol Ther* **13**, 694–698.

Browne, E.S., Wright, B.E., Porter, J.R. and Svec, F. (1992). Dehydroepiandrosterone: antiglucocorticoid action in mice. *Am J Med Sci* **303**, 366–371.

Budziszewska, B., Jaworska-Feil, L., Kajta, M. and Lason, W. (2000). Antidepressant drugs inhibit glucocorticoid receptor-mediated gene transcription – a possible mechanism. *Br J Pharmacol* **130**, 1385–1393.

Cameron, O.G., Addy, R.O. and Malitz, D. (1985). Effects of ACTH and prednisone on mood: incidence and time of onset. *Int J Psychiatry Med* **15**, 213–223..

Carroll, B.J., Feinberg, M., Greden, J.F. *et al.* (1981). A specific laboratory test for the diagnosis of melancholia. *Arch Gen Psychiatry* **38**, 15–22.

Casson, P., Santoro, N., Elkind-Hirsch, K. *et al.* (1998). Postmenopausal dehydroepiandrosterone administration increases free insulin-like growth factor-1 and decreases high-density lipoprotein: a six-month trial. *Fertility Sterility* **70**, 107–110.

Castillo-Richmond, A., Schneider, R., Alexander, C. *et al.* (2000). Effects of stress reduction on carotid atherosclerosis in hypertensive African Americans. *Stroke* **31**, 568–573.

Checkley, A.S., O'Dwyer, A.M., Raven, P., Taylor, N. and Lightman, S. (1994). Antidepressant effects of treatments with metyrapone and hydrocortisone. *Biol Psychiatry* **35**, 711.

Chiu, Y.J., Chi, A. and Reid, I.A. (1997). Cardiovascular and endocrine effects of acupuncture in hypertensive patients. *Clin Exp Hypertens* **19**, 1047–1063.

Chouinard, G., Belanger, M.C., Beauclair, L., Sultan, S. and Murphy, B.E. (1996). Potentiation of fluoxetine by aminoglutethimide, an adrenal steroid suppressant, in obsessive-compulsive disorder resistant to SSRIs: a case report. *Prog Neuropsychopharmacol Biol Psychiatry* **20**, 1067–1079.

Cleghorn, R.A. (1951). Adrenal cortical insufficiency: psychological and neurologic observations. *Can Med Assoc J* **65**, 449–454.

Cohen, S.I. (1980). Cushing's syndrome: a psychiatric study of 29 patients. *Br J Psychiatry* **136**, 120–124.

Coleman, D., Leiter, E. and Schwizer, R. (1982). Therapeutic effects of dehydroepiandrosterone in diabetic mice. *Diabetes* **31**, 830–833.

Cruess, D.G., Antoni, M.H., Kumar, M. *et al.* (1999). Cognitive-behavioral stress management buffers decreases in dehydroepiandrosterone sulfate (DHEA-S) and increases in the cortisol/DHEA-S ration and reduces mood disturbance and perceived stress among HIV-seropositive men. *Psychoneuroendocrinology* **24**, 537–549.

DeBattista, C., Posener, J.A., Kalehzan, B.M. and Schatzberg, A.F. (2000). Acute antidepressant effects of intravenous hydrocortisone and CRH in depressed patients: A double-blind, placebo-controlled study. *Am J Psychiatry* **157**, 1334–1337.

De Kloet, E.R., Vreugdenhil, E., Oitzl, M.S. and Joels, M. (1998). Brain corticosteroid receptor balance in health and disease. *Endocrinol Rev* **19**, 269–301.

Diamond, P., Cusan, L., Gomez, J.L., Belanger, A. and Labrie, F. (1996). Metabolic effects of 12-month percutaneous dehydroepiandrosterone replacement therapy in postmenopausal women. *J Endocrinol* **150**(Suppl), S43–50.

Dinan, T.G., Lavelle, E., Cooney, J. *et al.* (1997). Dexamethasone augmentation in treatment-resistant depression. *Acta Psychiatr Scand* **95**, 58–61.

Dong-Ho, H., Hansen, P., Chen, M. and Holloszy, J. (1998). DHEA treatment reduces fat accumulation and protects against insulin resistance in male rats. *J Gerontol* **53**, B19–B24.

Drugan, R.C., Basile, A.S., Ha, J.H. and Ferland, R.J. (1994). The protective effects of stress control may be mediated by increased brain levels of benzodiazepine receptor agonists. *Brain Res* **661**, 127–136.

Dubrovsky, B. (1991). Adrenal steroids and the physiopathology of a subset of depressive disorders. *Med Hypotheses* **36**, 300–305.

Dubrovsky, B. (1997). Natural steroids counteracting some actions of putative depressogenic steroids on the central nervous system: potential therapeutic benefits. *Med Hypotheses* **49**, 51–55.

Epel, E., McEwen, B. and Ickovics, J. (1998). Embodying psychological thriving: Physical thriving in response to stress. *J Soc Iss* **54**, 301–322.

Epel, E., Kiratli, J., Young, B. *et al.* (2000). Stress reduction for Type II diabetics reduces visceral adiposity. (in preparation).

Eriksen, H.R., Olff, M., Murison, R. and Ursin, H. (1999). The time dimension in stress responses: Relevance for survival and health. *Psychiatry Res* **85**, 39–50.

Escher, J., Hohmann, U., Anthenien, L. *et al.* (1993). Music during gastroscopy. *Schweiz Med Wochenschr* **123**, 1354–1358.

Fahrion, S., Norris, P., Green, E., Green, A. and Schnar, R. (1987). Biobehavioral treatment of essential hypertension. *Biofeed Self-Reg* **11**, 257–278.

Field, T., Morrow, C., Valdeon, C. *et al.* (1992). Massage reduces anxiety in child and adolescent psychiatric patients. *Child Adolesc* **31**, 125–131.

Field, T., Ironson, G., Scafidi, F. *et al.* (1996). Massage therapy reduces anxiety and enhances EEG pattern of alertness and math computations. *Int J Neurosci* **86**, 197–205.

Field, T., Hernandez-Reif, M., Seligman, S. *et al.* (1997). Juvenile rheumatoid arthritis: benefits from massage therapy. *J Pediatr Psychol* **22**, 607–617.

Field, T., Henteleff, T., Hernandez-Reif, M. *et al.* (1998a). Children with asthma have improved pulmonary functions after massage therapy. *J Pediatr* **132**, 854–858.

Field, T., Peck, M., Krugman, S. *et al.* (1998b). Burn injuries benefit from massage therapy. *J Burn Care Rehabil* **19**, 241–244.

Field, T., Schanberg, S., Kuhn, C. *et al.* (1998c). Bulimic adolescents benefit from massage therapy. *Adolescence* **33**, 555–563.

Gallois, P., Forzy, G. and Dhont, J. (1984). Hormonal changes during relaxation. *L'encephale* **10**, 79–82.

Geracioti, T.D., Jr, Orth, D.N., Ekhator, N.N., Blumenkopf, B. and Loosen, P.T. (1992). Serial cerebrospinal fluid corticotropin-releasing hormone concentrations in healthy and depressed humans. *J Clin Endocrinol Metab* **74**, 1325–1330.

Ghadirian, A.M., Englesmann, F., Dhar, V. *et al.* (1995). The psychotropic effects of inhibitors of steroid biosynthesis in depressed patients refractory to treatment. *Biol Psychiatry* **37**, 369–375.

Gifford, S. and Gunderson, J.G. (1970). Cushing's disease as a psychosomatic disorder: a selective review of the clinical and experimental literature and a report of ten cases. *Perspect Biol Med* **13**, 169–221.

Glaser, J.L., Brind, J.L., Vogelman, J.H. *et al.* (1992). Elevated serum dehydroepiandrosterone sulfate levels in practitioners of the Transcendental Meditation (TM) and TM-Sidhi programs. *J Behav Med* **15**, 327–341.

Gold, P.W. and Chrousos, G.P. (1985). Clinical studies with corticotropin releasing factor: implications for the diagnosis and pathophysiology of depression, Cushing's disease, and adrenal insufficiency. *Psychoneuroendocrinology* **10**, 401–419.

Gold, P.W. and Chrousos, G.P. (1999). The endocrinology of melancholic and atypical depression: relation to neurocircuitry and somatic consequences. *Proc Assoc Am Physicians* **111**, 22–34.

Goodwin, G.M., Muir, W.J., Seckl, J.R. *et al.* (1992). The effects of cortisol infusion upon hormone secretion from the anterior pituitary and subjective mood in depressive illness and in controls. *J Affect Disord* **26**, 73–83.

Goodyer, I.M., Herbert, J., Altham, P.M. *et al.* (1996). Adrenal secretion during major depression in 8- to 16-year-olds, I. Altered diurnal rhythms in salivary cortisol and dehydroepiandrosterone (DHEA) at presentation. *Psychol Med* **26**, 245–256.

Goodyer, I.M., Herbert, J. and Altham, P.M. (1998). Adrenal steroid secretion and major depression in 8- to 16-year-olds, III. Influence of cortisol/DHEA ratio at presentation on subsequent rates of disappointing life events and persistent major depression. *Psychol Med* **28**, 265–273.

Gordon, G.B., Bush, D.E. and Weisman, H.F. (1988). Reduction of atherosclerosis by administration of dehydroepiandrosterone. A study in the hypercholesterolemic New Zealand white rabbit with aortic intimal injury. *J Clin Invest* **82**, 712–720.

Greden, J.F., Gardner, R., King, D., Grunhaus, L., Carroll, B.J. and Kronfol, Z. (1983). Dexamethasone suppression tests in antidepressant treatment of melancholia. The process of normalization and test-retest reproducibility. *Arch Gen Psychiatry* **40**, 493–500.

Gutman, D.A., Owens, M.J., Skelton, K.H. *et al.* (2000). Behavioral, neuroendocrine, and pharmacokinetic observations on CRF-1-selective antagonist, R121919 in the rat. *Neuropsychopharmacology* **23**, S119.

Habib, K.E., Higley, J.D., Rice, C.J. *et al.* (2000). CRH type-1 receptor antagonism attenuates behavioral, endocrine and autonomic responses to stress in primates. *Neuropsychopharmacology* **23**, S119.

Hall, R.C., Popkin, M.K., Stickney, S.K. and Gardner, E.R. (1979). Presentation of the steroid psychoses. *J Nerv Ment Dis* **167**, 229–236.

Hamm, F.C. (1955). Adrenal surgery for psychosis associated with Cushing's syndrome. *Arch Surg* **71**, 617–619.

Haskett, R.F. (1985). Diagnostic categorization of psychiatric disturbance in Cushing's syndrome. *Am J Psychiatry* **142**, 911–916.

Hechter, O., Grossman, A. and Chatterton, R.T., Jr. (1997). Relationship of dehydroepiandrosterone and cortisol in disease. *Med Hypotheses* **49**, 85–91.

Herbert, J. (1997). Stress, the brain, and mental illness. *BMJ* **315**, 530–535.

Herbert, J. (1998). Neurosteroids, brain damage, and mental illness. *Exp Gerontol* **33**, 713–727.

Holsboer, F. (1988). Implications of altered limbic–hypothalamic–pituitary–adrenocortical (LHPA)-function for neurobiology of depression. *Acta Psychiatr Scand* **341**(Suppl.), 72–111.

Holsboer, F. (1999). The rationale for corticotropin-releasing hormone receptor (CRH-R) antagonists to treat depression and anxiety. *J Psychiatr Res* **33**, 181–214.

Holsboer, F. (2000). Molecular approaches and the CRH hypothesis of mood and anxiety disorders, CRF Antagonists, Held during the 2nd International Congress on Hormones, Brain and Neuropsychopharmacology. Rhodes, Greece.

Hu, Y., Cardounel, A., Gursoy, E., Anderson, P. and Kalimi, M. (2000). Anti-stress effects of dehydroepiandrosterone: protection of rats against repeated immobilization stress-induced weight loss, glucocorticoid receptor production, and lipid peroxidation. *Biochem Pharmacol* **59**, 753–762.

Iizuka, H., Kishimotor, A., Nakamura, J. and Mizukawa, R. (1996). Clinical effects of cortisol synthesis inhibition on treatment-resistant depression. *Nihon Shinkei Seishin Yakurigaku Zasshi* **16**, 33–36.

Ironson, G., Field, T., Scafidi, F. *et al.* (1996). Massage therapy is associated with enhancement of the immune system's cytotoxic capacity. *Int J Neurosci* **84**, 205–217.

Jeffcoate, W.J., Silverstone, J.T., Edwards, C.R. and Besser, G.M. (1979). Psychiatric manifestations of Cushing's syndrome: response to lowering of plasma cortisol. *Q J Med* **48**, 465–472.

Jevning, R., Wilson, A. and Davidson, J. (1978). Adrenocortical activity during meditation. *Horm Behav* **10**, 54–60.

Kalimi, M., Shafagoj, Y., Loria, R., Padgett, D. and Regelson, W. (1994). Anti-glucocorticoid effects of dehydroepiandrosterone (DHEA). *Mol Cell Biochem* **131**, 99–104.

Kamei, T., Toriumi, Y., Kimura, H. *et al.* (2000). Decrease in serum cortisol during yoga exercise is correlated with alpha wave activation. *Percept Mot Skills* **90**, 1027–1032.

Karst, H., de Kloet, E.R. and Joels, M. (1997). Effect of ORG 34116, a corticosteroid receptor antagonist, on hippocampal Ca2+ currents. *Eur J Pharmacol* **339**, 17–26.

Kathol, R.G. (1985). Etiologic implications of corticosteroid changes in affective disorder. *Psychiatr Med* **3**, 135–162.

Katz, S. and Morales, A.J. (1998). Dehydroepiandrosterone (DHEA) and DHEA-sulfate (DS) as therapeutic options in menopause. *Semin Reprod Endocrinol* **16**, 161–170.

Keenan, P.A., Jacobson, M.W., Soleymani, R.M. *et al.* (1996). The effect on memory of chronic prednisone treatment in patients with systemic disease. *Neurology* **47**, 1396–1402.

Kelly, W.F., Barnes, A.J., Cassar, J. *et al.* (1979). Cushing's syndrome due to adrenocortical carcinoma – a comprehensive clinical and biochemical study of patients treated by surgery and chemotherapy. *Acta Endocrinolol* **91**, 303–318.

Kelly, W.F., Checkley, S.A. and Bender, D.A. (1980). Cushing's syndrome, tryptophan and depression. *Br J Psychiatry* **136**, 125–132.

Kelly, W.F., Checkley, S.A., Bender, D.A. and Mashiter, K. (1983). Cushing's syndrome and depression – a prospective study of 26 patients. *Br J Psychiatry* **142**, 16–19.

Kelly, W.F., Kelly, M.J. and Faragher, B. (1996). A prospective study of psychiatric and psychological aspects of Cushing's syndrome. *Clin Endocrinol* **45**, 715–772.

Kho, H.G., Sweep, C.G., Chen, X., Rabsztyn, P.R. and Meuleman, E.J. (1999). The use of acupuncture in the treatment of erectile dysfunction. *Int J Impot Res* **11**, 41–46.

Kimonides, V.G., Spillantini, M.G., Sofroniew, M.V., Fawcett, J.W. and Herbert, J. (1999). Dehydroepiandrosterone antagonizes the neurotoxic effects of corticosterone and translocation of stress-activated protein kinase 3 in hippocampal primary cultures. *Neuroscience* **89**, 429–436.

Kling, M.A., Perini, G.I., Demitrack, M.A. *et al.* (1989). Stress-responsive neurohormonal systems and the symptom complex of affective illness. *Psychopharmacol Bull* **25**, 312–318.

Kling, M.A., Roy, A., Doran, A.R. *et al.* (1991). Cerebrospinal fluid immunoreactive corticotropin-releasing hormone and adrenocorticotropin secretion in Cushing's disease and major depression: potential clinical implications. *J Clin Endocrinol Metab* **72**, 260–271.

Kramlinger, K.G., Peterson, G.C., Watson, P.K. and Leonard, L.L. (1985). Metyrapone for depression and delirium secondary to Cushing's syndrome. *Psychosomatics* **26**, 67–71.

Kroboth, P.D., Salek, F.S., Pittenger, A.L., Fabian, T.J. and Frye, R.F. (1999). DHEA and DHEA-S: a review. *J Clin Pharmacol* **39**, 327–348.

Labrie, F., Diamond, P., Cusan, L., Gomez, J.L., Belanger, A. and Candas, B. (1997). Effect of 12-month dehydroepiandrosterone replacement therapy on bone, vagina, and endometrium in postmenopausal women. *J Clin Endocrinol Metab* **82**, 3498–3505.

Leblhuber, F., Windhager, E., Neubauer, C. *et al.* (1992). Antiglucocorticoid effects of DHEA-S in Alzheimer's disease [letter] [published erratum appears in *Am J Psychiatry* **149**, 1622]. *Am J Psychiatry* **149**, 1125–1126.

Leigh, H. and Kramer, S.I. (1984). The psychiatric manifestations of endocrine disease. *Adv Intern Med* **29**, 413–445.

Levine, A. and Mitty, H. (1988). Steroid content of the peripheral and adrenal vein in Cushing's syndrome due to adrenocortical adenoma and carcinoma. *J Urol* **140**, 11–15.

Li, K.L., Tung, S.C. and Wang, P.W. (1996). The effect of ketoconazole in pre-operative treatment in Cushing's syndrome: three cases report. *Chang Keng I Hsueh* **19**, 358–363.

Ling, M.H., Perry, P.J. and Tsuang, M.T. (1981). Side effects of corticosteroid therapy. Psychiatric aspects. *Arch Gen Psychiatry* **38**, 471–477.

Linthorst, A.C., Flachskamm, C., Hopkins, S.J. *et al.* (1997). Long-term intracerebroventricular infusion of corticotropin-releasing hormone alters neuroendocrine, neurochemical, autonomic, behavioral, and cytokine responses to a systemic inflammatory challenge. *J Neurosci* **17**, 4448–4460.

Littman, A.B., Fava, M., Halperin, P. *et al.* (1993). Physiologic benefits of a stress reduction program for healthy middle- aged Army officers. *J Psychosom Res* **37**, 345–354.

Lobo, A., Perez-Echeverria, M.J., Jimenez-Aznarez, A. and Sancho, M.A. (1988). Emotional disturbances in endocrine patients. Validity of the scaled version of the General Health Questionnaire (GHQ-28). *Br J Psychiatry* **152**, 807–812.

Lökk, J. (1998). Psychoendocrine concomitants in patients following a new design of a geriatric day-care unit. *Psychother Psychosom* **67**, 323–327.

Loli, P., Berselli, M.E. and Tagliaferri, M. (1986). Use of ketoconazole in the treatment of Cushing's syndrome. *J Clin Endocrinol Metab* **63**, 1365–1371.

Loosen, P.T. (1992). Psychiatric phenomenology in Cushing's disease. *Pharmacopsychiatry* **25**, 192–198.

Loria, R. (1997). Antiglucocorticoid function of androstenetriol. *Psychoneuroendocrinology* **22**, S103–S108.

Lustman, P., Griffith, L., Freedland, K., Kissel, S. and Clouse, R. (1998). Cognitive behavior therapy for depression in type 2 diabetes: A randomized controlled trial. *Ann Int Med* **129**, 613–621.

Maclean, C., Walton, K., Wenneberg, S. *et al.* (1997). Effects of the Transcendental Meditation program on adaptive mechanisms: Changes in hormone levels and respones to stress after 4 months of practice. *Psychoneuroendocrinology* **22**, 277–295.

Majewska, M.D. (1987). Steroids and brain activity. Essential dialogue between body and mind. *Biochem Pharmacol* **36**, 3781–3788.

Malison, R.T., Anand, A., Pelton, G.H. *et al.* (1999). Limited efficacy of ketocona-zole in treatment-refractory major depression. *J Clin Psychopharmacol* **19**, 466–470.

Mauri, M., Sinforiani, E., Bono, G. *et al.* (1993). Memory impairment in Cushing's disease. *Acta Neurol Scand* **87**, 52–55.

McCraty, R., Barrios-Choplin, B., Rozman, D., Atkinson, M. and Watkins, A.D. (1998). The impact of a new emotional self-management program on stress, emotions, heart rate variability, DHEA and cortisol. *Integr Physiol Behav Sci* **33**, 151–170.

McEwen, B.S. (1987). Glucocorticoid-biogenic amine interactions in relation to mood and behavior. *Biochem Pharmacol* **36**, 1755–1763.

McEwen, B. (1991). Non-genomic and genomic effects of steroids on neural activity. *Trends Pharm Sci* **12**, 141–147.

McEwen, B.S. (1997). Possible mechanisms for atrophy of the human hippocampus. *Mol Psychiatry* **2**, 255–262.

McEwen, B. (1998). Protective and damaging effects of stress mediators. *New Engl J Med* **338**, 171–179.

McEwen, B. (2000). Allostasis and allostatic load: Implications for neuropsy-chopharmacology. *Neuropsychopharmacology* **22**, 108–124.

McEwen, B. and Seeman, T. (1999). Protective and damaging effects of mediators of stress: Elaborating and testing the concepts of allostasis and allostatic load. *Ann NY Acad Sci* **896**, 30–47.

McEwen, B. and Stellar, E. (1993). Stress and the individual: Mechanisms leading to disease. *Arch Int Med* **153**, 2093–2191.

McEwen, B.S., Davis, P.G., Parsons, B. and Pfaff, D.W. (1979). The brain as target for steroid hormone action. *Ann Rev Neurosci* **2**, 65–112.

McEwen, B.S., Angulo, J., Cameron, H. and Chao, H.M. (1992). Paradoxical effects of adrenal steroids on the brain: Protection versus degeneration. *Biol Psychiatry* **31**, 177–199.

McGrady, A. and Horner, J. (1999). Role of mood in outcome of biofeedback assisted relaxation therapy in insulin dependent diabetes mellitus. *App Psychophysiol* **24**, 79–88.

McGrady, A., Woerner, M., Guillermo, A., Bernal, A. and Higgins, J. (1987). Effect of biofeedback-assisted relaxation on blood pressure and cortisol levels in normotensives and hypertensives. *J Behav Med* **10**, 301–310.

McKinney, C.H., Antoni, M.H., Kumar, M., Tims, F.C. and McCabe, P.M. (1997). Effects of guided imagery and music (GIM) therapy on mood and cortisol in healthy adults. *Health Psychol* **16**, 390–400.

Meador-Woodruff, J.H., Greden, J.F., Grunhaus, L. and Haskett, R.F. (1990). Severity of depression and hypothalamic-pituitary-adrenal axis dysregulation: identification of contributing factors. *Acta Psychiatr Scand* **81**, 364–371.

Michaels, R., Parra, J., McCann, D. and Vander, J. (1979). Renin, cortisol, and aldos-terone during transcendental meditation. *Psychosom Med* **41**, 50–54.

Miluk-Kolasa, B., Obminski, Z., Stupnicki, R. and Golec, L. (1994). Effects of music treatment on salivary cortisol in patients exposed to pre-surgical stress. *Exp Clin Endocrinol* **102**, 118–120.

Mockel, M., Rocker, L., Stork, T. *et al.* (1994). Immediate physiological responses of healthy volunteers to different types of music: cardiovascular, hormonal and mental changes [published erratum appears in *Eur J Appl Physiol* **69**, 274]. *Eur J Appl Physiol* **68**, 451–459.

Morales, A.J., Nolan, J.J., Nelson, J.C. and Yen, S.S. (1994). Effects of replacement dose of dehydroepiandrosterone in men and women of advancing age [published erratum appears in *J Clin Endocrinol Metab* **80**, 2799]. *J Clin Endocrinol Metab* **78**, 1360–1367.

Morales, A., Haubricht, R., Hwang, J., Asakura, H. and Yen, S. (1998). The effect of six months treatment with a 100 mg daily dose of dehydroepiandrosterone on circulating sex steroids, body composition and muscle strength in age advanced men and women. *Clin Endocrinol* **49**, 421–432.

Moxley, R.T., 3rd (1994). Potential for growth factor treatment of muscle disease. *Curr Opin Neurol* **7**, 427–434.

Murphy, B.E. (1991a). Steroids and depression. *J Steroid Biochem Mol Biol* **38**, 537–559.

Murphy, B.E. (1991b). Treatment of major depression with steroid suppressive drugs. *J Steroid Biochem Mol Biol* **39**, 239–244.

Murphy, B.E.P. (1997). Antiglucocorticoid therapies in major depression: A review. *Psychoneuroendocrinology* **22**, S215–S232.

Murphy, B.E.P. and Wolkowitz, O.M. (1993). The pathophysiologic significance of hypercorticism: antiglucocorticoid strategies. *Psychiat Ann* **23**, 682–690.

Murphy, B.E., Dhar, V., Ghadirian, A.M., Chouinard, G. and Keller, R. (1991). Response to steroid suppression in major depression resistant to antidepressant therapy. *J Clin Psychopharmacol* **11**, 121–126.

Murphy, B.E., Filipini, D. and Ghadirian, A.M. (1993). Possible use of glucocorticoid receptor antagonists in the treatment of major depression: preliminary results using RU 486. *J Psychiatry Neurosci* **18**, 209–213.

Murphy, B.E., Ghadirian, A.M. and Dhar, V. (1998). Neuroendocrine responses to inhibitors of steroid biosynthesis in patients with major depression resistant to antidepressant therapy. *Can J Psychiatry* **43**, 279–286.

Naber, D., Sand, P. and Heigl, B. (1996). Psychopathological and neuropsychological effects of 8–days' corticosteroid treatment. A prospective study. *Psychoneuroendocrinology* **21**, 25–31.

Nelson, J.C. and Davis, J.M. (1997). DST studies in psychotic depression: A meta-analysis. *Am J Psychiatry* **154**, 1497–1503.

Nemeroff, C.B. (1988). The role of corticotropin-releasing factor in the pathogenesis of major depression. *Pharmacopsychiatry* **21**, 76–82.

Nemeroff, C.B. (2000). Clinical studies on the role of CRF in mood and anxiety disorders, CRF Antagonists, Held during the 2nd International Congress on Hormones, Brain and Neuropsychopharmacology. Rhodes, Greece.

Nesbitt, L.T., Jr. (1995). Minimizing complications from systemic glucocorticosteroid use. *Dermatol Clin* **13**, 925–939.

Nestler, J.E., Barlascini, C.O., Clore, J.N. and Blackard, W.G. (1988). Dehydro-epiandrosterone reduces serum low density lipoprotein levels and body fat but does not alter insulin sensitivity in normal men. *J Clin Endocrinol Metab* **66**, 57–61.

Nieman, L., Chrousos, G. and Kellner, C. (1985). Successful treatment of Cushing's syndrome with the glucocorticoid antagonist RU486. *J Clin Endocrinol Metab* **61**, 536–540.

Nippoldt, T. and Sreekumaran Nair, K. (1998). Is there a case for DHEA replacement? *Balliere's Clin Endocrinol Metab* **12**, 507–520.

O'Dwyer, A.M., Lightman, S.L., Marks, M.N. and Checkley, S.A. (1995). Treatment of major depression with metyrapone and hydrocortisone. *J Affect Disord* **33**, 123–128.

Papolos, D.F., Edwards, E., Marmur, R., Lachman, H.M. and Henn, F.A. (1993). Effects of the antiglucocorticoid RU 38486 on the induction of learned helpless behavior in Sprague-Dawley rats. *Brain Res* **615**, 304–309.

Patchev, V.K. and Almeida, O.F.X. (1997). Daily DHEA or melatonin treatment prevents glucocorticoid-induced dysregulation of the hypothalamic–pituitary–adrenal axis, 2nd International Conference on Cortisol and Anti-cortisols, p. 46.

Pepin, M.C., Beaulieu, S. and Barden, N. (1990). Differential regulation by dexamethasone of glucocorticoid receptor messenger RNA concentrations in neuronal cultures derived from fetal rat hypothalamus and cerebral cortex. *Cell Mol Neurobiol* **10**, 227–235.

Pies, R. (1995). Differential diagnosis and treatment of steroid-induced affective syndromes. *Gen Hosp Psychiatry* **17**, 353–361.

Platania-Solazzo, A., Field, T.M., Blank, J. *et al.* (1992). Relaxation therapy reduces anxiety in child and adolescent psychiatric patients. *Acta Paedopsychiatr* **55**, 115–120.

Plihal, W., Krug, R., Pietrowsky, R., Fehm, H.L. and Born, J. (1996). Corticosteroid receptor mediated effects on mood in humans. *Psychoneuroendocrinology* **21**, 515–523.

Quarton, G.C., Clark, L.D., Cobb, S. and Bauer, W. (1955). Mental disturbances associated with ACTH and cortisone: A review of explanatory hypotheses. *Medicine* **34**, 13–50.

Raber, J. (1998). Detrimental effects of chronic hypothalamic-pituitary-adrenal activation: From obesity to memory deficits. *Mol Neurobiol* **18**, 1–22.

Ravaris, C.L., Sateia, M.J., Beroza, K.W., Noordsy, D.L. and Brinck-Johnsen, T. (1988). Effect of ketoconazole on a hypophysectomized, hypercortisolemic, psychotically depressed woman [letter]. *Arch Gen Psychiatry* **45**, 966–967.

Ravaris, C.L., Brinck-Johnsen, T. and Elliott, B. (1994). Clinical use of ketoconazole in hypercortisoluric depressives. *Biol Psychiatry* **35**, 679.

Raven, P.W., O'Dwyer, A.M., Taylor, N.F. and Checkley, S.A. (1996). The relationship between the effects of metyrapone treatment on depressed mood and urinary steroid profiles. *Psychoneuroendocrinol* **21**, 277–286.

Regestein, Q.R., Rose, L.I. and Williams, G.H. (1972). Psychopathology in Cushing's syndrome. *Arch Int Med* **130**, 114–117.

Reus, V.I. (1982). Pituitary-adrenal disinhibition as the independent variable in the assessment of behavioral symptoms. *Biol Psychiatry* **17**, 317–325.

Reus, V.I. (1985). Toward an understanding of cortisol dysregulation in major depression: A review of studies of the dexamethasone suppression test and urinary free-cortisol. *Psychiatr Med* **3**, 1–21.

Reus, V.I. and Wolkowitz, O.M. (1993). Behavioral effects of corticosteroid therapy. *Psychiatr Ann* **23**, 703–708.

Reus, V.I., Wolkowitz, O.M. and Frederick, S. (1997). Antiglucocorticoid treatments in psychiatry. *Psychoneuroendocrinology* **22**, S121–S124.

Ribeiro, S.C., Tandon, R., Grunhaus, L. and Greden, J.F. (1993). The DST as a predictor of outcome in depression: a meta-analysis. *Am J Psychiatry* **150**, 1618–1629.

Romeo, E., Strohle, A., Spalletta, G. *et al.* (1998). Effects of antidepressant treatment on neuroactive steroids in major depression. *Am J Psychiatry* **155**, 910–913.

Rosmond, R. and Björntorp, P. (2000). The hypothalamic-pituitary-adrenal axis activity as a predictor of cardiovascular disease, type 2 diabetes and stroke. *J Int Med* **247**, 188–197.

Ryu, H., Lee, H.S., Shin, Y.S. *et al.* (1996). Acute effect of qigong training on stress hormonal levels in man. *Am J Chin Med* **24**, 193–198.

Sapolsky, R. (1992). *Stress, the Aging Brain, and the Mechanisms of Neuron Death*, Bradford Books, Cambridge.

Sapolsky, R.M. (1993). Potential behavioral modification of glucocorticoid damage to the hippocampus. *Behav Brain Res* **57**, 175–182.

Sapolsky, R.M., Krey, L.C. and McEwen, B.S. (1986). The neuroendocrinology of stress and aging: the glucocorticoid cascade hypothesis. *Endocrinol Rev* **7**, 284–301.

Sapolsky, R., Uno, H., Rebert, C. and Finch, C. (1990). Hippocampal damage asociated with prolonged gluccocorticoid exposure in primates. *J Neurosci* **10**, 2897–2902.

Schulkin, J., McEwen, B.S. and Gold, P.W. (1994). Allostasis, amygdala, and anticipatory angst. *Neurosci Biobehav Rev* **18**, 385–396.

Seeman, T., Singer, B., Rowe, J., Horwitz, R. and McEwen, B. (1997). Price of adaptation – allostatic load and its health consequences. *Arch Int Med* **157**, 2259–2268.

Seeman, T., Singer, B., Rowe, J. and McEwen, B. (2001). Allostatic load as a marker of cumulative biological risk: MacArthur studies of successful aging. (*Submitted*).

Selye, H. (1956). *The Stress of Life*. McGraw-Hill, New York.

Sonino, N., Boscaro, M., Ambroso, G., Merola, G. and Mantero, G. (1986). Prolonged treatment of Cushing's disease with metyrapone and aminoglutethimide. *IRCS Med Sci* **14**, 485–486.

Sonino, N., Boscaro, M., Paoletta, A., Mantero, F. and Ziliotto, D. (1991). Ketoconazole treatment in Cushing's syndrome: experience in 34 patients. *Clin Endocrinol* **35**, 347–352.

Sonino, N., Fava, G.A., Belluardo, P., Girelli, M.E. and Boscaro, M. (1993). Course of depression in Cushing's syndrome: response to treatment and comparison with Graves' disease. *Horm Res* **39**, 202–206.

Sovner, R. and Fogelman, S. (1996). Ketoconazole therapy for atypical depression. *J Clin Psychiatry* **57**, 227–228.

Spencer, N., Poynter, M., Hennebold, J. *et al.* (1995). Does DHEA-S restore immune competence in aged animals through its capacity to function as a natural modulator of peroxisome activities? *Ann NY Acad Sci* **774**, 200–216.

Spillane, J.D. (1951). Nervous and mental disorders in Cushing's syndrome. *Brain* **74**, 72–94.

Stahl, F., Schnorr, D., Pilz, C. and Dorner, G. (1992). Dehydroepiandrosterone (DHEA) levels in patients with prostatic cancer, heart diseases and under surgery stress. *Exp Clin Endocrinol* **99**, 68–70.

Starkman, M., Gebarski, S., Berent, S. and Schteingart, D. (1992). Hippocampal formation volume, memory dysfunction, and cortisol levels in patients with Cushing's syndrome. *Biol Psychiatry* **32**, 756–765.

Starkman, M.N., Schteingart, D.E. and Schork, M.A. (1981). Depressed mood and other psychiatric manifestations of Cushing's syndrome: relationship to hormone levels. *Psychosom Med* **43**, 3–18.

Starkman, M.N., Schteingart, D.E. and Schork, M.A. (1986). Cushing's syndrome after treatment: changes in cortisol and ACTH levels, and amelioration of the depressive syndrome. *Psychiatry Res* **19**, 177–188.

Starkman, M.N., Giordani, B., Gebarski, S.S. *et al.* (1999). Decrease in cortisol reverses human hippocampal atrophy following treatment of Cushing's disease. *Biol Psychiatry* **46**, 1595–1602.

Sterling, P. and Eyer, J. (1988). Allostasis: A new paradigm to explain arousal pathology. In: Fisher, S. and Reason, J. (Eds), *Handbook of Life Stress: Cognition and Health*: John Wiley, Chichester, pp. 629–649.

Sudsuang, R., Chentazez, V. and Veluvan, K. (1991). Effect of Buddhist meditation on serum cortisol and total protein levels, blood pressure, pulse rate, lung volume and reaction time. *Physiol Behav* **50**, 543–548.

Svec, F. and Porter, J.R. (1998). The actions of exogenous dehydroepiandrosterone in experimental animals and humans. *Proc Soc Exp Biol Med* **218**, 174–191.

Taft, P., Martin, F.I.R. and Melick, R. (1970). Cushing's syndrome – a review of the response to treatment of 42 patients. *Austral Ann Med* **4**, 295–303.

Thakore, J.H. and Dinan, T. (1995). Cortisol synthesis inhibition: A new treatment strategy for the clinical and endocrine manifestations of depression. *Biol Psychiatry* **37**, 364–368.

Thase, M.E. (1994). Cognitive-behavioral therapy of severe unipolar depression. In: Nolen, W.A., Zohar, J., Roose, S.P. and Amsterdam, J.D. (Eds), *Refractory Depression: Current Strategies and Future Directions*. John Wiley, Chichester, pp. 269–296.

Thase, M., Simons, A. and Reynolds, C. (1993). Psychobiological correlates of poor response to cognitive behavior therapy: potential indications for antidepressant pharmacotherapy. *Psychopharmacol Bull* **29**, 293–301.

Tollefson, G.D., Haus, E., Garvey, M.J., Evans, M. and Tuason, V.B. (1990). 24 hour urinary dehydroepiandrosterone sulfate in unipolar depression treated with cognitive and/or pharmacotherapy. *Ann Clin Psychiatry* **2**, 39–45.

Trethowen, W.H. and Cobb, M. (1952). Neuropsychiatric aspects of Cushing's syndrome. *Arch Neurol Psychiatry* **67**, 283–309.

van der Lely, A.J., Foeken, K., van der Mast, R.C. and Lamberts, S.W. (1991). Rapid reversal of acute psychosis in the Cushing syndrome with the cortisol-receptor antagonist mifepristone (RU 486). *Ann Int Med* **114**, 143–144.

van Vollenhoven, R.F. (1997). Dehydroepiandrosterone: Uses and abuses. In: Kelley, W.N., Harris, Jr E.D., Ruddy, S. and Sledge, C.B. (Eds), *Textbook of Rheumatology, Vol. Update Series 25*. Saunders. Philadelphia, pp. 1–25.

Verhelst, J.A., Trainer, P.J., Howlett, T.A. *et al.* (1991). Short and long-term responses to metyrapone in the medical management of 91 patients with Cushing's syndrome. *Clin Endocrinol* **35**, 169–178.

Voigt, K.H., Bossert, S., Bretschneider, S., Bliestle, A. and Fehm, H.L. (1985). Disturbed cortisol secretion in man: contrasting Cushing's syndrome and endogenous depression. *Psychiatry Res* **15**, 341–350.

Walton, G. and Pugh, N. (1995). Stress, steroids, and 'ojas': Neuroendocrine mechanisms and current promise of ancient approaches to disease prevention. *Ind J Physiol Pharmacol* **39**, 3–34.

Walton, K.G., Pugh, N.D., Gelderloos, P. and Macrae, P. (1995). Stress reduction and preventing hypertension: preliminary support for a psychoneuroendocrine mechanism. *J Altern Complement Med* **1**, 263–283.

Welbourn, R.B., Montgomery, D.A.D. and Kennedy, T.L. (1971). The natural history of treated Cushing's syndrome. *Br J Surg* **58**, 1–16.

Whelan, T.B., Schteingart, D.E., Starkman, M.N. and Smith, A. (1980). Neuropsychological deficits in Cushing's syndrome. *J Nerv Ment Dis* **168**, 753–757.

Whitehouse, W., Dinges, D., Orne, E. *et al.* (1996). Psychosocial and immune effects of self-hypnosis training for stress management throughout the first semester of medical school. *Psychosom Med* **58**, 249–263.

Winokur, G., Black, D.W. and Nasrallah, A. (1987). DST nonsuppressor status: relationship to specific aspects of the depressive syndrome. *Biol Psychiatry* **22**, 360–368.

Wolf, O.T., Neumann, O., Hellhammer, D.H. *et al.* (1997). Effects of a two-week physiological dehydroepiandrosterone substitution on cognitive performance and well-being in healthy elderly women and men. *J Clin Endocrinol Metab* **82**, 2363–2367.

Wolkowitz, O.M. (1994). Prospective controlled studies of the behavioral and biological effects of exogenous corticosteroids. *Psychoneuroendocrinology* **19**, 233–255.

Wolkowitz, O.M. and Reus, V.I. (2000). Neuropsychiatric effects of Dehydroepiandrosterone (DHEA). In: Kalimi, M. and Regelson, W. (Eds), *Dehydroepiandrosterone (DHEA)*, Walter de Gruyter, Berlin, pp. 271–298..

Wolkowitz, O.M. and Reus, V.I. (1999). Treatment of depression with antiglucocorticoid drugs. *Psychosom Med* **61**, 698–711.

Wolkowitz, O., Sutton, M. and Koulu, M. (1986). Chronic corticosterone administration in rats: behavioral and biochemical evidence of increases in central dopaminergic activity. *Eur J Pharmacol* **122**, 329–338.

Wolkowitz, O.M., Rubinow, D., Doran, A.R. *et al.* (1990). Prednisone effects on neurochemistry and behavior. Preliminary findings. *Arch Gen Psychiatry* **47**, 963–968.

Wolkowitz, O.M., Reus, V.I., Manfredi, F. and Roberts, E. (1992). Antiglucocorticoid effects of DHEA-S in Alzheimer's Disease (Reply). *Am J Psychiatry* **149**, 1126.

Wolkowitz, O.M., Reus, V.I., Manfredi, F. *et al.* (1993). Ketoconazole treatment of hypercortisolemic depression. *Am J Psychiatry* **150**, 810–812.

Wolkowitz, O.M., Reus, V.I., Manfredi, F. *et al.* (1994). Antiglucocorticoid medication effects on specific depressive symptoms. *Biol Psychiatry* **35**, 678.

Wolkowitz, O., Reus, V., Robers, E., Manfredi, F. and Chan, T. (1995). Antidepressant and cognition-enhancing effects of DHEA in major depression. *Ann NY Acad Sci* **774**, 337–339.

Wolkowitz, O.M., Reus, V.I., Manfredi, F. *et al.* (1996). Dexamethasone for depression [letter]. *Am J Psychiatry* **153**, 1112.

Wolkowitz, O.M., Reus, V.I., Canick, J., Levin, B. and Lupien, S. (1997a). Glucocorticoid medication, memory and steroid psychosis in medical illness. *Ann NY Acad Sci* **823**, 81–96.

Wolkowitz, O.M., Reus, V.I., Roberts, E. *et al.* (1997b). Dehydroepiandrosterone (DHEA) treatment of depression. *Biol Psychiatry* **41**, 311–318.

Wolkowitz, O.M., Reus, V.I., Chan, T. *et al.* (1999a). Antiglucocorticoid treatment of depression: Double-blind ketoconazole. *Biol Psychiatry* **45**, 1070–1074.

Wolkowitz, O.M., Reus, V.I., Keebler, A. *et al.* (1999b). Double-blind treatment of major depression with dehydroepiandrosterone (DHEA). *Am J Psychiatry* **156**, 646–649.

Wolkowitz, O.M., Brizendine, L. and Reus, V.I. (2000a). The role of dehydroepiandrosterone (DHEA) in psychiatry. *Psychiatr Ann* **30**, 123–128.

Wolkowitz, O.M., Kramer, J., Reus, V.I. *et al.* (2000b). DHEA treatment of Alzheimer's Disease: a randomized, double-blind, placebo-controlled study, The 2nd International Congress on Hormones, Brain and Neuropsychopharmacology. Rhodes, Greece.

Wong, M.L., Kling, M.A., Munson, P.J. *et al.* (2000). Pronounced and sustained central hypernoradrenergic function in major depression with melancholic features: relation to hypercortisolism and corticotropin-releasing hormone. *Proc Natl Acad Sci USA* **97**, 325–330.

Xu, L., Holscher, C., Anwyl, R. and Rowan, M.J. (1998). Glucocorticoid receptor and protein/RNA synthesis-dependent mechanisms underlie the control of synaptic plasticity by stress. *Proc Natl Acad Sci USA* **95**, 3204–3208.

Zeiger, M.A., Fraker, D.L., Pass, H.I. *et al.* (1993). Effective reversibility of the signs and symptoms of hypercortisolism by bilateral adrenalectomy. *Surgery* **114**, 1138–1143.

Zobel, A.W., Nickel, T., Kunzel, H.E. *et al.* (2000). Effects of the high-affinity corticotropin-releasing hormone receptor 1 antagonist R121919 in major depression: the first 20 patients treated. *J Psychiatr Res* **34**, 171–181.

10

Hypothalamic–Pituitary–Adrenal Axis and Antidepressant Action

MARIE-THERESE WALSH[a] and TIMOTHY G. DINAN[b]

[a]*Department of Psychiatry, Royal College of Surgeons in Ireland, Dublin,*
[b]*Department of Clinical Pharmacology and Therapeutics, University College, Cork,*
Ireland

INTRODUCTION

Corticotrophin releasing hormone (CRH)-containing neurones in the paraventricular nucleus (medial parvocellular division) of the hypothalamus provide the central regulation of the hypothalamic–ptiuitary–adrenal axis (HPA) (Gray and Bingaman, 1996). CRH is a 41 amino acid peptide, which was characterized by Vale and colleagues (1981). Under basal conditions CRH is the dominant regulator of the axis (Arborelius *et al.*, 1999). Inputs to these neurones include classic neurotransmitters such as serotonin (5HT) and noradrenaline together with an opioid inhibitory input (Jessop, 1999). CRH acts through a CRH_1 receptor on the anterior pituitary and increases pro-opiomelanocortin (P0MC) gene expression and the release of both adrenocorticotrophic hormone (ACTH) and β-endorphin. In situations of stress many CRH-containing neurones co-express arginine vasopressin (AVP) (Scott and Dinan, 1998). This hormone, long associated with the posterior pituitary, is now known to play a key role in regulating the HPA axis. Studies in healthy subjects demonstrate that AVP acts through a V_{1b} receptor, synergising with CRH to bring about ACTH release from the anterior pituitary. This in turn regulates the release of cortisol from the adrenal cortex. The inability to activate the HPA axis in situations of stress, either physical or psychological, is incompatible with life.

Two types of cortisol binding site have been described in the brain. The type 1 receptor is indistinguishable from the peripheral mineralocorticoid receptor (MR) and is distributed principally in the septo-hippocampal region (Chao *et al.*, 1989). The type 2 or glucocorticoid receptor (GR) has a wider distribution and monitors stress-induced elevations in cortisol. It has approximately 10-fold lower affinity for cortisol than the type 1 receptor. Thus, animal studies show that while the type 1 receptors are occupied to a large extent under conditions of low circulating corticosteroid, the type 2 receptors have relatively low occupation under basal conditions, which increases dramatically when corticosteroid levels rise (Reul *et al.*, 1987a, b). These receptor systems provide negative feedback loops on cortisol synthesis at a limbic, hypothalamic and pituitary level. Feedback is defined on the basis of response rate, as immediate (within minutes), intermediate and delayed (within hours).

Studies of HPA function in major depression reveal numerous abnormalities, which are more pronounced in patients with melancholic features (Dinan, 1994). The following abnormalities are well documented: (1) 24h urinary free cortisol is enhanced (on average twice as high as in healthy controls) and serum cortisol levels are raised; (2) dexamethasone non-suppression is found in 40–70% of patients; (3) adrenal gland hyperplasia is reported; (4) release of ACTH in response to CRH challenge is blunted.

HPA HORMONES

Baseline measures

Several studies have examined baseline levels of the key HPA hormones in patients with depression. Plasma CRH levels have been investigated by Catalan *et al.* (1998). Thirty-six patients with either major depression or dysthymia, together with 17 healthy volunteers were recruited. Plasma cortisol and CRH concentrations were significantly higher in the patient group. Plasma cortisol and CRH concentrations correlated significantly, suggesting that the CRH is of hypothalamic origin. CRH immunoreactivity in the cerebrospinal fluid (CSF) is also increased in depression. Nemeroff's group, in a series of studies, have found consistently elevated CRH when depressives are compared with other diagnostic categories (Nemeroff *et al.*, 1984). In contrast, patients with atypical features of depression such as hyperphagia, hypersomnia and rejection sensitivity have below normal levels of CRH (Geracioti *et al.*, 1992).

In studies by van Londen and colleagues on 52 patients with major depression compared with 37 healthy controls (van Londen *et al.*, 1997), plasma concentrations of arginine vasopressin were higher in the depressed patients.

Several studies have found elevated plasma cortisol levels in depression. Single plasma samples are unreliable in detecting alterations even in Cushing's disease. However multiple sampling over a short time-frame is reported to increase the diagnostic reliability of cortisol in distinguishing depression from health. Halbreich *et al.* (1982) monitored cortisol between 1300h and 1600h and claim a high sensitivity for this approach.

Salivary cortisol is a convenient painless method of assessing cortisol. As in the case of plasma and urine, salivary cortisol is reported to be elevated in depression (Galard *et al.*, 1991). Depressed patients with an endogenous symptom complex had salivary cortisol and plasma ACTH measured. In healthy controls a strong correlation was established between plasma ACTH and salivary cortisol, but this relationship was lost in depression. Salivary cortisol was elevated in the depressives.

Baseline treatment effects

Treatment with fluoxetine decreases CRH levels in CSF (De Bellis *et al.*, 1993) and also decreases levels of arginine vasopressin. That elevated CRH is a state marker is also supported by a study in which the peptide was measured before and after a course of electroconvulsive therapy (ECT) (Nemeroff *et al.*, 1991). Nine patients with major depression and psychotic features were recruited. CSF concentrations of CRH, somatostatin and β-endorphin were measured. Concentrations of both CRH and β-endorphin decreased after ECT, while the concentration of somatostatin increased.

In response to treatment with conventional antidepressants plasma cortisol levels decrease (O'Keane *et al.*, 1992; Lesch, 1991) and similar decreases in urinary free cortisol are reported (Carroll *et al.*, 1976). Linkowski *et al.* (1987) monitored ACTH and cortisol concentrations at 15 min intervals in 11 men suffering from major depression and a healthy comparison group. During the acute phase of illness the patients had abnormally short rapid eye movement latencies, hypercortisolism, early timing of the nadirs of the ACTH-cortisol rhythms and shorter nocturnal periods of quiescent cortisol secretion. They were treated with either ECT or amitriptyline and after treatment, cortisol levels returned to normal due to a decrease in the magnitude of episodic pulses. Furthermore, the timing of the circadian rhythms of ACTH and cortisol as well as the duration of the quiescent period of cortisol secretion was normalized. The authors conclude that a disorder of circadian rhythmicity characterizes acute episodes of major depression and that this chronobiological abnormality as well as the hypersecretion of ACTH and cortisol are state rather than trait markers. Patients who fail to respond to treatment do not show such alterations.

Similarly, studies on a group of 37 depressed elderly inpatients and 25 healthy controls showed that amitriptyline significantly decreased CSF CRH levels in treatment responsive patients only (Heuser *et al.*, 1998). No effect was observed on vasopressin or somatostatin levels.

DYNAMIC HPA FUNCTION TESTS

Dexamethasone suppression test

The dexamethasone suppression test (DST) is a test of negative feedback inhibition within the HPA axis. It is the most extensively studied biological marker in psychiatry (APA Task Force, 1987). The standardized test consists of administering dexamethasone 1 mg at 2300 h and obtaining blood for cortisol estimation at 1600 h the following afternoon (Carroll, 1982). Non-suppression is usually defined as a cortisol level above 137 nmol/l (5 µg/dl). Most studies suggest that the test has 40–50% sensitivity and 70–90% specificity in the diagnosis of major depression.

Treatment and the DST

A recent meta-analysis has focused on the predictive value of the test (Ribeiro *et al.*, 1993). When studies in which a placebo was employed are examined non-suppressors were significantly less likely than suppressors to respond to placebo. Furthermore, suppressors responded better to antide-pressants than placebo, indicating the test does not usefully select patients who will respond to pharmacotherapy. Therefore, the baseline DST result is poorly predictive of outcome.

The test does provide a state dependent marker, as Carroll (1982) first reported. Effective treatment should normalize the response and persistent nonsuppression is associated with a poor outcome. Goldberg (1980) and Greden *et al.* (1980) who found that persistent nonsuppression, despite apparent clinical improvement, could serve as a marker of active underlying illness supported this observation. Subsequent studies comparing patients whose DST normalizes with those whose DST does not, indicate that persis-tent nonsuppression is associated with re-hospitalisation, suicide and recur-rence of severe symptoms (Holsboer *et al.*, 1982; Asnis *et al.*, 1986; Charles *et al.*, 1989).

CRH test

The CRH test is conducted by the intravenous administration of either ovine or human CRH and the monitoring of ACTH and cortisol output. Because of differing protein binding characteristics the response to ovine CRH is longer than that observed with the human variety. Numerous studies consis-tently demonstrate that ACTH output is blunted but cortisol output is normal following CRH administration in depression (Holsboer *et al.*, 1986; Amsterdam *et al.*, 1987; Ur *et al.*, 1992).

Treatment and the CRH test

Amsterdam *et al.* (1987) examined ovine CRH responses both before and during clinical recovery in depressed patients. Cumulative ACTH responses increased significantly during clinical recovery and were similar to those of normal subjects on recovery. Paradoxically, maximum and peak cortisol responses increased after recovery, suggesting that heightened adrenocortical responsiveness to ACTH during depression may take longer to normalize than abnormal pituitary responsiveness to CRH.

The test was found to be a good predictor of relapse in bipolar depression (Vieta *et al.*, 1997). The ACTH and cortisol response to 100 µg of human CRH was measured in 42 lithium-treated patients in remission from bipolar I disorder. Patients showed higher baseline and peak ACTH concentrations than healthy comparison subjects. A lower net area under the ACTH curve predicted depressive relapse within 6 months. The study suggests that the CRH test is potentially a good predictor of depressive relapse in remitted bipolar patients.

Combined dexamethasone–CRH test

When healthy volunteers are treated with dexamethasone prior to CRH infusion (dex-CRH test), release of ACTH is blunted and the extent of blunting is proportional to the dose of dexamethasone. Paradoxically, when depressives are pre-treated with dexamethasone they show enhanced response to CRH. The reason for this response is unclear but Holsboer (1995) suggests that vasopressin may be involved. An alternative explanation is that dexamethasone results in a build-up of ACTH in the pituitary. As there is enhanced forward drive in depression greater levels of ACTH are available for release on CRH challenge. Heuser *et al.* (1994) estimates the sensitivity of the test to be 80% in differentiating a healthy subject from a depressive. Deuschle *et al.* (1998) compared the association of the standard DST and the combined dexamethasone/corticotrophin releasing hormone (dex-CRH) challenge with parameters of diurnal cortisol profiles in 25 depressed patients and 33 age-matched healthy controls. While cortisol levels after the dex-CRH test were dependent upon minimal 24-hour cortisol and evening frequency of pulsatile cortisol release, post-DST levels were related to 24-hour mean cortisol. These researchers concluded that the dex-CRH test would allow more reliable inferences to be made with regard to the basal HPA activity than the DST test. Zobel *et al.* (1999) used the dex-CRH test to assess normalization of HPA regulation in patients in remission from major depression. In a sample group of 40 patients, the test was administered both after initiation of treatment and after remission, shortly before discharge. A high cortisol response on both occasions, or a substantially increased cortisol response at discharge, was found to be associated with a substantially increased risk of relapse. Thus it was concluded that the dex-CRH test is effective in predicting medium term outcome in patients with remitted depression. Use of the test has also implicated HPA axis dysregulation in panic disorder.

A study by Rybakowski and Twardowska (1999) used the dex-CRH test to compare 40 patients with bipolar (16) or unipolar (24) depression, both during a depressive episode and in remission, with 20 healthy controls.

Cortisol concentrations 16 hours after dexamethasone and cortisol release subsequent to CRH infusion were found to be significantly elevated in bipolar patients compared with both unipolar patients and controls. Unipolar patients with multiple depressive episodes had higher cortisol levels than controls after CRH infusion. In remission, bipolar patients had significantly higher cortisol levels after CRH infusion than unipolar patients, while first episode unipolar patients had lower cortisol levels both before and after CRH than control subjects. This study suggests that the dex-CRH test detects greater dysregulation of the HPA axis in depressives with bipolar disorder than in patients with unipolar depression. However, the dysregulation in unipolar depression may increase with repeated episodes.

Treatment and the dex-CRH test

The impact of amitriptyline on the dex-CRH test was assessed by Heuser *et al.* (1996). A total of 39 depressed inpatients, with a mean age of 69 years and a mean Hamilton depression score of 26 were recruited. The test was conducted at baseline and the end of weeks 1, 3 and 6 of treatment. Treatment consisted of amitriptyline 75 mg nocte. Overall there was a continuous drop in the severity of depression throughout the 6 weeks of treatment. The patients' mean steady-state plasma concentration of tricyclic (amitriptyline+nortriptyline) was 180 ng/ml. At baseline the patients had a profoundly abnormal HPA response, characterized by an exaggerated cortisol release in response to dex-CRH. The abnormality began to disappear after 1 week of treatment. Holsboer *et al.* (1995) examined dex-CRH responses during 5 weeks of treatment in 42 major depressives given trimipramine or trimipramine plus sleep deprivation or bright light therapy. For the total sample, the treatment non-responders had significantly greater ACTH secretion following CRH at both the beginning and end of the study. The test is therefore viewed as having predictive value in determining response.

Serotonin and the HPA

A significant serotoninergic input to the hypothalamus regulates CRH release and of the many 5HT receptors the 1A receptor seems dominant in this response (Dinan, 1997). Stimulation of these receptors in humans is known to not only activate the HPA axis but also to induce hypothermia. Lesch *et al.* (1990, 1991) used ipsapirone, the azaspirone, which acts as a partial agonist at the $5HT_{1A}$ receptor as a challenge in both depressives and healthy controls. Twenty-four subjects, 12 with unipolar depression and 12 matched healthy subjects were recruited. They were each given ipsapirone 0.3 mg/kg or placebo in random order. High basal cortisol levels were found in the depressives. The ACTH/cortisol and hypothermic responses were attenuated in patients with unipolar depression. The authors suggest that the impaired HPA response in depression may be due to a glucocorticoid-dependent subsensitivity of the postsynaptic $5HT_{1A}$ receptor or a defective post-receptor signalling pathway. Lesch et al. (1990) examined the impact of amitriptyline treatment on $5HT_{1A}$ induced hypothermia. Patients with major depression were chronically treated with amitriptyline, and temperature response to ipsapirone challenge was monitored before and after treatment. Amitriptyline caused further impairment in $5HT_{1A}$ mediated hypothermia. The study adds weight to the view that effective antidepressants down-regulate the $5HT_{1A}$ receptor during treatment. A study of fluoxetine, using a double-blind placebo-controlled design, in patients with obsessive compulsive disorder yielded similar findings (Lesch et al., 1991). The ability of ipsapirone (0.3 mg/kg) to induce hypothermia and ACTH/cortisol release was attenuated during fluoxetine challenge. More recent studies (Shiah et al., 1998) on eight patients with bipolar depression and 26 normal controls imply that there is a significant positive correlation between severity of depression as assessed by the Hamilton Depression Rating scores, and the hypothermic response to a single dose of ipsapirone (0.3 mg/kg). Serotonin acting drugs, for example fenfluramine, also impact on HPA activity. Schurmeyer et al. (1996) examined episodic secretion of ACTH and cortisol in six healthy volunteers under basal conditions and again during treatment with 20 and 60 mg fenfluramine given orally every 8 hours. While the lower dose had no effect on ACTH and cortisol secretion, the higher dose resulted in significant increases of mean plasma ACTH (+85%) and cortisol (+129%) levels as well as of urinary free cortisol secretion (+44%). Fenfluramine did not modulate the frequency, but increased the amplitudes of ACTH and cortisol secretory episodes. In addition, ACTH and cortisol responses to CRH were tested at the end of the sampling period but these remained unchanged. These authors concluded that fenfluramine stimulates the activity of the hypothalamic–pituitary– adrenal axis at a suprapituitary level by modulation of the amplitude of ACTH and cortisol secretory bursts. It has been suggested that the clinical efficacy of selective serotonin reuptake inhibitors depends on the ability to enhance serotonergic activity.

Synacthen tests

Thakore et al. (1997) recruited female patients fulfilling criteria for major depression, melancholic subtype. Subjects were treated with a selective serotonin reuptake inhibitor, either sertraline (50 mg) or paroxetine (20 mg). While depressed and after treatment, when again medication-free, patients underwent an ACTH test (tetracosactrin), 250 mg given as an intravenous bolus. Cortisol response to ACTH was measured as the level of cortisol post-ACTH relative to baseline. Treatment resulted in a significant drop in this value from 1633.3 ± 378.5 nmol/l (mean±SEM) to 595.1 ± 207.7 nmol/l. Successful pharmacological treatment of depression appears to be associated with a reduction in ACTH-induced cortisol release in drug-free patients. When baseline HPA characteristics of patients who relapse are compared with those who do not, significant differences are observed (O'Toole *et al.*, 1997). A group of patients, who required continuing treatment to hold their symptoms in abeyance, were compared with patients who were successfully tapered off medication without relapse. Relapsers had high baseline ACTH and cortisol together with enhanced cortisol response to ACTH. The authors suggest that abnormal baseline HPA measures increase the necessity for continuation treatment of depression.

Adrenal gland volume and antidepressants

Adrenal gland volume was measured using magnetic resonance imaging in 11 patients (nine adults and two adolescents) with major depression (Rubin *et al.* 1995). All subjects were assessed during the depressive episode and in full remission, when they were drug-free for at least 1 month. A group of healthy age- and sex-matched comparison subjects were also tested. Baseline ACTH and cortisol was measured, together with CRH and ACTH responses. Mean adrenal gland volume was approximately 70% larger in the depressives than healthy comparison subjects and reduced on average by 70% after treatment. Post-treatment, differences in adrenal volume were no longer present. Patients and healthy subjects had adrenal glands of similar volume. Baseline hormone measurements and responses to CRH or ACTH did not differ significantly between the two groups. The authors conclude that adrenal gland enlargement occurring during an episode of major depression is state-dependent, in that it reverts to the normal size range during remission.

THE HPA AXIS AND TREATMENT

Effective treatment of depression normalizes all HPA axis parameters at a hypothalamic, pituitary and adrenal level. Whatever the mode of effective treatment, ECT, selective serotonin reuptake inhibitors or tricyclic antidepressants all normalize HPA function, when producing a therapeutic effect. No compound incapable of normalizing the HPA axis has antidepressant properties. The sensitivity of the dex-CRH test has been exploited to assess HPA axis status in healthy individuals who are at high risk for psychiatric disorders because they have a first-degree relative with an affective illness. Holsboer *et al.* (1995) screened 431 consecutively admitted patients with depression and identified 35 families with one or more high-risk probands (HRPs). It was observed that the HRP group had cortisol levels intermediate between a healthy control group and a group of patients with an acute major depressive episode. To assess whether long-lasting disturbance of the HPA could be considered as a trait or vulnerability marker for depression, these researchers recently re-examined 14 of the 47 HRPs and found that their dex-CRH test results were surprisingly constant (Modell *et al.* 1998). This implies that disturbed HPA function could be regarded as a vulnerability marker, with a causal role for depression, rather than as an acquired change due to acute depressive illness.

It is generally assumed that standard antidepressants act by blocking the uptake of monoamines and consequently inducing receptor alterations (Schildkraut, 1965). However, they also exert important influences on glucocorticoid receptors. The effect of long-term imipramine treatment on glucocorticoid receptor immunoreactivity in various regions of the rat brain has been investigated (Kitayama *et al.*, 1988). A significant up-regulation of corticoid receptors was found on the noradrenergic locus coeruleus and the serotonin-containing neurons. A similar up-regulation occurs in the hypothalamus and hippocampus and thereby induces an increase in negative feedback, decreasing the overall activity of the HPA axis. These findings have been replicated in *in situ* hybridization studies, and the results have also been found to be applicable to the selective serotonin reuptake inhibitors (Pepin *et al.*, 1989).

Recent papers from the Max Planck Institute in Munich suggest that the HPA axis may be an appropriate target site for pharmacological interventions in depression (Barden *et al.*, 1995). Pepin *et al.* (1992a) used mouse cell lines to study the effects of desipramine on glucocorticoid receptor gene promoter activity and binding capacity. Transfection studies with a 2.7-kilobase glucocorticoid receptor gene promoter region fused to a chloramphenicol acetyltransferase reporter gene confirmed that desipramine produced a 50–200% increase in transcriptional activity. In cell lines derived from both neuronal and non-neuronal sources, there was a doubling of glucocorticoid receptor mRNA concentration after desipramine treatment, which corresponded to two-fold higher functional glucocorticoid binding capacity and increased glucocorticoid sensitivity. Further studies made use of a transgenic mouse model with impaired glucocorticoid receptor function (Pepin *et al.*, 1992b). These mice have a hyperactive HPA axis, as evidenced by elevated plasma corticosterone and ACTH levels. However, treatment of these animals with desipramine resulted in increased hypothalamic glucocorticoid receptor mRNA concentration and dexamethasone-binding activity with decreased plasma ACTH concentration and corticosterone levels (Pepin *et al.*, 1992c). These mice also had behavioural deficits indicative of cognitive impairment (Montkowski *et al.*, 1995). These, along with hormonal alterations, were abolished by long-term treatment with moclobemide, a reversible inhibitor of monoamine oxidase type A that acts clinically as an antidepressant.

More recently, the direct effects of long-term treatment with several antidepressants on glucocorticoid receptor binding and mRNA expression was examined in neuronal cultures prepared from hippocampi of rat fetuses

(Okugawa *et al.*, 1999). Both the tricyclic antidepressants desipramine and amitriptyline induced a biphasic stimulation of [³H]-dexamethasone binding by glucocorticoid receptor, with peaks at 2 and 10–14 days. Maximal effects for desipramine were observed at 14 days. The effects of 14-day treatment with desipramine required at least the first four-day exposure, and the first 10-day exposure was required for the full effect. Northern blot analysis of glucocorticoid receptor mRNA revealed that levels were significantly increased by 14-day treatment with desipramine, amitriptyline, mianserin, paroxetine and sulpiride, but not with haloperidol. Immunocytochemistry for GR revealed that two or 14-day treatment with desipramine significantly increased the number of GR-positive cells with dominant immunoreactivity in the nuclei of granule cell-like neurones or in perikarya of pyramidal cell- and granule cell-like neurones. These findings suggest that treatment with tricyclic antidepressants can lead directly to increased hippocampal gluco-corticoid receptor expression. Different classes of antidepressants are effective and they appear to act via up-regulation of glucocorticoid receptor gene transcription.

This action of antidepressants could account for their capacity to suppress HPA activity and may be of clinical importance. Heuser (1998), based on animal and patient studies, suggests that antidepressants could amplify feedback by glucocorticoids *in vivo*, and that this activity of antidepressants is essential for successful improvement of psychopathology (Heuser, 1998).

If the HPA axis is an appropriate target site for pharmacological inter-ventions in depression, as the recent papers from the Max Planck Institute suggest (Barden *et al.*, 1995; Barden, 1999), which aspects of HPA axis function may provide a suitable avenue for pharmacological manipulation in the management of depression?

Glucocorticoid synthesis inhibitors

The most extensively investigated site within the HPA for pharmacological intervention in the treatment of depression has been the adrenal cortex itself. Several investigators have made use of glucocorticoid synthesis inhibitors as potential antidepressants (Wolkowitz *et al.*, 1993; Thakore and Dinan, 1995; O'Dwyer *et al.*, 1995). Three synthesis inhibitors have been used in studies to date: (i) metyrapone, an 11 β-hydroxylase inhibitor; (ii) amino-glutethimide, which blocks the conversion of cholesterol to pregnenolone; and (iii) ketoconazole (an antifungal agent) that not only inhibits cortisol synthesis but also acts as a type 2 receptor antagonist.

Murphy and colleagues (1991, 1998) have provided the most extensive investigation of these agents. Following early indications that suppression of steroids may be efficacious in the treatment of otherwise treatment-resistant major depression (Murphy *et al.*, 1991), they have more recently reported on 20 patients with treatment-resistant major depression who were treated with either aminoglutethimide 250–1000 mg/day, ketoconazole 400–1200 mg/day or metyrapone 250–1000 mg/day (Murphy *et al.*, 1998). Most patients were treated for a total of 8 weeks. A response rate of around 50% was reported.

Thakore and Dinan (1995) used ketoconazole 400–600 mg/day for 4 weeks in eight severely depressed inpatients. Serotonergic responses were measured before and after treatment using the dexfenfluramine/prolactin stimulation test. Five of the eight patients showed an excellent response and three had a partial response to treatment. In all cases serotonergic responses were enhanced following ketoconazole treatment. Clinical improvement paralleled the decrease in cortisol levels.

At the Maudsley Hospital, O'Dwyer *et al.* (1995) conducted a single-blind study in eight depressed inpatients who received either metyrapone 1000–2000 mg/day together with hydrocortisone or placebo for 2 weeks. A crossover design was employed. The authors concluded that the metyrapone and hydrocortisone treatment resulted in an alleviation of depression, as evidenced by a decrease in Hamilton Depression Rating Scale (HDRS) scores. Wolkowitz *et al.* (1993) used ketoconazole 400–800 mg/day for 3–6 weeks in 10 patients with major depressive illness. A decrease of approximately 30% in HDRS scores was observed.

Less promising results were obtained by Amsterdam and Hornig-Rohan (1993) who found no response in 10 patients with refractory depression who were treated with ketoconazole.

Whether or not this strategy can yield a treatment for depression with benefits (at least for some patients) in excess of those provided by current antidepressants will not be answered by further small-scale studies. A full placebo-controlled study in an adequate sample size is necessary. A recent small double-blind placebo-controlled study (Wolkowitz *et al.*, 1999) examined the effect of 400–800 mg/day of ketoconazole on behavioural ratings in 20 medication-free depressed patients, eight of whom were hyper-cortisolaemic and twelve of whom were not. It was observed that ketoconazole, compared with placebo, was associated with improvements in depression ratings in the hypercortisolaemic, but not in the non-hypercorti-solaemic patients. These authors suggest that this study supports the idea that antiglucocorticoids have antidepressant activity in hypercortisolaemic depressed patients and that the data are consistent with a causal role of adrenocortical dysfunction in some depressed patients. They confirm the need for larger-scale trials.

CRH and arginine vasopressin

CRH and AVP antagonists are now available (Webster *et al.*, 1996) and may be of benefit in hypersecretory states such as melancholic depression.

Two subtypes of the CRH receptor have been identified and cloned in man (CRH$_1$ and CRH$_2$). Both receptors are adenylate cyclase-1 linked. Peptide analogues of CRH have been identified that antagonize the actions of CRH. Recently, nonpeptide antagonists have been developed, which offer the advantage of oral administration. Preliminary work with antalarmin, a novel pyrrolopyrimidine compound, suggests potential as an antidepressant. It acts as a CRH$_1$ receptor antagonist, displacing CRH from binding to the receptor in the anterior pituitary, frontal cortex and cerebellum, and potently inhibiting CRH$_1$-stimulated ACTH release

In depression, regulation of the HPA switches partly from CRH to AVP, with increased numbers of paraventricular cells co-expressing the latter peptide. AVP has three receptor subtypes, V_{1a}, V_{1b} and V_2. V_{1b} receptors are predominantly expressed on the pituitary and are coupled to phospholipase C (PLC). Mean plasma levels of AVP are higher in depressed patients than in healthy controls (van Londen *et al.*, 1997). A study on 48 patients with major depression and 30 healthy controls suggested that elevated AVP is associated with daytime psychomotor retardation and night-time motor activity in major depression (van Londen *et al.*, 1998). Stress up-regulates the number of AVP receptors on the anterior pituitary (Aguilera *et al.*, 1994), increasing the ACTH-releasing activity of AVP. Furthermore, ACTH secretion by AVP is less sensitive to glucocorticoid feedback inhibition than CRH-induced secretion (Abou-Samra *et al.*, 1986; Bilezijian *et al.*, 1987). Glucocorticoids actually increase the coupling of the AVP V_{1b} receptors to PLC (Rabadan-Diehl and Aguilera, 1998). This suggests a mechanism whereby AVP facilitates corticotroph responsiveness in the presence of elevated cortisol levels.

When patients with depression are given an intravenous infusion of CRH their ACTH responses are blunted. However, when both CRH and ddAVP are infused together, depressives and healthy volunteers have similar responses (Dinan *et al.*, 1999). This suggests that anterior pituitary AVP receptors are supersensitive in depression. To date no studies of AVP antagonists have been reported.

CONCLUSIONS

In the development of new antidepressants, a neuroendocrine strategy provides novel sites for possible antidepressant action. Since the development of the first antidepressants in the 1950s, pharmaceutical companies have targeted monoamine systems in a search for new compounds. While this approach has more recently resulted in a generation of compounds that are relatively safe in overdose and well tolerated, it has not yet produced compounds that act rapidly and are effective in more than 70% of cases. A change in target site from monoamines to the HPA axis may yield these added benefits. The results of placebo-controlled studies of agents that impact on the HPA axis are awaited.

REFERENCES

Abou-Samra, A.B., Catt, K.J. and Aguilera, G. (1986). Biphasic inhibition of adreno-corticotropin release by corticosterone in cultured anterior pituitary cells. *Endocrinology* **119**, 972–977.

Aguilera, G., Pham, Q. and Rabadan-Diehl, C. (1994). Regulation of pituitary vasopressin receptors during chronic stress: relationship to corticotroph responsiveness. *J Neuroendocrinol* **6**, 299–304.

American Psychiatric Association Task Force (1987). The dexamethasone suppression test: An overview of its current state in Psychiatry. *Am J Psychiatry* **144**, 1253–1262.

Amsterdam, J.D. and Hornig-Rohan, M. (1993). Adrenocortical activation and steroid suppression with ketoconazole in refractory depression. *Biol Psychiatry* **33**, 88A.

Amsterdam, J.D., Maisling, Winokur, G. *et al.* (1987). The CRH stimulation test before and after clinical recovery from depression. *J Affect Disord* **14**, 213–222.

Arborelius, L., Owens, M.J., Plotsky, P.M. and Nemeroff, C.B. (1999). The role of corticotropin-releasing factor in depression and anxiety disorders. *J Endocrinol* **160**, 1–12.

Asnis, G.M., Halbreich, U., Rabinowitz, H. *et al.* (1986). The dexamethasone suppression test (1 mg and 2 mg) in major depression: illness versus recovery. *J Clin Psychopharmacol* **6**, 294–296.

Barden, N., Reul., J.H.M. and Holsboer, F. (1995). Do antidepressants stabilise mood through actions on the hypothalamic–pituitary–adrenocortical system? *Trends Pharmacol Sci* **18**, 6–11.

Barden, N. (1999). Regulation of corticosteroid receptor gene expression in depression and antidepressant action. *J Psychiatry Neurosci* **24**, 25–39.

Bilezijian, L.M., Blount, A.M. and Vale, W.W. (1987). The cellular actions of vasopressin on corticotrophs of the anterior pituitary: resistance to glucocorticoid action. *Molec Endocrinol* **1**, 451–458.

Carroll, B.J. (1982). The dexamethasone suppression test for melancholia. *Br J Psychiatry* **140**, 292–304.

Carroll, B.J., Curtis, G.C., Davies, B.M. *et al.* (1976). Urinary free cortisol excretion in depression. *Psycholog Med* **6**, 43–51.

Catalan, R., Gallart, J.M., Castellanos, J.M. and Galard, R. (1998). Plasma corti-cotropin-releasing factor in depressive disorders. *Biol Psychiatry* **44**, 15–20.

Chao, H.M., Choo, P.H. and McEwen, B.S. (1989). Glucocorticoid and mineralocorticoid receptor mRNA expression in rat brain. *Neuroendocrinology* **50**, 365–371.

Charles, G.A., Schittecatte, M., Rush, A.J. *et al.* (1989). Persistent cortisol nonsuppression after clinical recovery predicts symptomatic relapse in unipolar depression. *J Affect Disord* **17**, 271–278.

De Bellis, M.D., Gold, P.W., Geraciotid, Listwak, S. and Kling, M.A. (1993). Fluoxetine significantly reduces CFS CRH and AVP concentrations in patients with major depression. *Am J Psychiatry* **150**, 656–657.

Deuschle, M., Schweiger, U., Gotthardt, U. *et al.* (1998). The combined dexamethasone/corticotropin-releasing hormone stimulation test is more closely associated with features of diurnal activity of the hypothalamo–pituitary–adrenocortical system than the dexamethasone suppression test. *Biol Psychiatry* **43**, 762–766.

Dinan, T.G. (1997). Serotonin and the regulation of hypothalamic–pituitary–adrenal axis function. *Life Sci* **58**, 1683–1693.

Dinan, T.D. (1994). Glucocorticoids and the genesis of depressive illness: A psychobiological model. *Br J Psychiatry* **164**, 365–371.

Dinan, T.G., Lavelle, E., Scott, L.V. *et al.* (1999). Desmopressin normalizes the blunted adrenocorticotropin response to corticotropin-releasing hormone in melancholic depression: evidence of enhanced vasopressinergic responsivity. *J Clin Endocrinol Metab* **84**, 2238–2240.

Galard, R., Gallart, J.M., Catalan, R. *et al.* (1991). Salivary cortisol levels and their correlation with plasma ACTH levels in depressed patients before and after the DST. *Am J Psychiatry* **148**, 505–508.

Geracioti, T.D., Orth, D.N. and Ekhator, N.N. (1992). Serial cerebrospinal fluid corticotropin-releasing hormone concentration in healthy and depressed humans. *J Clin Endocrinol Metab* **74**, 1325–1330.

Goldberg, I.K. (1980). Dexamethasone suppression tests in depression and response to treatment. *Lancet* **2**, 92.

Gray, T.S. and Bingaman, E.W. (1996). The amygdala: corticotropin-releasing factor, steroids and stress. *Crit Rev Neurobiol* **10**, 155–168.

Greden, J.F., Albala, A.A., Haskett, R.F. *et al.* (1980). Normalisation of dexamethosone suppression test: A laboratory index of recovery from endogenous depression. *Biol Psychiatry* **15**, 449–458.

Halbreich, U., Zumoff, B., Kream, J. and Fukushima, D.K. (1982). The mean 1300–1600 h plasma cortisol concentration as a diagnostic test for hypercortisolism. *J Clin Endocrinol Metab* **54**, 1262–1264.

Heuser, I. (1998). Anna-Monika-Prize paper. The hypothalamic–pituitary–adrenal system in depression. *Pharmacopsychiatry* **31**, 10–13.

Heuser, I., Bissette, G., Dettling, M. *et al.* (1998). Cerebrospinal fluid concentrations of corticotropin-releasing hormone, vasopressin, and somatostatin in depressed patients and healthy controls: response to amitriptyline treatment. *Depress Anxiety* **8**, 71–79.

Heuser, I.J.E., Schweiger, U., Gotthard, D.T. *et al.* (1996). Pituitary–adrenal–system regulation and psychopathology during amitriptyline treatment in elderly depressed patients and normal comparison subjects. *Am J Psychiatry* **153**, 93–99.

Heuser, I, Yassouridisa, G. and Holsboer, F. (1994). The combined dexamethasone: A refined laboratory test for psychiatric disorders. *J Psychiatr Res* **28**, 341–356.

Holsboer, F., Liebl, R.J. and Hofschuster, E. (1982). Repeated dexamethasone suppression tests during depressive illness. *J Affect Disord* **4**, 93–101.

Holsboer, F.H. (1995). Neuroendocrinology of mood disorders. In: Bloom, F.E. and Kuffer, D.J. (Eds), *Psychopharmacology: The Fourth Generation of Progress*, Raven Press, New York, pp. 957–970.

Holsboer, F., Gerken, A., Von Bardeleben, U. *et al.* (1986). Human corticotropin-releasing hormone in depression. *Biol Psychiatry* **21**, 609–611.

Holsboer, F., Lauer, C.J., Schreiber, W. and Krieg, J.C. (1995). Altered hypothalamic–pituitary–adrenocortical regulation in healthy subjects at high familial risk for affective disorders. *Neuroendocrinology* **62**, 340–347.

Kitayama, J.J., Janson, A.M., Cintra, A. *et al.* (1988). Effects of chronic imipramine treatment on glucocorticoid receptor immunoreactivity in various regions of the rat brain. Evidence for selective increases of glucocorticoid receptor immunoreactivity in the locus coeruleus and in 5-hydroxytryptamine nerve cell groups of the rostral ventromedial medulla. *J Neural Transmiss* **73**, 191–203.

Jessop, D.S. (1999). Central non-glucocorticoid inhibitors of the hypothalamo–pituitary–adrenal axis. *J Endocrinol* **160**, 169–180.

Lesch, K.P. (1991). 5-HT1A receptor responsivity in anxiety disorders and depression. *Prog Neuropsychopharmacol Biol Psychiatry* **15**, 723–733.

Lesch, K.P., Hoh, A., Schulte, H.M. *et al.* (1991). Long term fluoxetine treatment decreases 5-HT1A receptor responsivity in obsessive-compulsive disorder. *Psychopharmacology* **105**, 415–420.

Lesch, K.P., Mayer, S., Disselkamp-Tietzeh, *et al.* (1990). 5-HT1A receptor responsivity in unipolar depression: Evaluation of ipsapirone-induced ACTH in cortisol secretion in patients and controls. *Biol Psychiatry* **28**, 620–628.

Linkowski, P., Mendelwicz, J., Kerkhofs, M. *et al.* (1987). 24 hour profiles of adrenocorticotropin, cortisol and growth hormone in major depression: effect of antidepressant treatment. *J Clin Endocrinol Metab* **65**, 141–152.

Modell, S., Lauer, C.J., Schreiber, W. *et al.* (1998). Hormonal response pattern in the combined dex-CRH test is stable over time in subjects at high familial risk for affective disorders. *Neuropsychopharmacology* **18**, 253–262.

Montkowski, A., Barden, N., Wotjak, C. *et al.* (1995). Long~term antidepressant treatment reduces behavioural deficits in transgenic mice with impaired glucocorticoid receptor function. *J Neuroendocrinol* **7**, 841–845.

Murphy, B.E., Dhar, V., Ghadirian, A.M., Chouinard, G. and Keller, R. (1991). Response to steroid suppression in major depression resistant to antidepressant therapy. *J Clin Psychopharmacol* **11**, 121–126.

Murphy, B.E., Ghadirian, A.M. and Dhar, V. (1998). Neuroendocrine responses to inhibitors of steroid biosynthesis in patients with major depression resistant to antidepressant therapy. *Can J Psychiatry* **43**, 279–286.

Nemeroff, C.B., Owens, M.J., Bissette, G. *et al.* (1984). Elevated concentrations of CSF corticotropin-releasing factor-like immunoreactivity in depressed patients. *Science* **226**, 1342–1344.

Nemeroff, C.B,. Bissette, G., Akil, H. and Fink, M. (1991). Neuropeptide concentrations in the cerebrospinal fluid of depressed patients treated with electroconvulsive therapy: Corticotropin releasing factor, β-endorphin and somatostatin. *Br J Psychiatry* **158**, 59–63.

O'Dwyer, A.M., Lightman, S.L., Marks, M.N. and Checkley, S.A. (1995). Treatment of major depression with metyrapone and hydrocortisone. *J Affect Disord* **33**, 123–128.

O'Keane, V., McLoughlin, D. and Dinan, T.D. (1992). D-fenfluramine-induced prolactin and cortisol release in major depression: Response to treatment. *J Affect Disord* **26**, 143–150.

Okugawa, G., Omori, K. and Suzukawa, J. (1999). Long-term treatment with antidepressants increases glucocorticoid receptor binding and gene expression in cultured rat hippocampal neurones. *J Neuroendocrinol* **11**, 887–895.

O'Toole, S.M., Seckula, L.K. and Rubin, R.T. (1997). Pituitary–adrenal cortico axis measures as predictors of sustained remission in major depression. *Biol Psychiatry* **42**, 85–89.

Pepin, M.C., Beaulieu, S. and Barden, N. (1989). Antidepressants regulate glucocorticoid receptor messenger RNA concentrations in primary neuronal cultures. *Mol Brain Res* **6**, 77–83.

Pepin, M.C., Govindan, M.V. and Barden, N. (1992a). Increased glucocorticoid receptor gene promoter activity after antidepressant treatment. *Mol Pharmacol* **41**, 1016–1022.

Pepin, M.C., Pothier, F. and Barden, N. (1992b). Impaired type II glucocorticoid-receptor function in mice bearing antisense RNA transgene. *Nature* **355**, 725–728.

Pepin, M.C., Pothier, F. and Barden, N. (1992c). Antidepressant drug action in a transgenic mouse model of the endocrine changes seen in depression. *Mol Pharmacol* **42**, 991–995.

Rabadan-Diehi, C. and Aguilera, G. (1998). Glucocorticoids increase vasopressin V1b receptor coupling to phospholipase C. *Endocrinology* **139**, 3220–3226.

Reul, J.M., van den Bosch, F.R. and de Kloet, E.R. (1987a). Relative occupation of type-I and type-Il corticosteroid receptors in rat brain following stress and dexamethasone treatment: functional implications. *J Endocrinol* **115**, 459–467.

Reul, J.M., van den Bosch, F.R. and de Kloet, E.R. (1987b). Differential response of type I and type II corticosteroid receptors to changes in plasma steroid level and circadian rhythmicity. *Neuroendocrinology* **45**, 407–412.

Ribeiro, S.C.M., Tandon, R., Grunhaus, L. and Greden I.F. (1993). The DST as a predictor of outcome in depression: A meta-analysis. *Am J Psychiatry* **150**, 1618–1629.

Rubin, R.T., Phillips, J.J., Sadow, T.F. and McCracken, J.T. (1995). Adrenal gland volume in major depression: Increased during the depressive episode and decrease with successful treatment. *Arch Gen Psychiatry* **52**, 213–218.

Rybakowski, J.K. and Twardowska, K. (1999). The dexamethasone/corticotropin-releasing hormone test in depression in bipolar and unipolar affective illness. *J Psychiatr Res* **33**, 363–370.

Schildkraut, J.J. (1965). The catecholamine hypothesis of affective disorders: a review of supporting evidence. *Am J Psychiatry* **122**, 509–522.

Schurmeyer, T.H., Brademann, G. and von zur Muhlen, A. (1996). Effect of fenfluramine on episodic ACTH and cortisol secretion. *Clin Endocrinol* **45**, 39–45.

Scott, L.V. and Dinan, T.G. (1998). Vasopressin and the regulation of hypothalamic–pituitary–adrenal axis function: Implications for the pathophysiology of depression. *Life Sci* **62**, 1985–1998.

Scott, L.V. and Dinan, T.G. (1998). Urinary free cortisol excretion in chronic fatigue syndrome, major depression and in healthy volunteers. *J Affect Disord* **47**, 49–54.

Shiah, I.S., Yatham, L.N., Lam, R.W. Tam, E.M. and Zis, A.P. (1998). Cortisol, hypothermic, and behavioral responses to ipsapirone in patients with bipolar depression and normal controls. *Neuropsychobiology* **38**, 6–12.

Thakore, J.H., Barnes, C., Joyce, J. *et al.* (1997). The effects of antidepressant treatment on corticotropin-induced cortisol responses in patients with melancholic depression. *Psychiatry Res* **73**, 27–32.

Thakore, J.H. and Dinan, T.G. (1995). Cortisol synthesis inhibition: a new treatment strategy for the clinical and endocrine manifestations of depression. *Biol Psychiatry* **37**, 364–368.

Ur, E., Dinan, T.G., O'Keane, V. *et al.* (1992). Effect of metyrapone on the pituitary–adrenal axis and depression: Relation to dexamethasone suppressors status. *Neuroendocrinology* **56**, 533–539.

Vale, W., Spiess, J., Riviere, *et al.* (1981). Characterisation of a 41 residue ovine hypothalamic peptide that stimulates secretion of the corticotropin and beta-endorphin. *Science* **213**, 1394–1399.

van Londen, L., Goekoop, J.G., van Kempen, G.M. *et al.* (1997). Plasma levels of arginine vasopressin elevated in patients with major depression. *Neuropsychopharmacology* **17**, 284–292.

van Londen, L., Kerkhof, G.A., van den Berg, F. *et al.* (1998). Plasma arginine vasopressin and motor activity in major depression. *Biol Psychiatry* **43**, 196–204.

Vieta, E., Gasto, C., De Osaba, M.J.M. *et al.* (1997). Prediction of depressive relapse in remitted bipolar patients using corticotropin-releasing hormone challenge test. *Acta Psychiatr Scand* **95**, 205–211.

Webster, E.L., Lewis, D.B. and Torpy, D.J. (1996). *In vivo* and *in vitro* characterisation of antalarmin, a nonpeptide corticotropin-releasing hormone (CRH) receptor antagonist: suppression of pituitary ACTH release and peripheral inflammation. *Endocrinology* **137**, 5747–5750.

Wolkowitz, O.M., Reus, V.I., Manfredi, F., Ingbar, J., Brizendine, L. and Weingartner, H. (1993). Ketoconazole administration in hypercortisolemic depression. *Am J Psychiatry* **150**, 810–812.

Wolkowitz, O.M., Reus, V.I., Chan, T. *et al.* (1999). Antiglucocorticoid treatment of depression: double-blind ketoconazole. *Biol Psychiatry* **45**, 1070–1074.

Zobel, A.W., Yassouridis, A., Frieboes, R.M. and Holsboer, F. (1999). Prediction of medium-term outcome by cortisol response to the combined dexamethasone-CRH test in patients with remitted depression. *Am J Psychiatry* **156**, 949–951.

Index

ACTH, *see* Adrenocorticotrophic hormone
Acupuncture 195
Acute phase proteins 58
  antidepressant drugs and 169, 170
  in depression 10, 59, 158–160, 173
Addison's disease 186, 194
Adherence to treatment, *see* Compliance
      with treatment
Adipose tissue
  cortisol actions 72, 73, 74–75
  regulation 94–96
  sex steroid/growth hormone actions 73–74
  sympathetic activation and 74–75
Adrenal gland volume 6, 57–58, 220
Adrenergic receptors
  immune cells 57
  regulation by corticosteroids 28, 32
Adrenocorticotrophic hormone (ACTH) 3–4
  $5HT_{1A}$ agonist challenge and 218–219
  antidepressant therapy and 215, 216–217
  in depression 38, 215
  early life stress and 12, 14–15
  elevated levels 185
  receptors, in depression 6
  stimulation test (Synacthen test) 6,
      219–220
  stress response 35
Affective disorders
  early death and physical illness 88–91
  energy balance and 96–97
Age
  mortality in psychiatric disorders and 89
  natural killer (NK) cell activity and 157
Ageing
  atypical depression and 120–121
  maternal deprivation and 45
Aggressive behaviour 44
AIDS/HIV 167–168, 173, 196
Alcohol consumption 77
Alendronate 117–118
Allergies 58–59
Allostasis 182–184
Allostatic load 182–184, 198–199

antiglucocorticoid therapy and 194–195,
      199
  behavioural treatment approaches and
      195–198
  markers 183
  α-1-acid glycoprotein 159, 160
  α-1-antitrypsin 159, 160
Alzheimer's disease 56, 194
Aminoglutethimide 42, 222
  in Cushing's syndrome 186
  in depression 40, 223
  GR responses 222
  mechanism of action 188
Amitriptyline
  corticosteroid receptors and 27
  HPA axis function and 215, 218, 219
  plus spironolactone 42–43
Amygdala 2
Anabolic balance 183, 186, 187, 193
Androgens, elevated 79
Anger, ventricular arrhythmias and 138–139
Angina pectoris 131
Angiotensin converting enzyme blockers 141
Anorexia nervosa, osteoporosis and 115–116
Antalarmin (R121919/NBI30775) 224
Antibody synthesis 55, 172
Antidepressant drugs
  cardiovascular disease and 141–142
  corticosteroid receptors and 25–27,
      221–222
  CRH activity and 8, 15–16
  falls and fractures and 113–114
  glucose tolerance and 99–100
  HPA axis effects 40–42, 215, 216–225
  immunity and 168–169, 170–171
  see also individual agents
Antiglucocorticoid therapy 198, 222–223
  in Cushing's syndrome 185–186
  in depression 42–43, 187–195, 199
Antihypertensive drugs 140–141
Anxiety 68
  post-myocardial infarction 131
Apomorphine 29, 44